MEDICINE AND THE SAINTS

*Science, Islam, and the Colonial Encounter
in Morocco, 1877–1956*

T0256764

ELLEN J. AMSTER
FOREWORD BY RAJAE EL AOUED

UNIVERSITY OF TEXAS PRESS 🔻 *Austin*

Copyright © 2013 by the University of Texas Press
All rights reserved
Printed in the United States of America
First edition, 2013

Requests for permission to reproduce material from this work should be sent to:
    Permissions
    University of Texas Press
    P.O. Box 7819
    Austin, TX 78713-7819
    http://utpress.utexas.edu/index.php/rp-form

♾ The paper used in this book meets the minimum requirements of ANSI/NISO
Z39.48-1992 (R1997) (Permanence of Paper).

LIBRARY OF CONGRESS CATALOGING-IN-PUBLICATION DATA

Amster, Ellen J., 1970–
    Medicine and the saints : science, Islam, and the colonial encounter in Morocco,
1877–1956 / Ellen J. Amster ; foreword by Rajae El Aoued. — 1st ed.
        p.   cm.
    Includes bibliographical references and index.
    ISBN 978-0-292-76211-4
    1. Medicine—Morocco—History.   2. Health—Religious aspects—Islam.
3. Morocco—Colonization—History.   4. Islam and science—History.
5. Sufism—Morocco—History.   6. Muslim saints—Cult—Morocco.
I. Title.
    R653.M8A47   2013
    610.964—dc23

                                                        2012046686

doi:10.7560/745445

First paperback edition, 2014

MEDICINE AND THE SAINTS

FOR MY GRANDPARENTS MURIEL AND LEON FOLB,
WHO MADE IT POSSIBLE.

CONTENTS

I MUST SAY THAT I am deeply honored that Mme. Ellen Amster has asked me to write the foreword to her book about the history of the health system in Morocco.

This extensively researched work is a veritable mine of information for us and for the generations to come. It constitutes, henceforth, the authoritative reference on the subject. It permits us to understand the evolution of the Moroccan health service, its strengths and its weaknesses, and its impact on the health of the population.

In light of this past, and facing the contemporary challenges to health in Morocco today, what have we learned?

It is this question that I wish to address in this foreword, by connecting the historical past of the Institut National d'Hygiène du Maroc with the transformations it has undergone over the past century, and finally linking it to the future reserved for it as the consolidator of public health in Morocco.

THE HISTORY OF NEARLY A CENTURY OF THE INSTITUT NATIONAL D'HYGIÈNE

Inaugurated December 30, 1930, by the president of the Conseil Supérieur d'Hygiène de France, the Institut National d'Hygiène (INH) of Morocco has had from its inception the mission to address all problems of public health and hygiene, to monitor and control the propagation of transmissible diseases, and to provide information about the principles and methods of hygiene and prophylaxis to protect the health of the population of Morocco.

Having contributed to the eradication of numerous epidemic diseases and to the control of numerous maladies, the INH has seen its mission evolve over nearly a century (eighty years) toward developing expertise, the scientific and technical application of medical and environmental sanitation programs, biomedical research, and monitoring health safety.

CONSOLIDATION OF THE SYSTEM OF PUBLIC HEALTH AND MEDICINE IN MOROCCO

In Morocco, the system of public health and medicine is characterized by its intersectorality. Its continuous development has permitted considerable

Medicine and the Saints draws from diverse sources in the Arabic language and thus uses several strategies for transliteration.

For Arabic manuscripts and printed sources, I use the transliteration system for Modern Standard Arabic of the *International Journal of Middle East Studies*. Diacriticals are limited to the *ayn* and the *hamza*. For the convenience of the reader, lengthy Arabic passages are translated into English, but I have left individual words in Arabic where necessary for finer understanding, such as the distinction between *ʿilm* and *maʿrifa* as "knowledge."

The spelling of Moroccan names, places, and titles, and of words in the Moroccan colloquial dialect is influenced by the French language. I prefer to transliterate Moroccan Arabic names according to the MSA standards of *IJMES*, but where the person has chosen a French transliteration of his/her name for professional life (Aicha Ech-Channa, for example), or if he/she has a Berber name, I use French transliteration.

I conducted all but two interviews in Moroccan colloquial Arabic (*darija*), which contains medical terminology invented through the encounter with France ("hospital" is *spitar*, from the French *hôpital*, rather than the Arabic *mustashfa*, for example). These terms are left in the text, as are the occasional French words, to illustrate the code-switching inherent in Moroccan medical narratives. Like all Arabic colloquial dialects, Moroccan simplifies Arabic grammar and adds distinctive words. Thus I render direct citations in phonetic transcription rather than "correcting" them to Modern Standard Arabic.

Unless otherwise indicated, all translations from Arabic and French are my own.

ACKNOWLEDGMENTS

THIS BOOK IS THE PRODUCT OF many kindnesses great and small, and I would like to express my gratitude to those who aided me on the journey.

At the University of Pennsylvania, I would like to thank Steven Feierman, who opened my eyes to health and healing in Africa and showed me how to listen for missing voices. I would also like to thank Lynn Hunt, Lee Cassanelli, Lynn Lees, Achille Mbembe, Barbara von Schlegell, and Everett Rowson, who is eternally generous with his time and enthusiasm for all things Arabic and medieval.

In France, Lucette Valensi welcomed me to her seminar at the École des Hautes Études en Sciences Sociales, and Daniel Rivet opened his library and office. The staff of the Service Historique de l'Armée de Terre was extremely welcoming, and I received valuable assistance from Gilbert Bodinier and Samuel Gibiat. I would like to thank Noëlle Courtecuisse, Claude Lefebure, and Nelcya Delanoë for their generosity; Camille Gargar of the Val-de-Grâce Archives; and the staff of the Bibliothèque de l'École de Médecine at Odéon in Paris.

In Morocco, the faculty at Moulay Abdallah University in Fez graciously welcomed me as a student; I would like to thank Mohammed Bekraoui, M. Chafai al-Alawi, and the vice dean of arts and sciences at Fes-Saiss, Naguib Lahlou. In Rabat I found many generous helping hands, among them Saadia Boulhane, M. Bouamrani, and Muhammad Rushdie at the Bibliothèque Générale de Rabat, and Dr. La'rbi Idrissi and Dr. Hassan Taleb at the National Institute of Hygiene. Dr. Abdellatif Berbich welcomed me to the Académie du Royaume du Maroc, and Driss Moussaoui and A. Hamdoun hosted a wonderful conference on the history of medicine. In Fez, special thanks go to Najia Bouarfa, Mustapha Ajana, 'Abd al-Hafid al-'Alawi, Muhammad Zaim, Mustapha Murabit, and 'Ali Filali. From the Ministry of Public Health in Fez, Dr. Mohammed 'Alami Aroussi, Dr. Fouad Bouchareb, and Mr. Said 'Aqli were generous with their time. Finally, I would like to thank the Namrouch family of Fez, and especially Houda Namrouch. Houda patiently transcribed interviews and helped me translate them, accompanied me on visits, and helped to resolve a thousand daily problems. Without her kindness, this project would not have been possible.

For the conversion of my research to a finished book, I would especially like to thank Susan Miller, Nancy Gallagher, Patrice Petro, Julia Clancy-Smith, Justin Stearns, Daniel Sherman, and Mary Pickering for thoughtful and valuable commentary on the manuscript. I am indebted to the University of Wisconsin–Milwaukee for a Graduate School Research Committee Award and for faculty fellowships from the UWM Center for International Education and the Center for 21st Century Studies. Thanks also to my generous colleagues at the Institute for Research in the Humanities at University of Wisconsin–Madison, especially Susan Friedman and David Morgan.

I am also most fortunate to have a supportive and thoughtful circle of graduate colleagues, including Elizabeth Clement, Savita Nair, Mark Wilkens, Michael Kahan, Kirsten Wood, Michelle Rein, Michelle Zelinsky, Elisa von Joeden Forgey, Catherine Bogosian, Lauren Clay, Annemarie Stoner-Eby, Meltem Turköz, Joe Glicksberg, Akif Kirecci, Brian Caton, Alison MacKenzie, and Karim Tiro. Outside Penn, I have benefited from the wise counsel of Gregory Mann, Richard Fogarty, Diana Davis, Anne Marie Baylouny, Abdelhai Diouri, Sarah Farmer, Dale Eickelman, Susan Schaefer-Davis, Nabila Oulebsir, Sandy Sufian, and many others.

I would like to thank the granting institutions that supported my research and writing. The Mellon Foundation provided a dissertation grant for writing in 2000. In 1998–1999, I benefited from doctoral dissertation grants from the Fulbright-Hayes Program, the Chateaubriand Program of the Government of France, the Social Science Research Council International Dissertation Research Fellowship Program, and the American Institute of Maghreb Studies. This project was made possible also by several Foreign Language Area Studies Grants (FLAS) for Arabic language study at the University of Pennsylvania, the Arabic Language Institute in Fez, and Middlebury College.

Through a long and difficult process, my family has encouraged and sustained me. To them I dedicate this book, with love and gratitude.

MEDICINE AND THE SAINTS

COLONIAL EMBODIMENTS

IN 1907, A DOCTOR OF the French government was beaten to death by a Muslim mob in the Moroccan city of Marrakesh. After clubbing him to death and crushing his head, the crowd dragged the naked corpse of Dr. Émile Mauchamp by the neck through the city streets on a rope. This gruesome spectacle served as the pretext for the French invasion of Oujda in 1907 and the establishment of a French protectorate in Morocco in 1912. At his funeral, the French minister of Foreign Affairs eulogized Mauchamp as "civilization's martyr" to a fanatical Islamic hatred of science. But just before his death, rumors circulated in Marrakesh that the doctor prepared for an imminent French invasion by secretly poisoning his Muslim patients:

> [Mauchamp] belongs to a kind of French Christian freemasonry sworn to destroy the Muslims of Morocco. Savant and capable doctors like Mauchamp are chosen and sent among Moroccan populations. There, the doctors care for Arabs with the appearance of a great benevolence, curing them . . . gaining the confidence of all . . . but they have administered a subtle poison which acts two, three or four years later, and they will surely die.[1]

If we perform a historical autopsy, we find the viscera linking body to body politic. Poison is a way of knowing, a "French, Christian freemasonry" that will enter Muslim bodies to destroy Islam and undermine Moroccan independence, a knowing that annihilates both religion and biological life in Muslim bodies. Conquest appears a political and epistemological invasion, a clash of sovereignties inside a human body that is at once the field of battle and its prize. Colonialism, then, is a story of bodies, how ways of knowing become ways of being in bodies corporeal and political, a story of embodiments.

This book traces a history of colonial embodiment in Morocco through a series of medical encounters between the Islamic sultanate of Morocco and the Republic of France, 1877–1956. On the eve of colonialism, Frenchmen and Moroccans had very different ways of knowing the body. In a precolonial political imaginary derived from Islam, Moroccans invested sovereignty in God's Islamic community (*umma*) and negotiated authority through a human body known as contiguous with the land, Islamic history in Morocco, and temporal politics. Frenchmen constructed the republican citizen as a bounded, rational, and sovereign individual whose physicality constituted one dimension of his relationship to the state. Medicine reveals the Franco-Moroccan encounter, for it draws upon scientific paradigms (cosmologies), knowledge systems (hygiene and medical theory), and the technologies of physical intervention (therapeutics). As a social vehicle, the body is a mediator upon which to read ways of knowing and doing. A study of healing reveals the body's social logics, for a repair of the body usually entails a repair of society; as Jean Comaroff writes, "The body social and the body personal always exist in a mutually constitutive relationship."[2]

David Arnold has described colonial medicine as the hegemonic inscription of Foucauldian power/knowledge on the colonized body: "Colonialism used . . . the body as a site for the construction of its own authority, legitimacy and control."[3] Histories of colonial medicine illuminate how native bodies were invented as objects of scientific knowledge, racisms were naturalized, and health dictatorships were designed to sanitize, rationalize, and control native bodies. Yet the grand colonial medical schemes collapse in the social histories of colonial Africa and Asia, where unruly bodies eluded colonial control. Native patients often ran away from European hospitals, selectively used European cures while escaping (or ignoring) their ideological designs, or cheerfully extracted biomedical cures for re-integration within indigenous systems of healing. In the colonies, European medicine could not discipline colonized bodies, because it failed to constitute individual subjectivities. As Gyan Prakash notes, colonial biopower failed to create "self-subjecting individuals."[4]

Yet anthropologies of healing reveal strange reintegrations. Colonial terror is reborn as a healing dynamic between white and Indian residents of the Putamayo region in South America.[5] British biomedical technologies are renamed and circulate in an African semiotic field.[6] Colonial officers long absent from Sudan now reincarnate as possessing spirits in a women's Sudanese *zar* Islamic healing cult.[7] A South African "madman" wears precolonial cosmologies and global capitalism on his body as colorful bricolage.[8] Colonialism circulates in the viscera of postcolonial bodies, hidden in symbolic languages of corporeality and woven into traditional healing practice. Transformation comes not of inscribing knowledge but ingesting it, how people swallow new ways of knowing and use it to inhabit their bodies and the world.

Theories of embodiment allow us to move beyond the state to deconstruct the human as a meeting-place of social order and interior life. Pierre Bourdieu describes the human as a meeting of external space (home, town, polity) and internal space (emotion, thought, soul), a relationship mediated by the biological human body.[9] But Bourdieu assumes the body as a "pre-social base," a wet clay tablet onto which cultural modalities are inscribed as invisible habits (*habitus*), "[Where they] cannot be touched by voluntary, deliberate transformation, cannot even be made explicit."[10] Jean Comaroff attempts to restore individuals to agency with a more dynamic model of meaning creation; for example, the Tshidi create their biological/social bodies through healing practice in a "subject-object" encounter with the world.[11] Yet the actual biological body remains a clay tablet. It is the writing surface for the inscription of a socially produced knowledge.

The religious studies scholar Scott Kugle empowers the body through Sufism, the mystical approach in Islam. He adapts the phenomenology of Maurice Merleau-Ponty: "The concept of embodiment asserts that the body is not something residual, like a vehicle upon which the soul rides . . . [Plato] or something subsidiary to the mind . . . [Descartes]. Rather, the body is both the foundation for and product of the coming into being of a meaningful world, which is human being."[12] Islam articulates a human body radiant of meaning; God breathed of His spirit into clay to create Adam, a body that glows with reason, inspiration, and intuitive knowledge (*maʿrifa*), where breath (*nafas*) and soul (*nafs*) unite.[13] For Sufis, the human body speaks God's signs; it is the "locus of the manifestation of God's names and attributes—a theophany of the highest order."[14] The skin, hearing, and vision testify to God against their human owners in the Qur'an: "*They address their skins, 'How can you bear witness against us?' They answer, 'God has caused us to speak, as God causes all things to speak, for God created you in the first instance and you return inevitably to God!'*" (41:19–21). Kugle shows us the Islamic body as a signifier, a wellspring of meaning and the foundation of human subjectivity.

This book approaches embodiment as a historical and social process, a method aided by Foucault's biopolitics.[15] Foucault outlines the modern relationship of body to body politic, a modern art of governmentality called "liberalism." Liberalism claims to be natural, according to Foucault: "Nature is something that runs under, through [it] . . . It is, if you like, its indispensable hypodermis."[16] Thus, "Nature" ensures good laws, good government, and true political rights. Biopolitics are the "truth regime" that liberalism uses to extract Nature's truth from bodies, making the body a site of veridiction, of distinguishing the true from the false. Extended to empire, biopolitics are the effort to make colonized bodies speak, the mechanisms used to constitute the native body as a truth-teller whose "truth" defines the colonized as a political subject, determines his laws, and structures his governance. The biopolitical will to hegemony produced various historical examples in Africa and Asia of colonial health campaigns to destroy non-Western healing.[17] The colonizer demands, "Believe only our science, accept only our truth of your body, so that we may protect you, our state may expand, and our truth enter your very subjectivity." Biopolitics are also the state schemes created for subject populations as biological species, "It was the taking charge of life, more than the threat of death, that gave power its access even to the body."[18]

Yet postcolonial bodies escape; they are what Bruno Latour calls hybrids, the intermediate realities that defy a modern scientific understanding.[19] Therapy for postcolonial bodies demands a rethinking of modernity's categories, for the Moroccan body is *f-l-baynat*, "in the betweens," at the interstice between tradition and modernity, Occident and Orient, nature and culture.[20] Stefania Pandolfo describes modern Moroccan subjectivity as a cut, a fragmented narrative body caught between incommensurable worlds: "The epistemological 'cut'—the severing that defines a modernist position—is at the origin of a double exclusion . . . from 'culture' and the sense of community associated with it," and a "present" of "discrepant temporality."[21] The patient presents the doctor with a symptom of many dimensions, "discrepant and juxtaposed experiential registers . . . a bridge between worlds."[22] "Everything happens in the middle," writes Latour, but the reality of postcolonial bodies is inconceivable to a modern scientific mind. "It is the unthinkable, the unconscious of the moderns."[23]

If we allow an un-modern view, we find embodiment unfolding. The patient's pain renders visible a Moroccan digestion of modernity, the physical internalization of an epistemological, historical, and colonial war between French positivism and Sufi Islam to define the human being. This fragmenting pain bespeaks embodiment-as-process, a digestion of the experience of French colonialism and its forms of modernity; it is "the work of a subjectivity in the making."[24] This digestion and its historical origins are the subject of our study.

We begin in the nineteenth century with the slow implosion of the precolonial Moroccan state, the *makhzan*, and the reconstitutions of Morocco as a state and polity under French rule (1912–1956). The third of France's North African possessions after Algeria (1830) and Tunisia (1881), the French protectorate in Morocco (1912) was part of the French Third Republic's new mission to guide peoples of the empire to modernity through "association," a policy implemented by Morocco's first resident-general, Louis-Hubert-Gonzalve Lyautey (ruled 1912–1925). "Republican association" was a contradiction in terms, however, for French science progressed from an effort to contain Moroccan bodies to a refashioning of the Moroccan through his body. We trace the positivist ambitions of French colonial doctors, sociologists, philologists, and historians, a social history of the encounters and transformations occasioned by French medical interventions, and the ways that Moroccan nationalists ultimately appropriated a French model of modernity to invent the independent nation-state. We consider the legacy of colonial medicine in contemporary Moroccan health and healing through interviews with patients, doctors, and midwives in Fez, 1995–2000.

HEALING THE BODY, HEALING THE *UMMA*: MOROCCO AS A GEOPOLITICAL MORAL BODY

At first a distant African conquest of the Arab caliphates in the seventh century, Morocco developed its own unique history and Islamic spiritual tradition. The first Muslims in Berber Morocco were the invading armies of the Arab Umayyads, but Moroccan popular memory credits a blood descendant of the Prophet Muhammad with bringing Islam to Morocco, Idris b. 'Abd Allah (d. AD 793), and his son Idris II (d. 829). A blood descendant of 'Ali—the fourth caliph (Shi'ite imam) and blood cousin of the Prophet Muhammad—Idris I attempted unsuccessfully to overthrow the Abbasid state. Fleeing the Arabian Peninsula in 789, Idris founded a dynasty and state in North Africa entirely independent of the Abbasid administration. Though Sunni, Moroccans retain a reverence for the Prophet's blood descendants, the *shurafa'* (singular, *sharif*), and developed an indigenous Moroccan Sufi tradition uniting spiritual guidance with political leadership. Shi'ite and Sufi ideas unified in the figure of the Moroccan leader, who, like the Shi'ite imam and the Sufi *shaykh*, led from an intimate knowledge of God and His realities.

It is misleading to read Moroccan history in its kings, for the changing fortunes of North African dynasties inspired Ibn Khaldun's cyclical politics in the *Muqaddima*, and the limits of the sultan's state led nineteenth-century French observers to describe a *balad al-makhzan* ("land of the sultan's rule") and a *balad al-siba* ("land of insurrection"). The historian 'Abdallah Laroui describes the Moroccan state (*makhzan*; literally, "storehouse") as a contingent reality continuously negotiated between sultans, religious scholars (*'ulama'*), a commercial bourgeoisie, cities, tribes, and Sufi brotherhoods (*turuq*).[25] But anthropologists touch what historians cannot, the living of Islam as authority, *baraka*, "a mode of construing—emotionally, morally, intellectually—human experience, a cultural gloss on life."[26] Islam and the Moroccan polity were lived, imagined, and remembered in the body, a discursive and physical meeting-place of God, the polity, *shari'a* (religious law), and the soul. If Brinkley Messick describes Islamic textual domination of social reality as a "calligraphic state," then Morocco was a "geo-political moral body," a topographical landscape shaped by Islamic ways of knowing and healed and protected by Islamic knowers, the scholars (*'ulama'*) and the saints (*awliya'*).[27]

In precolonial Morocco, sovereignty arose from a Sufi Islamic conception of social corporeality. Moroccans recounted their local and collective histories through visiting shrines and practicing healing, forms of narrative that constructed Morocco as a great family tree. Branching from the generative body of Sultan Idris II to the tribes and cities of Morocco, God's healing mercies (*baraka*) flowed in water and human blood. Idris II became a Muslim "saint," or *wali*, the Friend of God whose knowledge of God restores His law to the Muslims, in their bodies and in the community (*umma*). As human bodies, the saints rooted God's mercy in the earth, dissolving the physical boundaries that separate individual souls from the Islamic *umma*. Chapter 1 shows how Sufi saints connected God's law in individual life to His law in social life through the body. The thaumaturgy of Moroccan saintly political leaders has been considered a facet of Weberian charisma and secondary to more "important" markers of social power like tribal affiliation, *sharifian* genealogy, or economic influence. But saintly healing betrays the essence of precolonial Moroccan political legitimacy. Saintly healing is the historical residue of a Sufi model

of popular sovereignty, an idea of popular politics that ultimately disappeared in Morocco between 1900 and 1930.

This interpretation is at odds with an existing literature on the Moroccan sultanate. For Elaine Combs-Schilling, the reigning 'Alawi dynasty
(1660–present) embodies the Prophet himself; the sultan is "the popular
representation of the collective [Moroccan] self," inscribed on living bodies in public Islamic rituals, sexual relations, birth, and death.[28] Other
scholars recognize the Moroccan monarch as a product of history who
emerged from colonial rule endowed with a new, absolutist power, the
"commander of the faithful, supreme representative of the nation" of the
1972 Moroccan Constitution, a sovereign who somehow transcends politics.[29] Abdellah Hammoudi attributes Moroccan authoritarianism to a
co-optation of the Sufi paradigm; the king absolutely dominates the Muslim citizen as the Sufi master ('arif) dominates the Sufi adept, eroding the
citizen's control over his own body (corps-propre) through a superior spiritual knowing.[30]

In contrast, this book contends that the king as "Moroccan sovereignty
embodied" is the invention of Sultan 'Abd al-Hafiz (ruled 1908–1912), a
construct made into administrative and legal reality by the 1912 Treaty
of Fez. Just as the Moroccan sultans adopted European sciences (engineering, medicine, architecture, water management) to enhance their state
power from 1660 to 1907, so 'Abd al-Hafiz strategically used French positivism to fight Muslim Sufi pretenders to his throne. Islamic saints historically challenged the sultans' authority, sometimes founding dynasties
(Almoravids, Almohads), leading jihad against invading foreign armies,
or ruling semiautonomous cities and regions (the Wazzaniyya). Using Islamic modernist thought (salafiyya) from the Muslim Orient, Sultan 'Abd
al-Hafiz and a circle of legal scholars discredited his Sufi rivals and their
forms of power by "redefining the real." Like French thinkers, Islamic
modernists defined truth as the "positive"—the empirical, the rational,
the verifiable, the true, and the visible. A new episteme changed political power, for "questions of epistemology are also questions of social order."[31] Sufi knowledge was suddenly recast as false and Sufi leaders became the scapegoats of Morocco's nationalist historical narrative—the
enemies of science, self-seeking charlatans, and the great collaborators
with the French occupier.[32]

The historical alliance of sultan-science-nationalism-salafiyya accounts
for Morocco's emergence from colonialism in 1956 as an Islamic monarchy rather than a secular Arab-socialist state like neighboring Algeria, Tu-

nisia, or Egypt. The 1912 Treaty of Fez decapitated the Muslim body politic and replaced its *makhzan* state with a French technocracy, a regime of science imposed over and against the Muslim body politic. In the king, Morocco retains an Islamic sovereignty re-embodied. In the Moroccan postcolonial state, a positive technocracy nationalized and Islamicized.

It is now a commonplace that the Islamic world adopted France as its model for scientific modernity. From Napoleon's invasion of Egypt in 1798, Muslim elites in the Ottoman Empire, Iran, North Africa, and Central Asia looked to France for massive modernization efforts (*tanzimat*), new militaries, medical schools, modern universities, and modern state bureaucracies.[33] Muslim intellectuals Rifaʿa al-Tahtawi, Taha Husayn, ʿAli Shariʿati, Ahmad Riza, Jamal al-Din al-Afghani, Muhammad ʿAbduh and others studied or lived in France and defined a self-conscious search for modernity through dialogues with French positivists. The Moroccan *salafis* Abu Shuʿayb al-Dukkali, ʿAllal al-Fasi, and Hasan al-Wazzani studied the rational social order of French and Islamic Comteans and envisioned its implementation for a modern Morocco. But in embracing French science as an unquestioned good, Islamic modernists have absorbed the French epistemological repugnance for Sufism and the Sufi path to knowledge. "*Salafi* anti-Sufism" derives not from Islam but from French positive science, an imperial episteme defined 1860–1900 against an Islamic and Sufi Other.[34]

AN EMPIRE OF POSITIVISM: MEDICINE AND THE FRENCH IMPERIAL NATION-STATE

In his [posthumous] work *La Sorcellerie au Maroc*, physician, secret agent, murder victim, and amateur ethnographer Émile Mauchamp cautions his reader, "If the documentary exposition of this work lacks poetry and grace . . . if it passes like a nausea of garbage, like an unchaste fetidity, it is because it is difficult to idealize garbage . . . As soon as one enters into the conceptions of Moroccan physiology and psychology . . . one must reconcile oneself to manipulating the naturalism of rubbish and latrines."[35] Like many of his Third-Republican contemporaries, Dr. Émile Mauchamp judged Islamic civilization by its sciences, particularly the medical sciences—physiology, anatomy, pathology, public health, pharmacy, and surgery. Medicine was the French yardstick of civilization in Muslim North Africa during the Third Republic (1870–1940) and reveals Greater France as an empire of positivism. France claimed not only to bring the benefits of science to empire but also its forms of knowledge, how to know oneself and the world. British imperialists defined essential difference in biological human races, but the French located civilization in the mind, in a rational ability to know.[36]

Imperial positivism illuminates the historical trajectory of the French civilizing mission in North Africa between 1830 and 1912. Alice Conklin locates the French "mission to civilize" in the republic of France and its boundless confidence in French superiority, mastery of nature, and a "perfectibility of humankind."[37] Yet historians have criticized the French Third Republic as racist, expansionist, and less benevolent than the military government in Algeria (1830–1871) or the monarchic "Royaume Arabe" of Napoleon III. Gérard Noiriel wonders that scientific racism should be elaborated after 1871, at the very moment when the Rights of Man were finally applied in France.[38] Gary Wilder finds no paradox in a racist republic, for Republican France was "never not an imperial nation-state." Created around a constitutive antinomy between universality and particularity, Republican France generated paradoxical outcomes for its colonized peoples, "social development without civil society, citizenship without culture, nationality without citizenship."[39] By 1902, France had abandoned direct rule and the assimilation of native peoples in favor of indirect rule and "association" with the colonized. Wilder attributes this policy shift to a rationalization of the French empire into a single juridico-political body, the interwar welfare state of Greater France.[40] Yet as Osama W. Abi-Mershed notes, assimilation and association shared the same underlying goal: to civilize, enlighten, unify, improve, and liberate the native through rational knowing.[41] The only true difference lay in method—how exactly to replace the native's irrational thought with a superior (French) rationality.

For a humane, rational, and modern imperialism, French colonial elites appropriated the ideas of Auguste Comte and *sociologie*, a "science of society." Émile Durkheim's *sociologie* offered colonial administrators an applied science through which to identify a society's evolution along a trajectory from the primitive to the civilized, a social laboratory for the classification of ethnographic "social facts." France thus became an "empire of facts,"[42] as policymakers used ethnography to design native education, medicine, cities, and laws uniquely tailored to the "Negro mind," the "Muslim mind,"[43] and the "Annamite mind." Alfred Le Chatelier, chair of "Muslim sociology and sociography" at the Collège de France, launched a Mission du Maroc to render Moroccan society as text, "ethno-graphy," thus constituting the archive from which to govern Morocco. The École Coloniale trained colonial administrators in *sociolo-*

gie to enable them to govern each society according to its culture and capacities, yet help peoples to evolve toward scientific method with hygiene,
roads, and public works—a persuasion through science to the liberation
of true thinking itself.

This book examines French empire through medicine, the French revolutionary science that became a "civilizing science" during the Third Republic. The revolutionary *idéologue* physicians of 1794 defined the human
being as a "finite, biologically-contrived entity" knowable and cultivable
through the scientific method—the Paris École de Médecine naturalized
the French rational self in observable anatomical phenomena—and hygienists such as Louis-René Villermé rendered human life in statistical ta-
bles.[44] Physicians designed state hygiene schemas to improve the citizen
and strengthen the national body, programs which doctor-legislators implemented as social-welfare legislation in the Third Republic.[45] Colonial
medicine had been a practicality for soldiers but became a pedagogy for
natives—hygiene to illustrate the public good, hospitals to demonstrate
the benevolent paternalism of French rule, and the laboratory to prove
the mechanical, biological, and universal truth of humanity.[46] Pasteurian biomedicine was an empire-wide network in which local knowledge
and metropolitan theory intertwined, where doctor-administrators circulated between colonial fields, metropolitan medical schools, and laboratory evidence. The imperial, transnational nature of the Pasteurian scientific community produced Charles Nicolle's typhus discoveries in French
Tunisia, Alphonse Laveran's isolation of the malaria parasite in French Algeria, and Alexandre Yersin's identification of a plague bacillus in French
Indochina.

But French colonial medicine was also torn by the internal contradictions of the French imperial nation-state itself. Pasteurian medicine was
the universal republic made flesh, an empirical science predicated upon
the universality of biological function in all human beings, a literal improvement of life by applying science to humanity. Pasteurian medicine
was also racial and particularizing, as colonial doctors elaborated exotic
pathologies from the ethnographically observed habits, morals, behavior,
and intellect of colonized peoples. The French compendia of "North African Pathology" were not merely topologies of disease organisms particular to the geographic region of Algeria-Tunisia-Morocco, they were also
articulations of Islam-as-pathology, corporeal manifestations of a "Muslim *mentalité*" on the biological body.

Chapter 2 traces the twining of French hygiene with *sociologie* in
North Africa from 1830 to 1900. In 1830, French doctors accepted Al-

gerian native physicians as fellow practitioners; by 1900, the same native healers were considered magicians and sorcerers. This rationalist critique was invented by French social scientists, *sociologues*, who used healing as a method of veridiction, "Tell me how you cure yourself, and I will tell you who you are." Magic betrayed the primitive mind trapped in the literal, visual, and sensory body, a Muslim *mentalité* incapable of abstract or conceptual thought. This colonially constructed Muslim mind became both the *mentalité indigène prémorbide* of the Algiers School of Psychiatry (1918) and a deformed "Muslim physiognomy" in the work of Algerian-French physician-legist Émile-Louis Bertherand.[47] In Morocco, doctors interrogated the Muslim body to reveal Islam's "truths" and to civilize the Muslim mind. Mauchamp claimed that French medicine would transform the Muslim through his body: "[Hygiene] will finish by impressing [the Moroccan], penetrating him, and fashioning him."[48]

The soldier, administrator, and colonial theorist Louis-Hubert-Gonzalve Lyautey invented the indirect-rule strategies codified in the interwar period by Minister of Colonies Albert Sarraut and the École Coloniale as "colonial humanism."[49] Lyautey advocated a peaceful conquest through science, a method he named *pénétration pacifique*, deploying four principles of action: *savoir, savoir-faire, savoir comment faire*, and *faire savoir*, ("knowing, knowing-how, knowing how to do, and making known").[50] Lyautey is often portrayed as a Catholic, royalist, anti-republican anti-intellectual, yet Lyautey theorized a Le Playist regeneration of France through a technocractic military-imperial French state in two articles published in the *Revue des Deux Mondes*.[51] Lyautey's field technique of collaborating with native elites attracted Minister of Foreign Affairs Théophile Delcassé, who wanted a *makhzan* strategy for the proposed Moroccan venture, and the scientifically minded Algerian *député* and leader of the École d'Alger, Eugène Étienne. Lyautey became the hero of the associationist colonial lobby of administrators from the AOF (Afrique Occidentale Française; French West Africa), the Union Coloniale Française, the Comité de l'Afrique Française, and their parliamentary group, the Parti Colonial. Lyautey implemented his vision as the founding resident-general of Morocco (1912–1925) and in France as director of the 1931 Paris Colonial Exhibition.

The treaty establishing the French protectorate in Morocco concretized Lyautey's vision and its internal contradictions. France was to modernize yet conserve, to incorporate Morocco to French empire yet preserve her sovereignty, to protect Islam with a positive science inherently hostile to it. Lyautey relied upon the physician to bridge these contradictions and to create Franco-Islamic social harmony, a colonial version of Third Republican *solidarisme*.[52] Instead, the French colonial welfare state broke apart at its seams of contradiction. The disjuncture between an ideal Moroccan-French social solidarity and a racially differentiating protectorate state came to crisis in the 1930s, as Moroccan nationalists reproached France for her failures and began to formulate an independent Moroccan modernity.

COLONIAL SCIENCE RE-EMBODIED, OR BECOMING ISLAMIC MODERN

One of the suspects to Mauchamp's murder was the Saharan jihadist, Islamic reformer, and leader of the Fadiliyya Sufi brotherhood Muhammad Mustapha Ma' al-'Aynayn Qaldami (1831–1910), the head of armed resistance against the French military in Mauritania.[53] When his "blue men of the desert" aimed their rifles at Mauchamp some months before the murder, the doctor complained afterwards, "[The governor] would do nothing and besides between a great saint like Ma el Ainin and myself there was no choice!"[54] But Ma' al-'Aynayn was already the last of a vanishing political idiom by 1907, a saintly, miracle-working Sufi Islamic leader like the Mahdi of Sudan or 'Abd al-Qadir in Algeria. Fighting saints disappeared in the twentieth century, to be replaced by self-styled modern and nationalist bourgeoisies who embraced Western political philosophy, industrialization, and the nation-state.[55] Embodied modernity did not make Moroccans into Frenchmen, but it did change Moroccan political authority; it made marabouts into nationalists.

The public spectacle of a French doctor's mutilated corpse in 1907 might suggest that Moroccans held little appreciation for French medical science and less for its practitioners. Yet European physicians, engineers, and army officers served the Moroccan court from the sixteenth century, and rural populations clamored for access to the new European sciences. Chapter 3 examines the complexities of French medicine on the eve of colonial conquest. Because the Moroccan public imagined sovereignty through the body, popular fears of imminent European territorial invasion and the concomitant loss of Moroccan self-determination took shape as medical rumor and collective symbolic violence to the body of a French doctor. After conquest, France used the body to co-opt Islamic authority in Morocco, both by reconstructing the Moroccan sultan as a sovereign ruler and by attempting to bring the *wali*'s saintly mediation to French scientific spaces.

In Moroccan cities, municipal hygiene forced a definition of the public: who is the citizen, what is the social body served by the protectorate state, how is sovereignty to be defined and located? Lyautey expected colonial medicine to generate a Franco-Moroccan civic culture, but colonial medicine produced instead state dysfunction and ultimately popular nationalism. Because a state not a republic provided health care to a patient who was not a citizen, Moroccans fought the imposed French medical state and hygienists treated Moroccans as a disease environment rather than a public to protect. Chapter 4 examines the dis-junctures of state-nation-body in French empire by following the social histories of malaria, plague, typhus, and typhoid in Moroccan cities. Through their biological bodies, Moroccans were able to assert themselves as political subjects and to contest the urban polity of which they were a part. Failed colonial urban hygiene politicized traditional Moroccan elites, who seized upon new French-created municipal government to demand promised scientific reforms, exact redress, and, ultimately, to question the legitimacy of French rule itself. Disease, not pamphlets, drove the public to the young Moroccan nationalists, who demanded a new polity through the suffering Muslim body itself.

In both French Republican and Moroccan Islamic contexts, the law defines the individual's capacities, the signs of his birth, life, and death, and the biological and ontological sources of his political rights. Chapter 5 shows how the male French doctor's quest for medical authority extended colonial technocracy into Muslim law, Muslim family life, and Moroccans' conceptions of their own bodies. Medical authority was also a gender question, for Muslim women made health decisions for the family, delivered babies, and provided expert legal evidence about women's bodies to Islamic courts. Women thus mediated how law and medicine met to constitute the Moroccan as juridical subject. But by offering a urine test for pregnancy, the Institut Pasteur relocated truth-telling from the Muslim soul to the French laboratory, the "essential characteristic of modern power."[56] In the laboratory, the body testified to scientists instead of to God, a new concept of truth that Moroccans themselves introduced to Islamic law courts.

Industrialization and urbanization progressed very rapidly in Morocco between 1915 and 1950, producing a food, disease, and housing crisis for which French authorities were entirely unprepared. To prevent a nationalist revolution and to protect its native industrial workforce, the French protectorate created a self-proclaimed "*médico-social*" welfare state after World War II, uniting the surveillance of individual bodies with the census, new housing, and maternal and infant health programs for Muslims. Paternalist France posed as patriarch to a modernizing Muslim family, sending Muslim girls to French "mother schools," opening maternity wards for Muslim women, and training natives as birth attendants to replace traditional midwives. Public health became the battleground between colonial authorities and Moroccan nationalists, who fought back with their own vision of state patriarchy.

Chapter 6 examines the biopolitical struggle between the colonial state and *salafi* nationalists to define the Moroccan nation and control the Muslim family. Moroccan nationalists framed colonialism as disease, yet even as they indicted the French civilizing mission, nationalists adopted the French language of scientific modernity. Moroccans reimagined the Muslim *umma* as a nation and targeted women as the polity's biological and cultural foundation. Amid clashing colonial-nationalist biopolitical schemes, the example of colonial obstetrics in Morocco suggests that the body itself remains a seat of individual human agency. In the Moroccan woman's collapsed pelvis and the Moroccan infant's kwashiorkor, the body itself testified, giving direct evidence against a failed state and a divided body politic.

Each chapter of the book addresses a different problem in the history of medicine and thus draws upon a range of sources and methodologies. The colonial is examined not in a linear narrative but as a series of medical encounters: international espionage and a doctor's murder (Chapter 3), disease and revolt in Moroccan cities (Chapter 4), a battle for authority between doctors and Muslim midwives (Chapter 5), and the search for national identity in the welfare state (Chapter 6). The sources are written and oral, French and Arabic: French military archives, municipal records, maps, French diplomatic archives, hospital records, medical photography, colonial ethnography, French medical journals and monographs, Arabic medical manuscripts, Moroccan Sufi hagiography, Moroccan newspapers, and my interviews with Moroccan herbalists, midwives, doctors, and patients in Fez, 1995–2000.

COLONIAL EMBODIMENT AND QUESTIONS OF MODERNITY

A considerable theoretical literature asks what colonialism teaches about modernity: if it was invented in the laboratory of the colonies and imported to the metropole, or the modern is a European self-construct defined against an un-modern non-West, or the elements that we call "modernity" are actually a collective invention of the world's peoples, or the

European modern is one in a multitude of modernities, or that modernity is a singular, universal project undertaken by various Western and non-Western societies in a self-conscious desire to be modern.[57] But as Bruno Latour insists, *We Have Never Been Modern*, because modernity's premise—the absolute separation of nature and culture—is impossible. Modernity is not only impossible, it is also blinkered, for a modern way of thinking cannot see the world as it truly is, full of hybrids. Why then would we—would anyone—wish to be modern?

Modernity offers a promise, a guarantee, that man can exact truth from nature and have sovereignty over himself as a citizen-subject. By separating nature and culture, science claims to perfectly translate Nature's truth, "it is not men who make Nature," and society is made by absolutely free beings, "human beings, and only human beings, are the ones who construct society and freely determine their own destiny."[58] To create truth and freedom, "There shall exist a complete separation between the natural world (constructed nevertheless by man) and the social world (sustained nevertheless by things)."[59] Yet man is hybrid, he is *the* hybrid by virtue of his body, a reality that the liberal political subject continually flees. Modernity is flight from the body, an internal self-mutilating cut to invent a modern citizen free of his body. The non-moderns are those enmeshed in bodies—the colonized, children, deviants, women—those whose unmastered corporeality excludes them from full political rights. These body-subjects are nature-culture contaminations unable to separate "what is knowledge from what is society," "For Them, Nature and Society, signs and things, are virtually coextensive. For Us they never should be."[60] Colonial modernity can only be conceived as the therapeutic rescue of Muslims, a replacement of Islamic epistemology by natural law and the liberating cutting-away of minds from bodies.

But if we take the body as a unit of analysis, we can both avoid and historicize modernity's epistemological cage. Embodiment offers a not-modern way of seeing, a subjectivity in and of the body. "The body is my point of view on the world," writes Merleau-Ponty, "I am the absolute source, my existence does not stem . . . from my physical and social environment; instead it moves out towards them and sustains them."[61] Healing is a beginning from which to recover being; as Victor Turner argues, the afflicted connect material and spiritual worlds in otherwise impossible combinations, overcoming mental categories to express "the act-of-being itself."[62] In Morocco, Vincent Crapanzano finds the Hamadsha Sufi order simultaneously treating "real" physical ailments and engaging history; the Hamadsha healers and patients "act out, albeit symbolically, the scars of their past."[63] This book offers a history of Moroccan politics and sovereignty through the body, a way to analyze the Islamic social discourses that currently challenge the legitimacy of postcolonial North African states. Bodies are what Timothy Mitchell has called the "unmanageable excess" of the modern, the repositories of nonmodernity that challenge us to rethink modernity itself.[64]

HEALING THE BODY, HEALING THE *UMMA*: SUFI SAINTS AND GOD'S LAW IN A CORPOREAL CITY OF VIRTUE

Ya Mawlay Yaʿqub
Daʿwini min al-habub
Fʾana gharib wa barrani.
(O Lord [Saint] Jacob
Cure me from the sore
For I am a stranger and an outsider.)
POPULAR FEZ SONG, REFERRING TO THE SHRINE OF MAWLAY YAʿQUB
NEAR FEZ, WHERE THE HOT SPRINGS PROVIDE RELIEF FROM A
VARIETY OF SKIN AILMENTS

AFTER A FAILED REVOLT AGAINST the Saʿdiyyan sultan ʿAbdallah II
(ruled 1613–1623), the city of Fez feared his vengeance and sent two mad
saints (*majdhubin*) to intercede on its behalf with the enraged ruler. When
the sultan received the two emissaries, Sidi Jallul bin al-Haj and Sidi
Masaʿud al-Sharrat, he scoffed, "The people of Fez couldn't find any to
mediate for them but these two shitters in their rags" (literally, "he who
evacuates his bowels").[1] Angered, Sidi Jallul replied, "By God, you will
not have a free hand [in Fez] for forty-one years," and the saints departed.
Suddenly, the sultan's stomach reversed and he vomited feces from his
mouth for several days, until he sent for the saints and begged their pardon. No sultan ruled in Fez for the period Sidi Jallul had predicted "until God brought" the ʿAlawi sultan Rashid. "And this story is true," concludes the court historian al-Ifrani, "for I heard it from many people, and
I summarize what was told to us."[2]

The vomiting sultan suggests a precolonial political imaginary in
which Sufi saints were "public healers," restoring bodies and the community to wholeness.[3] As al-Ifrani's chronicle suggests, this political vision
relied upon a way of knowing in which miracles, body experiences, and
the lives of the saints were history—not legends or symbols, but history,

accepted and integrated into the official text of a court scholar. Modern historians of Africa have illuminated alternate epistemologies to positivism and multiple ways of knowing the past; they ask us to "experience all these representations of reality as realities."[4] Sainthood was the essence of premodern Moroccan social reality, yet contemporary historians seldom include Islamic saints in the narrative of Moroccan history.[5] As Steven Feierman observes, historians tend to privilege the diachronic, stable, and linear—dynasties and colonial rule—the miraculous becomes unintelligible and therefore invisible to history.[6] What narrative might emerge, he wonders, were we to construct African history from purely African ways of knowing?

For the Moroccan historian al-Ifrani and his readers, the sultan's body obeyed a political authority derived from Sufi Islamic epistemology. In Islamic thought, the legitimate Muslim leader must be a reflection of the Prophet Muhammad and emulate his spiritual guardianship (*walaya*) and political power (*wilaya*) in the Muslim community (*umma*).[7] The Muhammadan Reality is knowledge of God, wrote the Sufi 'Abd al-Qadir al-Jilani; leadership is an "intellect ['aql] because it comprehends universal truths [*kulliyyat*], and a pen [*qalam*] because it is an instrument for the transmission of knowledge."[8] But because knowing could not be monopolized in an office, a kingdom, or even a sultan's body, the leader in Morocco was often not the sultan, nor indeed a single person.

As the Moroccan jurist 'Abd al-Qadir al-Fasi (1598–1680) observed, leadership in Morocco was of two separable elements: a limited, temporal sultanate and a continuous, spiritual imamate.[9] The cities and tribes of Morocco invested the sultan with temporal authority through a legal contract of rule, a *bay'a*, defining him as the servant of God's *umma* who must respect the people's rights.[10] Spiritual leadership, the imamate, flowed from direct knowledge (*ma'rifa*) of God's reality (*haqiqa*), a diffuse, mobile, invisible, esoteric, Gnostic knowing superior to and outside the mechanisms of state control. The *awliya'*, (singular, *wali*), translated variously as "Friends of God," "People of [His] Right Hand," or "Islamic saints," were knowers (*'arifun*) among the people—jurists, tribesmen, Sufis, merchants, physicians, beggars, craftsmen, sultans, women, and others—who achieved intimacy with God. The public validated saints by recognizing their miracles, visiting them in life and death, and narrating their lives in healing. Miracle-working saints sometimes contended with the sultans for political power, directed military action and war, created states or quasi states, governed territory, collected taxes, and negotiated trade agreements.

The vomiting sultan reveals this political vision as reliant upon a human body obedient to God and active in worldly politics. The Sufi Muhya ad-Din ibn 'Arabi described its cosmological system; the human body is a microcosm of the human city and a parallel realm for God's "divine system for the reform (*islah*) of the human kingdoms."[11] As God appointed the human soul to be His Vice-Regent on Earth, so He created the human body as a citadel for its residence. As a just ruler produces a harmonious city, so a just soul produces a harmonious body; an unjust soul will provoke the body's members to revolt. So it was that the stomach of Sultan 'Abdallah II rose against tyranny in the two citadels—Fez and his own person—to uphold God's law in the two realms. The Qur'an warns man that his body will testify to God on the Day of Judgment: "*That day shall We set a seal on their mouths, but their hands will speak to Us and their feet bear witness to all that they did*" (36:65). In Fez in 1623, we find Qur'anic promise fulfilled: a body testified to God in order to restore God's law to man and society. Michel Chodkiewicz has argued that Moroccan saints concretized Sufism's abstractions through their human personalities,[12] but it was the body that grounded Sufi knowing in social reality. It was the body-as-space that allowed saints to act in the world and heal the *umma* as a geopolitical entity.

Fez illustrates an elusive concept: the Sufi polity. The ideal Islamic polity, the City of Virtue, *al-madina al-fadila*, was first articulated by the Islamic philosopher al-Farabi. But al-Farabi envisioned a city of reason, not a Sufi city of saintly miracles. Contemporary scholars of Islamic political theory also give little thought to Sufism, which they consider an individual and contemplative path to God.[13] Yet the Fez of al-Ifrani's text exemplified al-Farabi's virtuous city: a man could realize his full perfection only in society, the law was God's law, and a knower of God (*'arif*) guaranteed the application of His laws. Indeed, the knower (*'arif*) could be at once political and "beyond this earthly world."[14] As Sufi knowing was shared among many *awliya'*, authority was decentralized, rendering the sultan the people's executor. The human body was thus the means by which God's law entered into human life, not the source of "evil inclinations" or "enslavement" for the soul.[15]

But this Sufi polity was challenged in the early twentieth century, when the threat of foreign invasion led a Moroccan sultan, his court officials, and some legal scholars to consider a different idea of truth. To defend Morocco against European colonialism, the sultan's court adopted European scientific and military reforms and Islamic modernist *salafiyya* philosophy from the Orient (Mashriq). Predicated upon a positive theory of knowledge, *salafiyya* proved useful to Sultan ʿAbd al-Hafiz (ruled 1908–1912) for the consolidation of his central state power. With its war on saintly intermediaries (*wasaʾit*) and invisible knowledge, *salafiyya* empowered the sultan to discredit saintly critics and rivals. In 1909, Sultan ʿAbd al-Hafiz executed a Sufi saint, marking the definitive triumph of sultans over saints, of positivism over *batini* knowing, and a new imagining of social corporeality in Morocco.

UNITING TWO MODELS OF POLITICAL LEGITIMACY: THE *SHARIF* AND THE SUFI *QUTB*

We raise to degrees those whom We will, and above every possessor of knowledge is One more knowing.
QURʾAN 12:76

What was the role of saints in Moroccan politics on the eve of the French protectorate? Ernest Gellner has argued that tribal society produces saints functionally to mediate disputes in the absence of a central state authority, whereas Clifford Geertz sees saintly *baraka* (blessing) as a Weberian charisma possessed by saints and sultans to varying degrees.[16] Vincent Cornell offers an alternative: the Jazuliyya Sufi order synthesized a uniquely Moroccan and Islamic conception of political sovereignty in the sixteenth century, a precolonial Moroccan political identity fundamentally unlike nationalism or *salafiyya* Islamic reform.[17] This chapter considers the social, geographic, spatial, and temporal aspects of Jazulite sovereignty, an Islamic *umma* imagined in and through the human body.

The philosophical basis of Moroccan political sovereignty developed as a blend of *sharifian* Hasanid Shiʾism and Jazulite Sufism. In other words, Moroccans had two ways of envisioning political leadership, both of which emulate the Prophet Muhammad. After the Prophet died in 632, the Islamic world battled over how to replace him. A refugee from the conflict fled to Morocco in 789, Idris ibn ʿAbd Allah, a blood descendant of the Prophet Muhammad through his grandson al-Hasan (d. 669).

The oldest model of political authority in Morocco is thus "sharifism," a notion that blood descent from the Prophet imparts both a privileged knowledge of God's realities and the legitimacy to rule. Although the Umayyads invaded Morocco, Idris I created a unified Islamic state under his rule in 789 and Moroccans credit his lineage, the Idrisids (789–921), with the introduction of the Arabic language and Islam to Morocco.[18] After being overthrown by the Zanata Berbers in 921, the Idrisids continued to claim the throne by promoting a sharifian model of leadership and celebrations for the Prophet's birthday (*mawlid*).[19]

A newer model of leadership came from Sufism and the Moroccan Sufi Muhammad ibn Sulayman al-Jazuli (d. 1465). Sufi thinkers prior to al-Jazuli conceived the Friend of God, the *wali*, as a person who reflected the "Muhammadan way" through his direct knowledge (*ma'rifa*) of God. Muhya ad-Din ibn al-'Arabi (d. 1240) believed that the *wali* could come to mirror the divine archetype of the Perfect Man and be a human expression of the divine Word in the universe.[20] 'Abd al-Karim al-Jili (d. 1402–3) argued that the Prophet Muhammad never died, but is an eternal living reality who returns in each generation to guide the people in the guise of an "axial saint" (*qutb*).[21] Muhammad al-Jazuli argued that because the Sufi *qutb* mastered both exoteric and esoteric spheres of knowledge, he was the ideal political leader: "By virtue of the Truth (*haqiqa*), he becomes a leader of men, who assent [to his guidance] by carrying out what he asks them to do."[22]

Al-Jazuli thus fused sultanic and saintly authority, temporal and spiritual leadership, with a theory of knowledge. The Jazuliyya argued that the axial saint, like Muhammad, reached the "point of complete knowledge" at which all truth and guidance converged. According to a Jazulite *shaykh*:

> The Terrain of Safety is the "point of complete knowledge" (*nuqtat al-'ilm al-kamali*) that legitimizes the sainthood of authority, *wilaya*. The "city" (*madina*) of this dominion is Muhammad, the "gate" (*bab*) of the city is the Prophet's cousin and son-in-law 'Ali, the founder of the Sufi Way, and the "key" (*miftah*) to the gate is the Generative Saint (*al-ghawth*) or Axis of the Age (*qutb az-zaman*). This person stands alone as the successor to the Prophet.[23]

Al-Jazuli reconciled the *sharif* and the *qutb* socially by uniting the fragmented Moroccan Sufi brotherhoods into a single network and a universal spiritual path. Idrisids entered or founded Sufi orders with Jazulite doctrine, like the 'Isawa of Meknes, and al-Jazuli praised the Prophet's lineage with his book of prayer, *Dala'il al-khayrat wa shawariq al-anwar fi dhikr as-salat 'ala an-nabi al-mukhtar* (Tokens of blessings and advents of illumination in the invocation of prayers on behalf of the chosen Prophet). Finally, al-Jazuli encouraged his followers to visit Moroccan saints when the hajj pilgrimage to Mecca was impossible.[24] This Jazulite notion, that a visit to the saints of Morocco could replace a visit to the Ka'ba, helped to create a local Moroccan spiritual authority generated by the *baraka* (blessing) of local saints.

The Sa'adiyyan sultans appropriated Jazulite ideas in the sixteenth century, when Sultan Muhammad al-Qa'im (1509–1517) led Moroccan armies to victory over Portuguese invaders. His son Muhammad ash-Shaykh "al-Mahdi" (1548–1557) united Morocco under Sa'adiyyan leadership in 1549 and portrayed himself as a saintly renewer of religion (*mahdi*).[25] Quite rightly, al-Mahdi saw the Jazuliyya as potential political rivals, but the Jazulite *shaykh* al-Wazzani explicitly renounced political ambition: "Rather than fearing the *qutb*, the just Islamic ruler should welcome this saint and cleave to him. Comparing the state to a tree . . . the *qutb* is the water that brings the state to life."[26] For most of Moroccan history, the saints left political rule to the sultans, but in moments of dynastic conflict, foreign invasion, and social crisis, *mahdis* and Sufi saints rose to lead the people in jihad and a renewal of religion.

The Jazuliyya thus provided the root metaphor of the Moroccan leader as Knower, but the human body provided the space for his knowing to enter the world. Consider the words of al-Jazuli: "The fully actualized Jazulite sheikh (*ash-shaykh al-wasil*) has arrived at the station of direct perception (*maqam al-mushahada*) . . . When he returns to humankind he has illumination (*anwar*), sciences (*'ulum*) and laws (*ahkam*)."[27] Knowing is spatial, for the *wali* is in the place of prophethood, an axis around whom reality revolves (*qutb*), a sanctuary for the believer (*maqam*),[28] and a doorway to the divine: "The saint is a door and visiting them is a key and loving them is entry, for if you loved them, they love you, and if they love you they choose you, they help you arrive at the goal, and they raise you to your Lord."[29] It is the saint's location in space as a body that allows him to mediate between divine and material worlds, to bind men to God (*murabit*, he who binds/connects). It is for this reason that pilgrims touched saints' bodies for cure, swallowed their saliva, ate earth from their graves, and slept in their tombs, for the *wali*'s body was an opening to God in the world.

TELLING HISTORY ON THE GRAVES: SAINT SHRINES AS A TOPOGRAPHICAL MAP OF THE PAST

The saints were thus literal tent stakes, anchoring a floating map of miraculous events on the Moroccan landscape with their bodies. Mircea Eliade has argued that the hierophanic miracle is a breaking-through from divine to terrestrial reality, rendering historical time legible as sacred space.[30] As Christian pilgrims read the Bible in the stained-glass pictograms of medieval cathedrals, so Moroccans read a history of God's presence on a landscape defined by the graves of His saints. The *awliya'* were people of different times and places whose knowing opened the world to God's miraculous grace (*baraka*). By visiting their graves, pilgrims connected discrete moments in time to form a topographical map of the past, a geographic Moroccan *umma*. As the Moroccan public remembered the past in pilgrimage, so the sultans tried to manipulate public memory by both building and destroying buildings on *wali* graves. To illustrate such politics, we consider a short history of the graves of Idris I and Idris II.

The grave of Idris I on Zarhun mountain became a rallying point for the political ambitions of his descendants, the Idrisids. As blood descendants of the Prophet Muhammad, the Idrisids used their ancestor Idris I to claim the throne lost in 921, a challenge to which the Berber dynasties were especially vulnerable. The Berber Marinids (1256–1465), for example, had no blood tie to the Prophet and thus only an insecure claim to power.[31] Trying to force the people to forget Idris I and the Idrisids, the Marinid sultan 'Uthman II (1310–1331) used his armies to chase pilgrims from Idris's grave, as the chronicler Abu Hasan 'Ali al-Jazna'i recounted:

> Idris—may God be pleased with him—was buried outside the gate of Walili. And the people have been determined to visit his tomb. There they cry out their needs to God and are heard (by Him). His body appeared in its shroud in the year 718H/A.D. 1318. So people streamed to it from every part of the Maghrib, causing fears of a riot. Our lord, Abu Sa'id 'Uthman b. Ya'qub b. 'Abd al-Haqq—may God accept his deeds—sent an army to drive them away from that place, and to put an end to the disturbances.[32]

To build their own legitimacy, the Marinids used the body of Idris II to reinvent themselves as his political heirs. In 1437, the Marinids "discovered" the unblemished corpse of Idris II perfumed with amber and untouched by decay, which they reburied in a magnificent shrine in the city of Fez.[33] The "Mawlay Idris" shrine-mosque thus became a center of visitation, and Idris II the patron *wali* of Fez after five hundred years of obscurity. The Marinids also promoted a written history of Morocco and commissioned scholarly histories of Fez, *Rawd al-Qirtas* (Garden of Papers; 1326) and *Zahrat al-As* (The Myrtle Flower; 1360), chronicles which

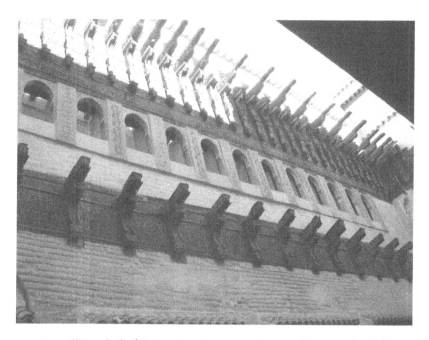

FIGURE 1.1. Water clock of Bu Inania madrasa, one of many edifices constructed by the Marinids in Fez to enhance their political legitimacy. (Author photograph.)

highlight Idris II as the builder of Fez. The Marinids presented themselves as his heirs by constructing magnificent Fez mosques, fountains, and *madrasat*.[34]

Two hundred years later, when the sharifian ʿAlawiyyin (1661–present) came to power, Sultan Ismaʿil (1672–1727) found the city of Fez fiercely resistant to his policies. To replace Fez as a sacred site and to supplant the Marinids with his own dynasty, Ismaʿil built a mosque and madrasa complex at the tomb of Idris I on Zarhun mountain and prayed there himself.[35] Ismaʿil hoped that the new shrine would remind the people of his place in the Prophet's lineage and draw pilgrims' devotion away from Idris II in favor of Idris I, thus shifting the sacred center of Morocco from Fez to Zarhun mountain.

Despite the sultans' efforts, Moroccans interpreted the shrines, saints, and Idrisids for themselves. Oral traditions across Morocco recount that as the Idrisids fell from power, an Idrisid child fled to their region and found refuge with a local family, who hid him from enemy soldiers. Over time the sharifian child became so mixed with the family's own sons that the whole family was known as *shurafa'*. A French sociologist recorded one such narrative in the Habt region near Marrakesh in 1911:

> At the moment of the persecution of the Idrisids by Musa ibn Abi-l-ʿAfiya, in 317 A.H. (929 A.D.) . . . a *sharif* Idrisi who was still a child, pursued by enemy soldiers who wanted to kill him, took refuge in the house of a *baqqal* (oil and soap merchant) of the Ghezaoua. Summoned by the pursuers to hand over the young *sharif*, the *baqqal*, to save a descendant of the Prophet, gave one of his own sons to the soldiers. Later, after the persecution of the Idrisids ended, the *baqqal* revealed to the *sharif*, whom he raised with his own sons, his real origin . . . The *Awlad al-Baqqal* [Children of the *baqqal*] quickly became the object of veneration of all the people of the country.[36]

This oral tradition reveals a merging of the Moroccan body politic with the human body, a human tree branching from Fez to other cities and tribes, transmitting the Prophet's *baraka* from the Idrisids to local lineages across Morocco. The tree is an image of the Sufi chain of spiritual learning (*silsila*), but the people used the generative human body of

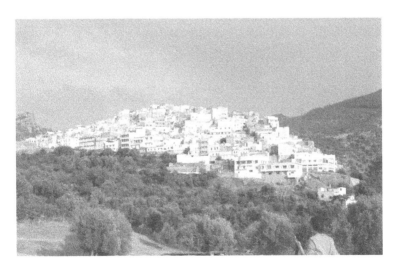

FIGURE 1.2. City-shrine-tomb of Idris I, Mawlay Idris az-Zarhun.

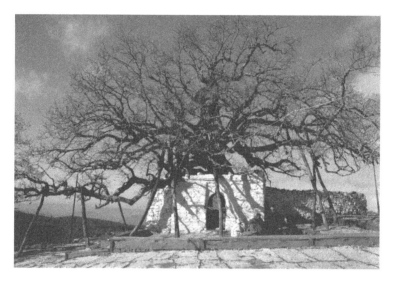

FIGURE 1.3. The shrine-body of Mawlay ʿAbd al-Salam ibn Mashish, which is also an actual tree. (Peter Sanders Photography.)

Idris II to join the Sufi tree with the Prophet's family tree, a popular synthesis of sharifian and Sufi authority. An actual tree grows from the grave of the Idrisid and axial saint ʿAbd as-Salam ibn Mashish (d. 1228), a literal and metaphorical expression of his corporeal and spiritual power (see Fig. 1.3). As saints' bodies were vehicles for articulating Moroccan history, so suffering bodies were places for God's spiritual guidance (*walaya*) to renew itself in individual human life.

THE BODY AS ARCHIVE: IDRIS II AND THE ʿAZAMI CURE FOR BU ZELLUM

In 1999, I sat behind a desk in a state medical clinic in the Lamtiyyin neighborhood of Fez and interviewed four elderly local residents. After a rousing critique of today's health service, one man volunteered that his family cures "Bu Zellum," a shooting pain from the base of the spine down the leg caused by "a blocked artery in the leg" or "a constriction of the intestines":

> We have an illness, because we are *shurafaʾ* and our ancestor is Sidi Yahya, the son of this Mawlay Idris, he is our ancestor. And we have a

wahmy [spiritual, psychological] illness, they call it Bu Zellum. We cure it. It strikes here (showing base of the spine), in this joint here.

To treat Bu Zellum, the patient must visit the tomb of Sidi Yahya in the Sanhaja region and consult one of his descendants from the 'Azami tribe. Each patient has "his plant" in the open countryside (*khalaa*, empty place, undomesticated land), which "lights up the night like burning embers" to the 'Azami, who mark it with ashes or wheat chaff.[37] The next day, the 'Azami return to the plant and cut its stem, thus "cutting the vein" for the patient:

> At dawn, we get up and go out to that plant, we spend the night with it, we say we are going to cut [Bu Zellum] by means of it (*ghadi naqtao biha*) to so-and-so, for example. We put that plant in front of us, and we read *al-Fatiha* over it [the opening verse of the Qur'an] . . . They say, "In the name of God the Beneficent, the Merciful, praises to God the Lord of Worlds," to the end of the verse. Then we say, "I cut it for so-and-so, son of [his mother's name]." And they cut that stem with a knife, and he is cured, by the permission of God.[38]

When I inquired why the 'Azami are able to cure this pain, the answer was a history of the early Islamic state in Morocco:

> E: Why does that thing work?
> M: What do you mean?
> E: What is the means [of operation]? How does it work?
> M: That *baraka* . . . Our grandfather, he is Sidi Yahya, the son of Mawlay Idris. Because Mawlay Idris the second left twelve sons . . . It is a historical question. When the rule of the Idrisids disappeared, the Idrisids began to escape. Our ancestor came, escaped to this area, here to the region of Taounat. To one mountain. There he lived, there he had children. There now there is still a tribe, how big! Big! It is called the *shurafa'* 'Azamiyyin.

I began to regard the Moroccan body as an archive, a repository of a lost form of political authority. Saintly healing has often been marginalized by Peter Brown's "two-tiered model of religious piety," which posits that a supreme being is grasped only by an orthodox elite, whereas the masses need an anthropolatrous cult of the saints in order to understand and approach divinity.[39] But as scholars of Sufism argue, theoretical Islamic concepts become "activated" when experienced, built, and enacted in the sensory world. Reciting the Qur'an releases God's word to energize the phenomenal world. The pilgrim realizes the full reality of the Ka'ba as the axis of the universe when he circumambulates it physically on his own two feet.[40]

In the 'Azami cure, we see the patient live God's mercy in his own body and connect his personal life to a larger history of the Moroccan *umma*. The 'Azami link the sufferer to the Prophet Muhammad through healing; as Idris II reflected the Prophet, so Sidi Yahya reflects Idris II. The cure connects layers of reality otherwise fragmented in temporal life—politics, geography, history, the soul, and God—restoring the individual's integration to a divine cosmological and moral order. Hasan al-Yusi (d. 1691) called the saints "a medicine and a cure,"[41] for as the scholars write, the saint "connects the various layers of reality to each other,"[42] he is the "object of [God's] self-awareness,"[43] and His means in the world.[44]

The cure also locates Moroccan identity in geographic space, for the patient must access *baraka* through the *wali*'s body or its topographical projection—a tomb, a tree, a spring. Sidi Yahya's buried body transforms Taounat mountain into a living extension of his soul, a wellspring of 'Azami identity. Saints' bodies also planted and thus legitimized other collective identities. Each guild in Fez had its patron *wali*; for example, weavers visited the grave of Sidi 'Ali al-M'salih, a weaver who miraculously produced great volumes of cloth in a single day.[45] The *jaysh* military tribes that the sultans brought to Fez explained their presence in the city as a miracle of their tribal *wali*, Sidi Qasim. The Shararda *jaysh* troops discovered a miraculous "second tomb" for Sidi Qasim on the grounds of their Fez fort (*qasba al-shararda*), thereby planting their identity in Fez.[46] A saint's shrine was thus simultaneously an environment for tribes, guilds, and villages to collect memory (a *milieu de mémoire*),[47] an opening to divine grace in the world, and a chronological point on the geographic Moroccan map of history.

Saints heal by actualizing the human body as the meeting place of divinity and materiality. In Sufi thought, the body is both a clay vessel for divine spirit (*ruh*) and an isthmus (*barzakh*) between the "oceans of God and the cosmos."[48] The Qur'an alludes to human bodies as sites of God's revelation (*ayat*), "*We will show them Our Signs in the horizons, and within themselves*" (41:53) and of His reflection (*tashbih*); God has a "face" (2:115) and "two hands," and created Adam in His own image.[49] The human body is fragile yet contains the Omnipotent, according to the

Hadith *qudsi*: "My earth and My heaven do not encompass Me, but the heart of My servant does encompass Me." Unlike the Christian rejection of the flesh, the Muslim body can hold God, according to the Hadith *qudsi*:

> Nothing draws My servant near to Me like the performance of what I prescribe for him as religious duty . . . So that, when I love him, I become the ear by which he hears, his eye by which he sees, his hand by which he grasps, and the foot by which he walks. Thus, by Me he hears; by Me he sees; by Me he grasps and by Me he walks.[50]

A human body existing simultaneously in several planes of reality is suggested by emanationist Islamic cosmology and colonial ethnography collected in 1926 in Marrakesh:

> Stars are the celestial doubles of human beings, *jinn* familiars are their underground doubles, and the leaves of the Trees of Paradise are their doubles in Paradise. When human beings are sick, the genie double is sick with the same sickness, his star pales and the leaf of the Tree of Paradise yellows and curls. At the hour of death, the genie dies first, the star falls from the sky as a shooting star and the leaf detaches from the Tree of Paradise.[51]

Extending the tree metaphor, we find a human body bridging the boundaries of multiple worlds, with roots in the earth, a trunk in human society, and leaves in paradise. The body itself thus links the operation of God's law in individual life to His law in society, a relationship we examine in a social history of the city of Fez. Our source is the three-volume hagiographical compendium of the Moroccan scholar Muhammad ibn Ja'far al-Kattani, *Kitab salwat al-anfas wa muhadathat al-akyas bi man uqbira min al-'ulama' wa al-sulaha' bi Fas* (Entertainment of the souls and discourse of the sagacious concerning the scholars and righteous persons buried in Fez), a late nineteenth-century aggregate of written and oral memory about the Fez saints (*awliya'*). Read in light of contemporary healing narratives, colonial ethnography, and the Fez urban landscape, the *Salwa* blurs the human city and the human body. The Knowers animate and illuminate the city's soil, model social virtue for the city's residents, and open a channel between spirit and matter with the key of Sufi knowing.

THE BEATING HEART OF MAWLAY IDRIS:
THE CITY OF FEZ AS A BODY OF KNOWLEDGE

Orientalists describe the Islamic city as a social reflection of Islamic law, but al-Kattani describes Fez as a living being brought into existence by prayer, the collective wish of the Muslims to be the city described in the Qur'an: "*God will bring forth a community whom God loves and who love God, humble toward those who believe and powerful against those who reject, who struggle in the path of God and fear nobody's reproach*" (5:54).[52] In al-Kattani's *Salwa*, Fez is a *zawiya* (Sufi lodge) often visited by the Prophet Muhammad, a city His saints protect from tyranny: "[In Fez] the arrogant one will find people who break his force, and his power will vanish because of their power."[53] The saints mediate the city's ecosystem, causing rain to fall and plants to spring from the earth. Without their knowledge, "afflictions would flow forth onto the people of the earth like an inundation" and the people would be "blind like beasts."[54] Science (*'ilm*) flows from the city and its inhabitants; it "wells from the chests of its people" and "gushes forth from the city walls," a flood opened by the builder of Fez, Idris II.[55]

In al-Kattani's text, Idris II is a Muhammadan figure who called upon God to make Fez "a house of knowledge (*'ilm*) and law, the recitation of Your Book and may she uphold Your limits, and may her people be faithful adherents of the Sunna."[56] "Mawlay" (Lord) Idris brought Islam to the people as sciences (*'ulum*), law (*shari'a*) and truth (*haqiqa*): "The root of the tree of religion was confirmed, and her branches stretched to the sky. Through his *baraka*, the people of Morocco knew that of which they had been ignorant . . . and God set things to rights through him."[57] Idris II's buried body infuses the earth with his knowing. Healing narratives depict Idris II as a beating heart and the city waters as his circulatory system, carrying God's blessing (*baraka*) to the city's mosques on the waters of the River Fez. A Fez resident told me this *baraka* cured him of typhus: "And I put my legs into that pool of water [at the Bou Inania madrasa] and it works very quickly, like magic, and my Lord gives me life, and here I am standing up, my daughter."[58] A French physician recorded a cure at Bab Lufa, the tiny waterspout projecting from the wall of Mawlay Idris's shrine (see Fig. 1.4):

> An inscription in kufic characters engraved on the cup indicates that the fountain is a *habous* property [*waqf*, inalienable religious property] of Moulay Idriss. The patient takes the cup with the right hand, says "In the

name of God," (Bismillah), drinks three swallows of water and thanks God (Alhamdulilla). Then he recites: "May the *baraka* of this water of venerated Moulay Idriss expand in me, may God accord it to me, cure me and give me good health. May the will of God be done, of God the Healer" . . . The patient lights an olive oil lamp next to the fountain called "menara." . . . If the patient can't be transported, his family takes a bottle of water from Bab Loufa, which he drinks, then rubs the area of his body where the problem is.[59]

Fez topography recapitulates the history of the Moroccan Islamic state in microcosm, a history grounded by bodies. The construction of Fez fell to Idris II after his father's death in 793. Idris II invited Muslims from Cordova in Andalusian Spain and refugees from Qarawan in Tunisia; thus, Fez is divided between the Qarawiyyin and the Andalusiyyin districts. According to the Maliki school of Islamic law, the dead should be buried in cemeteries outside the city walls, and most Fassis were buried at the Bab Ftuh and Bab Guisa portals. Exceptional people were buried in-

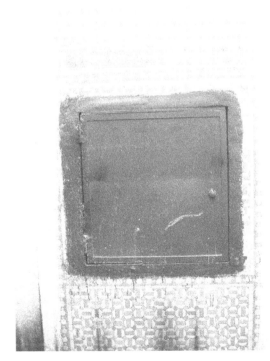

FIGURE 1.4. The fountain of Bab Lufa at Mawlay Idris mosque, today covered with a metal door. The tilework reads: "Drink here and wrath disappears / Become skilled by the name of God in visitation and prayer." (Author photograph.)

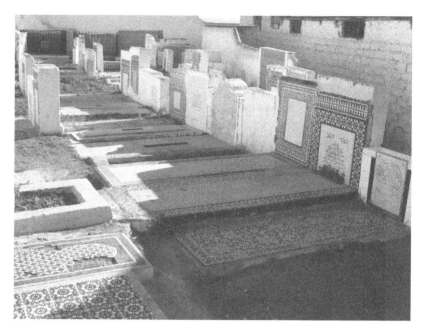

FIGURE 1.5. Most Fez residents were buried outside the city walls, but Sufi orders and saintly families like the Wazzani had sepulchral gardens, or *rawdat*, like this one in the Lamtiyyin neighborhood. (Author photograph.)

side the city walls in the floors of homes or in the private sepulchral gardens (*rawdat*) created for *shurafa'* and Sufi brotherhoods (Fig. 1.5). The streets of Fez thus literally contain its history.

The urban space resembles an organic being, growing and changing with the souls buried in its streets. A buried *wali* body could grow into a shrine, a mosque, a Sufi lodge (*zawiya*), or an entire city quarter. The body of Sidi Ahmad al-Shawi (Fig. 1.6) has become a city quarter, that of Sidi al-Khayyat (Fig. 1.7) a community mosque, and that of Sidi Qasim ibn Rahmun (d. 1733) a Sufi lodge.[60] The street layout of Fez reflects an organic progress of urban expansion rather than an intentional state design (Fig. 1.8), because the people created the city with their prayers. Prayer creates physical reality, as 'Abd al-'Aziz ad-Dabbagh wrote in "Al-Ibriz": "The hearts of the people of our lord Muhammad have a great importance with God, and even if they gathered together in a place where no one was buried and they thought a *wali* was there and asked God for something in that place, indeed God would hurry to respond to them."[61]

For example, through faith (*niya*), the people brought a man to Fez

FIGURE 1.6. The grave of Sidi Ahmad al-Shawi has become a neighborhood, here announced by a plaque over the archway. (Author photograph.)

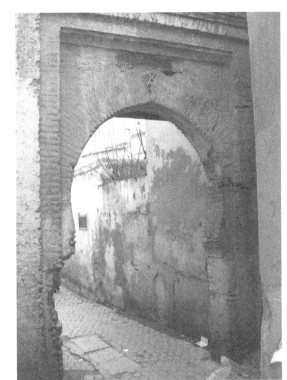

FIGURE 1.7. Sidi al-Khayyat has become a mosque. His grave is fenced here. (Author photograph.)

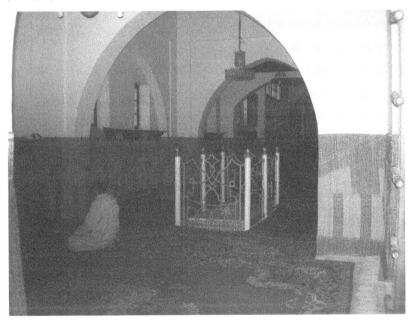

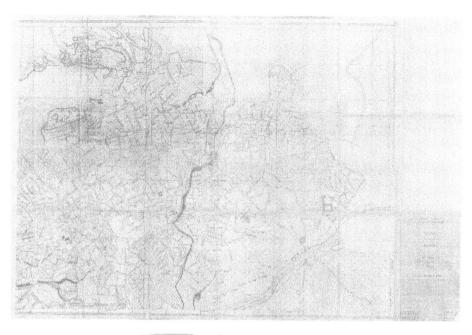

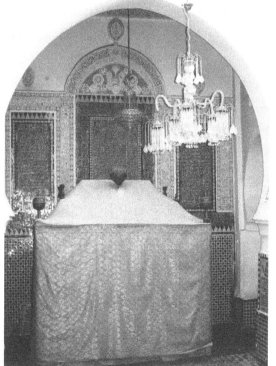

FIGURE 1.8. The street layout of Fez does not reflect a state-directed design, as can be seen in this map from 1960. (Archives of the Fez Municipality.)

FIGURE 1.9. The *khulwa* (prayer place) of ʿAbd al Qadir al-Jilani in Fez. The actual al-Jilani is buried in Baghdad, but by constructing this grave, the people have grounded al-Jilani's spiritual presence in Fez. Many Fez residents are now buried here beside "al-Jilani," thus validating his constructed body with actual physical bodies. (Author photograph.)

who never set foot in Morocco, the Baghdad Sufi 'Abd al-Qadir al-Jilani, founder of the Qadiriyya Sufi order. The people repeatedly clashed with the Fez *qadi* (judge) Muhammad al-'Arabi Burdala over "visiting" al-Jilani. Pilgrims attributed a pillar of the Qarawiyyin mosque to al-Jilani and left him offerings there, until the *qadi* had the pillar destroyed in order to prevent "heresy." Al-Kattani also protested, "Shaykh Mawlana 'Abd al-Qadir . . . never entered Morocco . . . So how is it possible that it is said he reached the city of Fez and worshipped God in some of its places? This is clearly lies, but the Fassis claim that some of them saw the *shaykh* in this place, and some of them believe that . . . he came to it after his death supernaturally."[62] But the people's prayers ultimately triumphed over scholars and judges in the urban space. The people washed themselves at a collecting drain in Tiyaliyyin street asking al-Jilani for cure, and today there is a grave and shrine for al-Jilani in this spot. With prayer, the people created an embodiment for al-Jilani in Fez; there is now a grave and prayer-place (*khulwa*) for his soul to inhabit (see fig. 1.9).

The people of Fez imagined the city space as a meeting-place of spirit and matter, a mirror of the human body. The *Salwa* describes Fez as a revolving spiral, spinning out from the grave of Idris II to the neighborhoods and peripheral gardens; he is the spiritual, geographic, and cosmological axis (*qutb*) around whom the city and its inhabitants revolve.[63] The *Salwa* thus articulates a cartographic imaginary entirely different from the spatial map drawn by the French in 1913, for it is a world organized and animated by the spiritual energy of saints (see Fig. 1.10). Al-Kattani writes of the saints as "caliphs" of the Prophet, "swimmers in his light, which spreads out from his ocean," "a refuge for those who fear, a place for sinners to find peace . . . doors to God on earth."[64] Their bodies provide openings in the skin of reality, making mundane city spaces into points of God's grace.[65] Burial reunites the saint's flesh with its primordial origin, the clay into which God breathed of His spirit. Al-Kattani writes, "Permission is given to take earth from saints' graves to ask for cure . . . because it is musk and under it is musk."[66] The city space of Fez joins the individual to the social, its perfumed earth is a thin membrane between the souls of the people and the collective Muslim *umma*.

Knowing illuminates Fez; her axial saints draw knowing from the founding Jazulite *shaykhs* of Morocco and her scholars master all domains of knowledge, acquiring learning even from the *jinn*.[67] The Fez scholars are Sufi-jurists who reconcile the "visible sciences" (the "sciences of evidence": *fiqh*, hadith, *tafsir*, grammar) with the intuitive (Sufi) knowing of God (*ma'rifa*). In the story of his own great-grandfather, al-Kattani illustrates the natural compatibility of esoteric and rational knowledge:

Once [The *wali* Sidi al-Walid ibn Hashim al-Kattani] came to our ancestor [Sidi al-Taʿa ibn Idris al-Kattani (d. 1848)] and said, "Give me a piece
of bread and two pieces of *khaliʿa* [dried meat]." He refused, for he understood this request as a sign that two of his children would die: "By God
and the *shariʿa*, I won't give you anything." And he said to him, "You
must! And I won't go until I have taken them." He gave the [*khaliʿa*],
and his tears fell onto his beard, and [the *wali*] took them and gave him
two hats. He said, "Take these two in place of what you took from me;
they are for the *wali* and the scholar which will be in each generation of
your descendants until the day of judgment . . ." A few days later, his son
Ismaʿil died of the plague, his most beloved son, and one of his daughters
died . . . what the *wali* spoke of came to pass.[68]

The scholar (*ʿalim*) and Sufi saint (*ʿarif*) are the two faces of a Knower
who upholds God's law in all dimensions of reality. This duality is illustrated by the career of the Qarawiyyin scholar Hasan al-Yusi (d. 1691).
The jurist al-Yusi wrote two formal epistles chiding the ʿAlawi sultan

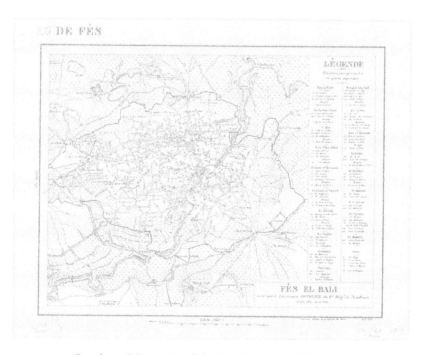

FIGURE 1.10. French spatial mapping of the city of Fez in 1913. (American
Geographical Society Library, University of Wisconsin–Milwaukee Libraries.)

Isma'il for his despotic policies, which he claimed violated the sultan's contract of rule (*bay'a*): "[Your laws] eat the flesh of the subjects, drink their blood, suck their bones and brains, leaving them neither religion nor the world."[69] In an oral tradition collected by Clifford Geertz in the 1970s near Sefrou, al-Yusi is remembered as a saint who visits the sultan's palace. In that narrative, when a worker falls ill while building for Sultan Isma'il, the sultan orders the man to be sealed alive inside the unfinished wall. The man's fellows come in secret to complain to al-Yusi, who calmly breaks every dish in the palace. When the sultan arrives to demand an explanation, al-Yusi asks, "Well, which is better—the pottery of Allah or the pottery of clay?" Furious, the sultan commands al-Yusi to leave his city, and the saint exits the city gates to pitch his tent in the graveyard beside the city walls. Al-Yusi says, "Tell [the sultan] that I have left your city and I have entered God's." When the enraged sultan arrives on horseback to force his departure, al-Yusi responds, "I went out of your city and am in the City of God, the Great and Holy." When the mounted Isma'il charges al-Yusi, the royal steed's legs sink into the earth. Isma'il cries, "God has reformed me! God has reformed me! I am sorry! Give me pardon!"[70]

This oral narrative of al-Yusi as a miracle-working saint is not mythology but an alternate expression of the Knower as the guardian of God's law.[71] In both narratives, al-Yusi uses his knowledge to correct the sultan, protect the community of Muslims, and restore the true balance of spiritual and temporal power. He reprimands Sultan Isma'il for elevating his own political law (*wilaya*) above God's guidance (*walaya*), and al-Yusi insists that the Muslims are sovereign over themselves. In the formal epistle, al-Yusi warns Isma'il that he has broken his legal contract and so the Muslims now have the right to revolt against him. In the *wali* story, al-Yusi breaks the sultan's law literally by smashing his plates, contrasting God's eternal kingdom with fragile kingly power. He leaves "your city" of man-made walls for the graveyard, the city of the souls, the eternal "City of God." The dead act as a jury, judging Isma'il guilty and dragging him down for God's punishment. As both jurist and saint, al-Yusi defends a sovereign Muslim *umma* and confirms the right of the Muslims to revolt against unjust rule.

In al-Kattani's *Salwa*, the *awliya'* also show the people how to relate to one another in society, inhabit God's City, and live the Prophet's hadith, "God the Highest said, loving Me requires love of each other, loving Me requires cooperation, loving Me requires advising one other."[72] The *awliya'* invite the people to righteousness and punish evildoers, even within their own bodies. If a criminal approached the *wali* Abu Ya'za, he would find the body part used to perform evil acts streaked with black lines.[73] Blindness, vomiting, and pain would strike the villain who came to harm the innocent: "Indeed, a group of assassins wanted to extract some of the people from the shrine of [Ahmad ibn Yahya al-Lamti (d. 1572)], who sought refuge with him. When the killer approached the shrine, a sickness seized him in his belly. His intestines felt as though they had been cut, and he gave up his plan, and this terrible pain remained until he died."[74] It is God who punishes, but the *wali* acts as a voice for His will. Such was the encounter between the treasonous son of Sultan Isma'il, Hafid, and the *wali* Masa' al-Khayr al-Masmudi (d. 1705) in the streets of Fez Jadid:

> [Hafid] ordered that [the *wali*] be seized and brought to him . . . He asked, "Are you really a *murabit*?" And al-Masmudi said, "If God has said so!" And the son of the sultan said, "And do you know God?" He said, "Yes." He said, "By what do you know Him?" And he said, "I know that He is the one who ordered you to be killed, and He offers no blood money [*dia*] for you!" And after that day Mawlay Hafid was assassinated in Fez Jadid, because he wanted to revolt against his father and [the sultan] knew this.[75]

In al-Kattani's text, the *awliya'* bring the Qur'an to life and fulfill the Qur'anic promise of God's immanence: "*Indeed We have created man, and We know whatever thoughts his inner self develops, and We are closer to him than [his] jugular vein*" (50:16). The *wali* tells men news of the unseen; al-Masmudi shouted "Good afternoon" to passersby: "The people understood this as a sign that the people of goodness were going and goodness went with them, because in the afternoon the light is fading, and nothing remains after it but darkness."[76] If Ahmad ibn 'Umar al-Sharif al-Bahlul (d. 1655) gave a man a straw bag, the recipient knew that he would soon die. Many of these *awliya'* were *majdhub* (*majnun, bahlul*), the "unruly Friends of God" whose nakedness, bizarre speech, and antinomian behavior defy religious law and social convention. Sidi Ahasayn al-Aqra' al-Fallusi (d. 1845) called the people to blindness and hunger and hit them in the eye or mouth with spittle. Sidi al-Waryaghli (d. 1748) "could not differentiate between heat and cold, giving and withholding, and let fall all obligation."[77] Scholars have attempted to explain the *majnun* as a madman suffering from organic illness, as one possessed, or as a radical ascetic, but the solution lies in a Sufi understanding of the human body.[78]

Because the human being is a meeting-point of the divine and mate-

rial worlds, as the soul merges with God, the body becomes an open channel for His will. In a 1998 interview, a ninety-five-year-old Fez resident
named My Khaddouj explained that her father (d. 1920s) was *majnun*,
possessed by believing (Muslim) *jinn*:

> For seven years he ate bread, and he ate *jawi* [an herb used as incense],
> and he drank tea with saffron . . . The people who are in him (*an-nas li*
> *fihi*), those things, that is what they wanted. The believers that were in
> him, that's what they ate . . . From God. Those [*jinn*] that are from God.
> [He was one of] the people of rotation (*an-nuba*). And whoever the turn
> comes to, and he who has the key, he opens the door.[79]

Her family were blood descendants of the Prophet, but the "key" un-
locking between the divine and the physical world was her father's direct
knowing (*ma'rifa*) of God. Her son remarked:

> That is just like some part of the newspaper from God . . . And when he
> finds a woman, he says, Hey man! Man! Show your face, he says this to
> the woman. And when he finds a man, he tells him, hide your face . . . He
> had *baraka* in him . . . For example, you came, and he knew you. What
> was in your mind, he will tell you.[80]

He prayed in the mosques, and the people came with illness, sterility, and
other wishes, "When they opened the door of Mawlay Idris [mosque], you
find the slaves of God . . . so the people followed him, and they grabbed
at him":

> A lot of sick people came to him. See, you came with your dress on like
> that, wearing clothes, and you come, you tell him, pray with me. She takes
> off her clothes, and she wraps herself in her *haik* [*hijab*, cloak], and she
> goes naked. They acquire houses, they acquire clothes, they acquire things
> . . . He even spit money out of his mouth.

One night he invited the neighbors to his home for his own funeral, did
his ablutions, prepared his shroud, and sent for his daughter and her
baby son:

> At ten o'clock at night, he invited them, and the Lord of Faith took his
> faith [he died]. They let the word be spread . . . That night they [washed
> his body] in rosewater and orange flower water, they made a new *gha-*

sil [platform for washing the dead] for him . . . And the guardians and the police, they told people, not like that, you all want to tear him apart. And when they covered him again with a *qiswa*, and they were pushing with their shoulders, and then they pulled off his clothes until he was left with only the shroud. And the slaves of God were out of their minds. Just the youths were holding him up, from hand to hand.[81]

Death of either the ego or the biological body does not interrupt the *wali*'s guidance, as al-Jazuli wrote: "The knowers of God (*al-'arifun*) are a folk who work righteousness . . . [thus] they are freed [from material constraints] . . . they die; when they die they come back [to God] and live [again]; when they live, they speak with the Living who never dies."[82]

The saint is a healer because he can see the junction of body and soul, what Toshihiko Izutsu calls *qadar*, "an extremely delicate state in which an archetype is about to actualize itself in the form of a concretely existent thing. To know *qadar*, therefore, is to peep into the ineffable mystery of Being."[83] "*Shaykh* of the age" al-'Arabi ibn Ahmad al-Darqawi (d. 1823) reached "a position of breaking and healing." His son 'Ali (d. 1857) cured a man by reading the Qur'an over water and having him drink it, "By God, the moment I drank that water the illness left me like a hair pulled gently from dough."[84] The *awliya'* visit the sick in their sleep as the soul wanders from its bodily container. The companion of a *wali* wrote, "I was sick in my eyes until I could hardly see; then I saw Sidi Muhammad [ibn 'Abd al-Wahid al-Kattani (d. 1872)] in my dreams and he wiped my eyes; I awoke [cured]."[85] Only through bodily experience can the human soul realize its full potential in the world,[86] thus the people experienced Berber saint Abu Ya'za by "tasting" his knowing (*ma'rifa*) with their senses: "Anyone who saw [Abu Ya'za] became blind from the light of his face, and among those who became blind through the sight of him are the *shaykh* Abu Madiyan. No one was able to see until he wiped his face with the cloth of Abu Ya'za, then he would return to sight. Then he would become blind, and the people of Morocco asked for rain by means of him, and they would draw water."[87] Vision expresses the soul's journey; the raw *walaya* of Abu Ya'za obliterates the adept's sight until he reconciles inner (*batini*) and manifest (*zahiri*) reality in the Sufi way (*tariqa*), becoming a person of insight (*basir*). Blindness also expresses the soul's arrival to God, for the Sufi master Abu Madiyan "would become blind, and the people of Morocco asked for rain by means of him, and they would draw water."

Because pilgrims associated healing with saints, saintly persons were invented at the sites of purely medical cures. Patients with oto-rhinolaryngological problems, gynecological disorders, muscular pain, and skin lesions immersed themselves in the hot, sulfurated waters of a mineral spring near Fez, which the people named Mawlay Ya'qub ("Saint Jacob").[88] This "saint" never existed, but has a shrine, as does his "daughter," the eponymous Lalla Shafiyya, or "Lady Cure."[89] In a similar process of invention, the *maristan* (hospital) for the mentally ill built by the Marinids, Bab al-Faraj, or "Door of Relief," was corrupted in the popular vernacular to "Sidi Frej," or "Saint Frej." Al-Kattani objects:

> Near Suq al-'Attarin and Suq al-Henna is the place where the people sick in spirit are—the insane. This place is designated by the name Sidi Frej although there is no person with that name buried there, nor any tomb. This house was built by a Sultan to bring together the sick Muslims who had no protection, and it was given the name "Bab al-Faraj" because the sick found relief for their ills.[90]

Invented saints suggest a larger view of healing as the social, spiritual, and worldly restoration of God's law, rather than the mechanical repair of a purely material human body.

DISSECTION AND THE DIVINE:
AUTOPSY AS A PATH TO SUFI ILLUMINATION

Yet how can spiritual healing can be reconciled with "Greco-Islamic medicine," the rationalist medicine inherited by the Islamic world from Hellenic Greece? Many famous Galenic physicians of the Islamic medieval period served the Moroccan court, among them Ibn Bajja (Avempace), who was vizier to Sultan Yahya ibn Tashfin and became governor of Fez (d. 1138); Abu Bakr Ibn Tufayl, personal physician and minister to Sultan Abu Ya'qub Yusuf in 1182; and Ibn Rushd (Averroes), who succeeded his friend Ibn Tufayl at court.[91] Abu Marwan ibn Zohr (Avenzoar) dedicated his *Al-Iqtisad* to his Almohad patron, Sultan Ibrahim ibn Yusuf. Even Abu 'Imran Musa ibn Maymun al-Qurtubi (Maimonides) lived briefly in Fez.[92] Morocco produced its own impressive physicians, including 'Abd al-Qasim ibn Muhammad al-Ghassani, the pharmacologist 'Abd al-Qadir ibn Shaqrun al-Maknassi, 'Abd as-Salam al-'Alami, and the medical dynasties of the al-Fasi and the Adarraq. In this section, we will see that the larger cosmological vision developed in Islamic medicine greatly surpassed that of its Greek intellectual ancestors.

The physician and minister Abu Bakr Ibn Tufayl describes his own journey to God through medicine with a philosophical novel, *Hayy ibn Yaqzan*. The title character, Hayy, is born alone on a desert island and easily gains mastery over the animals with superior human reason. But Hayy is helpless to prevent the death of his beloved, a doe that suckled him as an infant. In an attempt to save her, Hayy quickly performs a dissection of her lifeless corpse. Lifting the pericardium from the heart, Hayy suddenly realizes the existence of the soul: "He soon dropped the body and thought no more of it, knowing that the mother who had nursed him . . . could only be that being which had departed."[93] From pathological anatomy, Hayy quickly deduces the emanationist structure of the universe, the existence of God, and a Sufi discipline through which he arrives at direct communion with the divine.[94] Ibn Tufayl thus presents the human condition as a cycle of reason and *haqiqa*; the God-given qualities of reason and love drive man to scientific inquiry, and science leads man to God through His creation. Rational medicine was Ibn Tufayl's own path to God, as he tells his Almohad patron, "I want only to bring you along the paths in which I have preceded you and let you swim in the sea I have just crossed."[95]

But contemporary scholars have been unable to reconcile Islam and Galenic medicine, practically speaking. Michael Dols and Lawrence Conrad dismiss saintly healing as an import from foreign sciences or an artifact of pre-Islamic paganism.[96] Anthropologists explain away saintly healing as social ritual rather than "real" medicine for "real" disease; blood is a means to separate social groups, cautery is a rite, pharmacology is a symbol.[97] Or a medical pluralism model is used; vertical spiritual healing addresses "godly" diseases, while horizontal medicine addresses "worldly" ones.[98] But Moroccan saintly healing was science, if by science we understand an organized intervention based on a paradigmatic understanding of the universe. Moroccans deployed an Islamic cosmological model that accommodated both Sufi and Galenic ways of knowing. Although these were distinct styles of knowledge, Sufism and Galenism intersected in the human body and its therapeutic cure.

The physician and philosopher Ibn Sina used Greek science to give the Qur'an a physics and a geography.[99] He thus created what Thomas Kuhn terms a "scientific paradigm," a framework through which scientists formulate the questions of research, describe the objects of the world and their relationships, and establish standards for evidence and proof.[100] The Islamic paradigm presents the universe as an emanation of the Divine Intelligence, a set of hierarchically organized forms projected onto the world of matter. An illustration of how Islamic physicians located Galenic medicine within Islamic cosmology may be seen in a pharmacological compendium popular in Morocco in 1900, the *Tadhkira awla al-albab wa al-jamia' li'ajbi al-'ajab* of the Ottoman physician Dawud ibn 'Umar al-Antaki (d. 1599).[101]

Al-Antaki's anatomy and physiology are purely Galenic. He compares man to the physical world; man is composed of the humors blood (like air), phlegm (like water), yellow bile (like fire), and black bile (like earth). Change is produced by temperature and humidity: "All compounds require heat to refine, and humidity to facilitate the doing, and cold to thicken, and dryness to preserve the form."[102] He analogizes digestion to cooking and nutrition, and generation to Aristotelian "powers" that attract and repulse humors in the body.[103] Reason, memory, and sense perception are motivated by mechanical powers, not a soul; "natural power" directs the beating of the heart, "animal power" moves the body, and "psychological power" draws from the sensory organs. Each remedy in his pharmaceutical dictionary has an extensive empirical description, for example: "*Jar an-nahar* [neighbor of the river]: It is called thus because it only exists in the water or near it. It is like chard except it is fuzzy with prickly roots and seven leaves . . . It is cold and dry in the second degree and blocks diarrhea and blood and cuts thirst when drunk. It solves tumors when applied topically and mends wounds when it is moist or dry. It harms the nerves but sugar corrects this."[104]

Yet al-Antaki locates medicine within a larger, cosmological hierarchy of the sciences. The greatest sciences are the six of divinity: the necessary existence of God, the principles of existing things, proof of the Creator, classification of the concepts, states of the soul after separation from the body, and "the unseen (*al-samayat*), the field of prophecy and the day of judgment."[105] The next most excellent science is mathematics, because it treats pure forms that are free of matter. The other sciences follow in degree of engagement with the material: music, engineering, chemistry, biology, and medicine. The most degraded are the "sciences connected to the self of a person": kingship, psychology, and city planning. Al-Antaki calls the person who organizes the perceptible (*zahiri*) world using reason "the sultan,"[106] but the direct knower of God who thereby transforms the laws of nature is "the *mufad*": "As for the invisible (*bataniyya*) science, evidence of its presence is indicated by great proofs [miracles] and it is the power of prophecy, and that person is the *mufad*, and he has the power of abstract matters which distinguishes him from ordinary men."[107]

Sufis and physicians thus agreed that direct knowing of God opens the secret of the physical universe.[108] The Qur'an speaks of the world revealing God: "*And He has made everything in the Heavens and everything on Earth . . . These are certainly Signs for people who reflect* (45:13)."[109] But only the intuitive knower can interpret God's signs in nature: "*Such metaphors—We devise them for humanity, but only those with knowledge understand them* (29:43)."

Galenic and Sufi paths of inquiry were thus different, but physicians validated Sufi healing as parallel practice.[110] Al-Antaki presents illness as an organic disorder caused by mechanical blockage and imbalances of heat and humidity: "[*Yarqan,* jaundice]: Its cause is the weakness of the attraction of the spleen, so it pushes what belongs to it to the belly and yellows the skin by that humor [yellow bile]. And black jaundice is if [black bile] is pushed to the mouth of the stomach. [It causes] hunger and profuse excrement. [The remedy], clean the spleen from whatever was in it before and open the blockage by bloodletting."[111] Yet al-Antaki also has a section of his book devoted to Qur'anic amulet writing (*'ilm al-harf*) and provides charts showing the "body, spirit, self, heart, and intelligence" of each Arabic letter, days of the week ruled by *jinn,* and the correspondences between planets, numbers, body parts, elements, and letters.[112] Al-Antaki includes these as "sciences related to medicine" because he conceived of a cosmological human body much greater than the material entity of Galenic medicine.[113]

"*Jinn* disease," the notion that *jinn* cause illness, lies at the intersection of Galenic and Sufi conceptions of the body. The *jinn* are a race "*created from the fire of a scorching wind*" (15:27) who live parallel to man on earth[114] and strike men out of jealousy or "when humans accidentally harm or hurt them by urinating on them, by pouring hot water on them, or by killing some of them."[115] *Jinn* and Galen meet in the blood; Sufis describe a "lower soul" (*nafs*),[116] and Galenic physicians an "animal soul" that regulates respiration, heartbeat, growth, nutrition, and appetite. The Hanbali jurist Ibn Taymiyya synthesized Galenic and Sufi physiology: "The *Jinn* most certainly do have an effect on humans according to the Prophet's clear statement in the following authentic narration, 'Verily Satan flows in the blood stream of Adam's descendants.' For, in the blood is the *ether* known to doctors as the 'animal soul' which is emitted by the heart and which moves throughout the body giving it life."[117]

The vast field of applied Moroccan medical practice defies simplification to one theoretical system; healing involved interventions at different levels of the body. The *wali* opened the transcendent world directly, as al-Kattani wrote, "Through sight of [the *awliya'*], God enlivens the dead hearts like a downpour of rain enlivens the dead earth, hardened chests are opened and difficult matters become simple."[118] But the *wali* could localize God's *baraka* in the patient's body; thus, a second intervention captured divine form in a physical substance. Water was thought to retain the forms of words; thus, the saliva of a *talib*, *sharif*, or Sufi after prayer was applied to the body as medicine or Qur'anic verses were dissolved in water and drunk.[119] A third level targeted the *jinn* through exorcism or *'ilm al-harf* (the science of the letter, amulet-writing).[120] Finally, Galenic therapies addressed the purely physical and humoral aspects of imbalance and climate.

The Moroccan body was thus "overdetermined," a site of intersecting scientific frames within an Islamic cosmology. Moroccans lived a Jazulite idea of sovereignty not simply by using Jazulite texts as cures, though birthing mothers were washed with water over which al-Jazuli's *Dala'il al-khayrat* had been recited in order to relieve the pain of childbirth, and children were dedicated to a *wali* by shaving their heads, an imitation of the induction ceremony for adepts to the Jazulite order.[121] Rather, Moroccans lived Jazulite sovereignty in saintly healing itself. The moment of cure affirmed the saint as an opening between divine and material worlds and a manifestation of God's love for His *umma*. Although Sufism was not necessarily medicine, it affirmed man as a soul and body, locating him in cosmological, historical, social, and physical space.

THE HERESY TRIAL OF AL-KATTANI: KILLING SAINTS WITH A POSITIVE WAY OF KNOWING

In 1909, the Moroccan sultan 'Abd al-Hafiz had the Sufi leader Muhammad ibn 'Abd al-Kabir al-Kattani publicly humiliated, whipped to death, and his corpse dumped into an unmarked grave. Historically, the sultans displayed their power on the bodies of criminals and staked their severed heads to the city gates, but al-Kattani's death was not punishment for an actual crime. Al-Kattani's 1896 heresy trial and 1909 state execution symbolized the consolidation of a state ontological war against Sufi epistemology and its diffuse model of political sovereignty. European intrusions over the nineteenth century had created a dangerous rift between the weak sultanate (*makhzan*) and outspoken Islamic scholars, who demanded that the sultan lead a jihad against foreign invaders. The sultan resolved this crisis by adopting *salafiyya*, the rationalist Islamic reform movement elaborated in the Orient by the intellectuals Muhammad 'Abduh (1849–1905) and Jamal al-Din al-Afghani (1839–1897). *Salafiyya* provided a means for Islamic scholars and the state to join forces, use European science, and reimagine sovereignty from a positive way of knowing.[122]

Reform was an urgent matter in Morocco after the European powers defeated the Moroccan armies in 1844 and 1860, forcing the sultans to accept ruinous trade concessions, the jurisdiction of European courts over Muslim and Jewish commercial agents of European powers ("protégés"), punitive war reparations, and a set of expensive military and economic reforms. The *'ulama'* criticized the sultan for allowing both European law to govern Moroccan society and European armies to occupy Moroccan cities, for incurring millions of francs in foreign debt, and for failing to address famine, drought, and epidemics. After 1860, many of the *'ulama'* began to focus on the survival of Morocco without the sultanate, preparing for its inevitable demise.[123]

In British-occupied Egypt in 1899, the jurist Muhammad 'Abduh confronted a similar colonizing landscape; a sphere, ever expanding, of European civil law in Egyptian society, and another sphere, ever shrinking, of Islamic *shari'a* in Muslim life.[124] 'Abduh responded by reconciling the *shari'a* with secular law. The true Islam of the *salaf* (first Islamic community) encompassed the products of reason, he argued, but the Islamic world had stagnated due to lazy scholarship, foreign contaminations, tyrannical political authorities, and the "doctrinal heresies" of Shi'ism and Sufism. Reform (*islah*) consisted of replacing the scholar of imitation with a new cleric of modern science, whose progressive *ijtihad* (Islamic legal interpretations) would realize Islam as a Comtean social order.[125] The intellectual Jamal al-Din al-Afghani responded to new Western sciences by redefining them as Islamic. Al-Afghani argued that Islam was a rational religion of proofs—"Everywhere [the Qur'an] addresses itself to reason"[126]—and science, "the only true ruler of the world."[127] 'Abduh and al-Afghani inspired popular parliamentary revolutions across the Middle East and North Africa in the early twentieth century.

Oriental *salafiyya* found enthusiastic reception among Moroccan ministers, *nizam* soldiers, and *'ulama'*. The Moroccan scholar and minister Abu Shu'ayb al-Dukkali studied at al-Azhar University in Cairo and became a pioneer of *salafiyya* in Morocco. Ibrahim al-Tadili (d. 1894) founded a *salafi* Islamic university in Rabat upon his return from Egypt. The *salafi* journals *Al Manar*, *Al Ahram*, and *Al Mu'ayyad* circulated in Moroccan intellectual circles. Muhammad al-Hajwi advocated using 'Abduh's modern reform of Islamic law to defend Moroccan society: "We lack a true system of laws; if the foreigner occupies our country, nothing will limit his action; we will be at the mercy of his autocratic whims."[128]

On the fringes of Morocco in Algeria and the Sahara, the Sanusiyya, Qadiriyya, and Fadiliyya Sufi orders waged jihad against French colonial invaders, but they mobilized a traditional idea of Islamic renewal (*tajdid*),

not *salafiyya*.[129] Historically, the Moroccan renewers of religion were millenarian *mahdis* like the Almohads and Almoravids, or scholars who returned to the Qur'an and Sunna for a fresh Islamic legal interpretation
(*ijtihad*).[130] Moroccan Sufi-jurists like Ahmad ibn Idris (1749–1837) rejected both Wahhabi and *salafi* paths to Islamic renewal; he criticized especially *salafi* attacks on sainthood and the *salafi* reliance on reason alone
for *ijtihad*.[131] The hubristic use of reason could pervert God's law, warned
the Moroccan scholar Hasan al-Yusi, for "God organizes the causes, and
the consequences are of His wisdom"; God orders natural phenomena
as "custom" (*'adat*), which He may break in miracle as He wills.[132] The
North African Sufi jihadist Muhammad b. 'Ali al-Sanusi agreed that absolute natural laws were a "heresy of causes."[133]

Only the Fez Sufi Muhammad ibn 'Abd al-Kabir al-Kattani (d. 1909)
synthesized Sufi and *salafi* ideas for a "Sufi modern": "To do so he synthesized the Islamic mystical, rationalist and legal doctrines and tried to reconcile the universal Islamic concept of *tajdid* (renewal of religion) with local Moroccan concepts of political and religious power and authority."[134]
Like the *salafis*, al-Kattani envisioned a modern clergy who would educate
the people, interpret law, and draft a constitution, but he saw the reforming cleric as a Sufi *shaykh*, not a jurist. He insisted that esoteric knowledge
retain an equal footing with reason for interpretation of the law: "*Ijtihad* is factual in the two realms and neither realm is more valuable than
the other, for *haqiqa* without *shari'a* is as useless as is *shari'a* without *haqiqa*."[135] Man experienced discovery both in the empirical world, "written by the hand of the divine being on a stone or a leaf," and directly from
God, "[he] hears the Voice [say it]."[136] Al-Kattani thus defended the esoteric knowing of Sufi sainthood; indeed, he extended the Sufi saint into
the realm of the sultan's legal administration.

At first both *salafi* and Sufi modern reforms were welcome at court, but
after a series of self-styled thaumaturgical saints led rural rebellion against
the sultan, as the mystic and opportunist Jilali ibn Idris al-Zarhuni "Bu
Himara" did in 1902–1909, the sultanate attacked sainthood and asserted
human state power (*wilaya*) over saintly knowing (*walaya*).[137] The assault
focused on the scholarly voice of saintly *walaya*, al-Kattani.

The attack on al-Kattani began with the regent Ahmad b. Musa (ruled
1894–1900), who accused him of "enticing foolish minds" and "seduc-
ing the common people" with extravagant claims for the spiritual benefits of his Sufi order's special prayer (*wird*).[138] The regent prodded the *qadi*
of Fez to action: "Whoever appears in an ecstatic state must, by law, sub-
mit his words and deeds to measure on the scale of *shari'a*"; the Fez schol-

ars reluctantly agreed that "if interpreted in their external meaning [*ala zahiriha*]," al-Kattani's claims were indeed blasphemous.[139] In October of 1896, the *makhzan* closed the Kattaniyya *zawiya* for "doctrinal corruption." But after a critical military ally of the sultan's government openly supported al-Kattani, the heresy charges were dropped and al-Kattani was invited to join the Qarawiyyin mosque-university hadith council.

Al-Kattani's ability to reconcile Moroccan Sufism with secular science gained wide appeal, and rural populations, *'ulama'*, and bureaucrats of the sultan's new administrations joined the Kattaniyya brotherhood. Al-Kattani's Sufi modernism was so popular that the sultan's brother 'Abd al-Hafiz (ruled 1908–1912) solicited al-Kattani's support for his bid for the throne.[140] In 1907, the Fez *'ulama'* declared the reigning sultan, 'Abd al-'Aziz (r. 1900–1907), to be in violation of his *bay'a*, and the people of Fez broke their oath of allegiance to him from December 28, 1907, to January 4, 1908.[141] The Fez scholars proclaimed 'Abd al-Hafiz sultan on January 4, 1908, and presented him with a *bay'a* of fourteen conditions, including recognition of popular sovereignty, expulsion of foreign agents, and the creation of a parliament, which he refused.[142] After 'Abd al-Hafiz received a traditional *bay'a*, he set about eliminating all challengers to his power, including his former ally Muhammad ibn 'Abd al-Kabir al-Kattani.

Salafiyya served 'Abd al-Hafiz by discrediting Sufi knowing; the sultan no longer had to bow to saintly critique, only to reason and the power of men. *Salafiyya* recast saints as charlatans who faked thaumaturgy and miracles to dupe an ignorant public.[143] Yet the sultan also refused the *salafi* idea of popular sovereignty; the Tangier-based *salafi* newspaper *Lisan al-Maghrib* proposed a draft constitution for Morocco in 1908 adapted from the Ottoman Constitution of 1876, "His Majesty cannot long refuse his people the benefits of a constitution and a parliament."[144] 'Abd al-Hafiz was vulnerable to critique, for he continued his brother's hated policies.[145] But he created his legitimacy by denouncing al-Kattani as a heretic, at once discrediting saints, embracing positive science, and frightening the editors of *Lisan al-Maghrib* into leaving Morocco for Syria in 1909.

'Abd al-Hafiz began by criticizing al-Kattani for the ecstatic singing, dancing, and music of his Sufi brotherhood's prayer sessions, a position popular with *salafi* jurists like Abu Shu'ayb al-Dukkali, the head of the Qarawiyyin hadith council. Identifying Kattaniyya prayer itself as sedition, the sultan closed the Kattaniyya lodges, imprisoned Kattaniyya disciples, and accused al-Kattani of inciting civil unrest, "creat[ing] *fitna* among the Muslims and involv[ing] himself in [activities] that do not receive the blessing [of God]."[146]

'Abd al-Hafiz used the human body to assert himself as a sovereign king, claiming the body as the domain of his earthly law, not God's. No miracle rescued the saintly al-Kattani from a savage beating death, and the whip demonstrated the powerlessness of saintly knowing before the sultan's brute power. The sultan paraded his victory by amputating al-Kattani's disciples' hands and having the bloody stumps rubbed with salt, their mutilated survival a public testimony to the sultan's supremacy.[147] The sultan carved his personal law on al-Kattani by destroying his body, exacting personal revenge from a subject who "above all had struck the sovereign in the very body of his power."[148]

'Abd al-Hafiz presented a new concept of the Moroccan sultan as the political sovereign and biological embodiment of the Prophet's authority. But the people rejected him as a usurper and rose in a series of armed revolts behind five pretenders to the throne in the years 1909–1911. Surrounded by hostile tribal armies in Fez in 1911, 'Abd al-Hafiz called upon France to liberate him and accord him recognition as the ruler of Morocco. The French sent troops to Fez, an operation that ended in the 1912 treaty establishing a French protectorate in Morocco. One person, 'Abd al-Hafiz, signed the treaty with France on behalf of Morocco. To make possible the delegation of the Moroccan administration, state, economy, territory, and subjects to a foreign power, Article 3 of the treaty located Moroccan sovereignty in the person and throne of the sultan: "[France] prend l'engagement de prêter un constant appui à Sa Majesté chérifienne contre tout danger qui menacerait sa personne ou son trône ou qui compromettrait la tranquillité de ses États." (France pledges to lend constant support to His Chérifien Majesty against all dangers that may threaten his person or his throne or would compromise the stability of his state.) France thus validated what Moroccans would not: the sultan as the embodiment of Moroccan political sovereignty itself.

IN MOROCCO, SAINTS WERE a means to imagine the body politic, remember the past, and map a narrative of memory onto the landscape. As the Fez *qadi* 'Iyad wrote, "I love the stories of the scholars and their good works more than *fiqh* because they are the literature of the people."[149] Saints were so fundamental to the Moroccan concept of history that Jews also recounted the past through "Jewish saints,"[150] and Muslims and Jews often visited the same saintly graves.[151] As the historian Neil Kodesh has argued, such alternate ways of knowing suggest a political body transcending the king's court, a "construct of knowledge" that exists "beyond the royal gaze."[152]

In Morocco, the people constructed themselves as a sovereign Islamic *umma*, a geopolitical moral body, through saints and the human body. As the meeting-place of divinity and materiality, the cosmological human body was a place for the Moroccan saint to connect (*murabit*, "he who connects") "the gatherer of that which is divided, [who] brings the Prophet and the Sufi adept together."[153] "Healing" was the saint's restoration of God's law to men and to society, parallel realms simultaneously inhabited by the human being. What remains of this alternate Islamic Moroccan *umma* are contemporary illness narratives and fragments of healing practices at the tombs of the saints, historical artifacts of a Sufi way of politics.

The disappearance of saints as political leaders is a story of Islamic modernist thought (*salafiyya*), first deployed by Sultan 'Abd al-Hafiz and later adopted by the protectorate agreement and the Moroccan nationalist movement. Esoteric knowing had always challenged the sultan's earthly power, but concessions to the Europeans over the nineteenth century further weakened royal legitimacy. Islamic scholars divested Sultan 'Abd al-'Aziz of his throne, but his brother Sultan 'Abd al-Hafiz cleverly adopted rationalist *salafi* ideas to strengthen his rule. The sultan found *salafi* thought more conducive than Sufi modernism to the consolidation of his absolutist state power.

As guardians of the Islamic *umma*, Muslim scholars chose a variety of responses to the French conquest in 1912. *Salafi* scholars like Abu Shu'ayb al-Dukkali, Muhammad al-Hajwi, and Muhammad ibn al-'Arabi al-'Alawi entered the French protectorate's "Chérifien" government as state functionaries, because they believed Islamic renewal lay with new sciences and European-style state reforms. Traditional Sufi scholars rejected the protectorate agreement and either continued jihad, as did the sons of Ma' al-'Aynayn, Ahmad al-Hiba and Murabbih Rabbuh,[154] or else they abandoned the sultanate altogether and focused on preserving Islam among the believers. The author of the *Salwa*, Muhammad ibn Ja'far al-Kattani, left Morocco for Mecca in 1905 and called upon individual Muslims in his *Nasihat Ahl al-Islam* (Advice to the People of Islam, 1908) to maintain Islam in their private lives.

With the collapse of the City of God as a body politic, there remained only the City of God of the human body, as a last refuge for knowing Him, receiving healing from Him, and obtaining the worldly guidance of His saintly friends.

MEDICINE AND THE *MISSION CIVILISATRICE*: A CIVILIZING SCIENCE AND THE FRENCH SOCIOLOGY OF ISLAM IN ALGERIA AND MOROCCO, 1830–1912

IN 1883, THE FRENCH ORIENTALIST and philologist Ernest Renan announced a revolutionary position: Islam killed science, "Islamism and science . . . The ambivalence contained in these words: Arab science, Arab philosophy, Arab Art, Muslim science, Muslim civilization. In killing science, Islam killed itself and condemned itself to a complete inferiority in the world."[1] The Third Republic (1870–1940), the moment when the Rights of Man were finally applied in France, was also the era of French imperial expansion and scientific racism. This was not a contradiction, for the French Republic was simultaneously universalist and racist, delineating the irrational, the primitive, and the undeveloped for "civilizing" and exclusion from full political rights as French citizens.[2]

Renan's 1883 lecture illustrates the modality of the Third Republican civilizing mission—a positivist idea of science and its relationship to society. The French colonial lobby appropriated ideas from Auguste Comte, Émile Durkheim, and Ernest Renan to define France's imperial mission in the world. France would bring positive knowledge, Comte's liberatory path for all humanity, and apply it according to Durkheim's "science of society" (*sociologie*), which would measure a society's level of evolutionary progress according to its categories of thought. Each colonized society could be located along a path from the primitive to the civilized and governed according to its cultural particularities. Science would promote social evolution, and medicine was considered one of these "civilizing sciences."

A positive, republican idea of science influenced French Islamic policy in the empire and the medical service created under Resident General Hubert Lyautey in Morocco (1912–1925). Edmund Burke has argued that Lyautey drew upon the ethnography of military *bureaux-arabes* officers, a local "sociology of non-sociologists" uninfluenced by the currents of metropolitan thought.[3] But Lyautey's protectorate was a technocracy dependent upon the ideologies, instruments, and practices of French science. The Algerian *député* and colonial leader Eugène Étienne argued that *sociologie* would ensure a rational, benevolent, and modern colonial rule, the "science of man modeled on the sciences of nature."[4] Alfred Le Chatelier, the first chair of *sociologie et sociographie musulmane* at the Collège de France (1902) launched the Mission du Maroc, which Lyautey institutionalized as the protectorate's Section Sociologique for native affairs.[5] Native *sociologie* was the method used to describe, divide, and administer French Morocco.

This idea of science also explains both the shift in French colonial policy from assimilation to association and the radical change in French hygiene policy for North Africa. Early French hygienists in Algeria (1830–1870) argued that Algerians could be improved and assimilated to France through public works, intermarriage, and education, because physicians understood the human mind, the human body, the law, and the environment to form a single economy. But after *sociologie* defined human difference in the mind, French doctors saw Muslim Moroccans as primitives incapable of participating in a republic or perceiving the physical world rationally. French ethnographers in Algeria and Morocco provided an archive of "social facts" through which Lyautey's administration knew Muslim minds and bodies; a Qur'anic healing amulet was no longer a local historical accident but irrefutable evidence of a hidden and irrational Muslim *mentalité*.[6] Medicine and *sociologie* became intertwined; healing provided social artifacts for sociologists, and sociologists provided a racial theory to inform the study of Moroccan pathology.

HYGIENE IN THE SERVICE OF POLITICS: *ACCLIMATEMENT* AND COLONIALISM IN ALGERIA

The central question for France in 1830 was whether to colonize Algeria with civilian settlers or to rule the territory indirectly through native elites. Could Frenchmen "acclimate," or survive and reproduce, in the Algerian climate? The hygienists Dr. Jean-Christian-Marc-François-Joseph Boudin, Dr. Joanny-André-Napoléon Périer, and Dr. Émile-Louis Bertherand advanced radically different answers: Boudin advocated indirect rule, Périer the assimilation of Muslims to France, and Bertherand a regime of racial apartheid. The flexibility of French hygiene to divergent colonial agendas demonstrates the fluidity of a French nineteenth-century medicine in transition from the humoralism of Hippocrates and Galen to the bacteriology of Louis Pasteur and Patrick Manson, not a triumphant science that conquered Africa for France.[7] But more importantly, politics—rather than medical realities—ultimately determined French hygiene policy for Algeria. From a multitude of medical voices, colonial and metropolitan actors selected one theory and guaranteed its victory through law and institutions.[8]

Boudin, a chief physician of hospitals in Algeria and a later president of the Société d'Anthropologie, declared the Algerian climate too dangerous for French settlement.[9] Citing a mortality rate in Algeria eight times that of the metropole, Boudin considered French *acclimatement* in Algeria to be impossible. Between 1837 and 1846, the death rate for Frenchmen in the territory was 77.8 per thousand men, and deaths so exceeded births that Boudin predicted the extinction of the French race in Algeria within twelve years.[10] The Chamber of Deputies consulted Boudin's work in 1847 when considering a massive proposal for settling French workers as an agricultural peasantry on Algerian lands, and Boudin's findings were debated in *L'Union*, in *La Gazette Médicale*, and at the Academy of Medicine.[11]

The July Monarchy (1830–1848) came to the rescue of colonial interests by commissioning an encyclopedic study of the animals, plants, waters, landscape, history, architecture, and population of Algeria, the multivolume *Exploration scientifique de l'Algérie* of 1840–1842. This mission of botanists, zoologists, painters, philologists, geologists, et al. grew from an environmental colonial movement that promoted the settling of French people in the French empire. By demonstrating the survival of exotic animal species in the metropolitan *jardins d'acclimatement*, the founder of the Société Zoologique d'Acclimatation, Isidore Geoffrey Saint-Hilaire (1805–1861), argued that human organisms could also adapt morphologically and physiologically to exotic colonial environments.[12]

The physician of the *Exploration scientifique de l'Algérie*, Joanny-André-Napoléon Périer, used this climatic and environmental model of man to defend French settlement in Algeria and the assimilation of Algerian Muslims to France. In *De l'Acclimatement en Algérie* (1845) and *De l'Hygiène en Algérie* (1847), Périer argued that Frenchmen could simultaneously master and adapt to the Algerian environment.[13] Man was a product of his geography, "some [persons] have a nature like mountainous country, humid and covered with forests, others are like dry soil," and as the Baron de Montesquieu connected legal systems to climatic zones, so Périer described "democratic forms of power in the North, aristocratic in the South, political in the East."[14] But Périer envisioned a dynamic interplay between the human intellect, soil, forests, water, and atmosphere: man could improve the landscape (and himself) through agriculture. Like man, the environment was salubrious if cultivated and dangerous if abandoned; Algeria was a land "fecund and rich by nature" that "war and barbarism" had allowed to become swamp, "a source of miasmatic infection, the principal source of maladies."[15] In this sickly Algerian atmosphere, the Frenchman underwent a Lamarckian degeneration: "After many years, [a Frenchman] acquires the skin color of the natives, he accepts their customs and even their way of thinking."[16] France must therefore organize this social-moral-human-environmental economy in order to rescue Algeria and implant the French race.

Périer thus envisioned the French civilizing mission as grand public works—environmental management, sanitation, and irrigation—and as the intermarriage of Algerians and Frenchmen. As the Franks and Gauls had blended to produce the French, so Algerians and Frenchmen would interbreed to create a new people of French mind and Algerian physique. Legislation and education would facilitate a reconciliation of the Qur'an and the Gospels until "the day will come when . . . tired of battling, surprised by the similarities, [we] will enter finally into a truly religious career of conciliation and progress for all."[17] In Périer's theory of hygiene, human differences were mutable; the Negro, Arab, and Caucasian were not essentially different races, but climatic variants on a single human type. Périer thus adapted the "anthropological school of environmentalist monogenism" of Isidore Saint-Hilaire and Armand de Quatrefages—the notion that race was fluid because all human beings descended from a single ancestor—in order to promote French settlement in Algeria.[18]

Périer's environmentalism resonated with the followers of the utopian socialist Claude Henri de Rouvroy, Comte de Saint-Simon (1760–1825) and with the *royaume arabe* (Arab kingdom) policy of Emperor Louis-Napoléon III (ruled 1852–1870). Saint-Simonians sought the regeneration of France in a coupling of France with the Muslim Orient, for "the birth of the modern society: technological and industrial in its economic enterprises, peaceful and spiritual in its socio-political relations."[19] Colonial cadres from the École Polytechnique, the Paris École de Médecine, and military *bureaux-arabes* implemented Saint-Simonian schemes in education, social engineering, and grand public works.[20]

FRENCH PHYSICIANS AND MUSLIM *ATIBA'*, 1830–1870

On the ground in the 1830 invasion of Algiers, French military physicians encountered a disease environment that defied all known medical theories. Frenchmen suffered staggering morbidity from cholera and dysentery: 16,482 of 204,397 French troops died, 224,822 were hospitalized in the first five years, and in one year the entire army cycled through the hospital three times.[21] Doctors accompanied Marshal Thomas Robert Bugeaud's gradual conquest of Algerian territory (1840–1871) and three surgeons ministered to conquered territory in 1844; by 1846, each *bureau-arabe* had its own physician. M. G. Worms, physician to the Constantine campaign, admitted, "Neither the Turks, nor the African population which trembled beneath them, were visited by such calamities."[22] Confronted with the limitations of their own medicine, French doctors opened themselves to using native therapies. As Worms wrote, "I was brought, relative to epidemic disease in Algeria, to views and medical practice diametrically opposed to those . . . of the school from which graduate the majority of military health officers."[23]

French doctors were receptive to Arab medicine in part because the French medicine of 1830–1870 was not yet well-differentiated from the humoralism of Galen and the climatology of Hippocrates. Historians date modern medicine in France from the Revolution of 1789, the dissolution of medical guilds and the establishment of three *écoles de santé* in 1794, and the enacting of medical professionalization legislation in 1803,[24] but until Pasteur's discoveries in the 1880s, actual French medical practice changed slowly. French doctors continued to bleed patients, to prescribe "hot" remedies for "cold" sickness, and to speak of Galenic temperaments and environmental balance: "General and local bloodletting, cupping-glasses the length of the vertebral column, long lukewarm baths and opium, such are the means which Dr. Saiget, surgeon major of the hospital of Oran, used in the treatment of tetanus patients [1839]."[25] The École de Médecine in Paris was renowned for its new clinical approach to the study of disease, but the Paris school tended to produce new nosologies rather than new therapies.[26]

In the field, French doctors met *atiba'* (singular, *tabib*), Muslim physicians who held an *ijaza* (certificate) in philosophic medicine, often from a mosque-university like the Qarawiyyin in Fez.[27] Although the Qarawiyyin was not a medical school, it kept a library of more than 30,000 volumes, among them the *Qanun fi at-Tibb* and *Manthuma* of Ibn Sina, the *Tadhkira* of Dawud al-Antaki, the *Tadhkira* of al-Siyuti, the *Al-Kamil* of ar-Razi, the *Mufradat* of Ibn al-Baytar, and two works by Moroccan physicians: the *Hayat al-hayawan* of ad-Damiri and the *Hadiyat al-maqbulat* of al-Marrakashi.[28] Students primarily memorized university manuscripts in *ragaz* poetry meter but also purchased printed books; the lithographic printing press was introduced to Fez in 1864.[29] In the rural countryside,

Dr. Henri Cenac observed of the functioning of medical dynasties, "The T'bib is the professor of the son destined to replace him," and *atiba'* families often made their own nosologies in a family clinical notebook, a copy of a classical medical manuscript annotated with case histories.[30] Medical texts were accessible to scholars in mosques, *zawiyat*, or private libraries.[31] As the land voyage to Mecca of the Moroccan scholar al-'Ayashi illustrates, rural peoples often solicited learned hajj pilgrims to share their manuscripts, and copies were made by scribes for local mosque libraries.[32]

The *tabib* received a certificate of competence (*ijaza*) from his medical master attesting to his knowledge, good character, and benevolent care of the poor. The 1832 *ijaza* of the Fez *tabib* Muhammad Kahhak was drawn by the *qadi* of Fez and signed by seventy Fez residents—*shurafa'*, shopkeepers, barber-surgeons (*hajjam*), and *atiba'*:

> The physicians and the scarificators [barber-surgeons] recognize that he is expert in the medical arts and in knowledge of the humors, the equilibrium of which is the source of the good function of the human body . . . that he fulfills the conditions required by works of medicine: knowledge of the nature of medicines, plants, herbs, trees, minerals . . . the art of curing wounds, sewing together torn tissues, setting bones . . . how to identify different varieties of urine collected in crystal receptacles . . . That he knows the amount of blood to collect . . . and he knows the veins to cut, that he knows in which cases to administer a purge and when an astringent . . . Hence total and complete license is attributed to him, conferring on him the right to exercise the profession of doctor.[33]

In 1865 in Batna, Kabylia, the physician Cenac observed, "The *tabib* devotes himself entirely to medicine, owns land farmed by tenants and is exempt from all corvée labor"; he grows herbal medicines and asks a fee proportional to the means of the patient.[34] Patients placed their tents around the *tabib*, forming a mobile hospital with "hygiene conditions we seek to realize in our cities."

"One of the most remarkable points of native therapy," wrote Dr. Rique, "is the extreme facility with which they cure wounds."[35] The *tabib*'s poultice of henna and melted butter did not ferment in the flesh like powdered lead, the coagulant used in French military surgery. Drs. Giscard (1834) and Arutin (1842) admired how *atiba'* set fractures, cauterized blood vessels with a hot knife, and sutured wounds with dried camel nerves.[36] In Tangier, Dr. Dulac saw *atiba'* perform cystotomies with "a knife with a

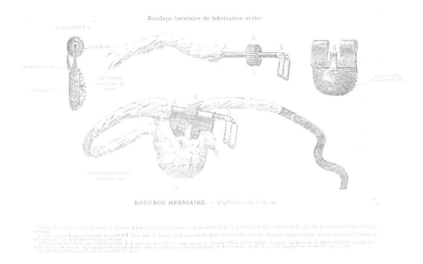

FIGURE 2.1. Hernia truss of native Muslim manufacture. Note the use of a metal gear to tighten the truss. (Lucien Raynaud, *Étude sur l'hygiène et la médecine au Maroc* [1902].)

thin pointed blade with which to penetrate the bladder, and a blunt hook to find the bladder stone."[37] *Atiba'* also couched for the cataract, a procedure which restores partial vision to the eye by displacing the clouded lens with a needle: "I presented to them a Cataract box, and they designated the Scarpa needle as the instrument that . . . penetrates the eye across the transparent cornea. To hear these Moors, many cataract patients were operated upon with success."[38]

The similarity of French and North African treatment regimens suggests similar underlying notions about the etiology of disease. Both treated cholera with heat: Algerians fed patients boiling olive-oil drinks and placed hot rocks on the flesh, and French doctors prescribed hot tea, vigorous alcohol rubs, opium, and forced marches to "reanimate the body's heat." Heating originates in a Galenic view of cholera as caused by a humoral imbalance rather than an external bacterial agent; cholera is a "cold" sickness occasioned by excessive cold and dry black bile. Neither group clearly understood contagion, though Algerians fled the sick and buried the cholera dead immediately, whereas French doctors 1849–1859 disagreed about whether cholera was transmitted by human contact or "poisoned air."[39]

The key difference between French and Algerian medicines lay in the use of statistics. French military physicians in Algeria compiled morbidity data for the cholera epidemics of 1849–1851. Dr. Vedrenes observed cholera's contagion: "It is remarkable that the two squadrons on the exterior of our bivouac . . . were the first cases of the malady that night. Born at the two extremes of our camp, the epidemic slowly entered the squadrons of the center and became general. This fact demonstrates the infectious nature of cholera."[40] Yet French doctors freely adopted native remedies; Vedrenes reasoned that "the Hottentots, the Negroes, the Indians, and the Eskimos" rubbed hot oils on the body, so why shouldn't he?[41]

Despite their equanimity, French doctors did not consider North African medicine equal to their own. Muslim patients consulted an array of popular healers, herbalists, midwives, barber-surgeons, and "sorcerers," visited Muslim saint shrines, and read "Medicine of the Prophet" collections of aphorisms, herbal remedies, hadith, and legal opinions. French doctors did not condone such practices, but neither did they consider them the essence of native medicine. Vedrenes noted: "When the Moroccan *tabib* has exhausted all his medical remedies and knowledge he has recourse to religion to cure the patient: thus he writes on a piece of paper some Qur'anic verses accompanied by cabalistic signs, he burns it and has the patient swallow the cinders . . . Finally, as a last resort, he sends the patient to the tomb of some marabout renowned for miraculous cures where he must sacrifice a cow, sheep, goat or some chickens."[42] Religious cures were what they were in Europe, wrote Cenac, "Like their European counterparts, there are those who believe it, those who doubt, and skeptics":

> Those who doubt say, "If it doesn't help, it doesn't hurt either." . . . The skeptics laugh, "My wife thinks it protects her from the evil eye." . . . If you object to the same individual that his sons . . . and his purebred horses have their contingent of amulets around their necks, his response is invariable, "These were put on at home; I do not want to force anyone to share my incredulity. My sons can take them off when they reach the age of reason, if such is their desire."[43]

French doctors in the field suggested using *atiba'* as subaltern agents of the French medical corps in Algeria. After training twelve *atiba'* in smallpox vaccination, one doctor proposed an *atiba'* medical corps to the Ministry of War: "They seemed to have a great interest in our demonstrations, and one of them took the blade to vaccinate an Arab child."[44] When Dr. Dumas observed natives fleeing his Orléansville hospital and overdosing on medications, he mixed mercury into a native syphilis preparation called "l'hashba" and had traditional native apothecaries distribute it.[45]

On August 3, 1880, the president of the republic authorized the École de Médecine in Algiers to grant a certificate of French medicine to *atiba*'.[46] But the French Algerian military and civilian administrations rejected all efforts to include *atiba*' in the French colonial medical service. From the multiple medical voices in Algeria, colonial authorities selected those of brothers Alphonse and Émile-Louis Bertherand, the hygienists of segregation and racial pathology, to ensure a French monopoly on "modern" medicine.

ISLAM AS PATHOLOGY: ÉMILE-LOUIS BERTHERAND AND THE HYGIENE OF RACE

Race theorists, French settlers, and the Société d'Anthropologie rejected Périer's environmental hygiene and assimilation theories, finding their champion in Émile-Louis Bertherand, a *bureaux-arabes* doctor (1848–1853) who became a medical-legal expert at Algiers courts, an editor of Algerian medical journals, and the founder of the Société Protectrice de l'Enfance Algérienne.[47] Bertherand argued that native Algerians were culturally and physiologically different from Europeans because Islamic despotism, law, family, religion, custom, sexuality, superstitions, and vicious habits had deformed native physiology. Bertherand thus shifted the source of disease from the environment to society and provided a scientific justification for racial hierarchy in Algeria.[48] "The Algerian question is above all one of hygiene and anthropology," he wrote, and only secondarily of "inhospitable climes."[49]

Bertherand explained the deaths of French colonists in Algeria as a consequence of social degeneration and climatic unsuitability. Colonists died because they were poor specimens—anemic factory workers and ignorant Norman peasants of excessive height, fatty diet, dissolute alcoholic habits, and moral laxity.[50] In their stead, he advocated a colonial society eugenically engineered by the hygienist, from the cultivation of land to the scientific breeding of French colonial children.[51] Bertherand recommended that short, darker-skinned Mediterranean orphans of Public Assistance be used to settle Algeria, where the colonial state could educate them, marry them to each other, and grant them lands to farm: "These young people, disciplined early in hygiene with a lifestyle appropriate to the climate, would conserve practical ideas ensuring fruitful work and good health . . . Is it not thus that Bugeaud's military colonies found success, with a formally disciplined existence?"[52]

For Bertherand, the indigenous races of Algeria ("Arabs, Kabyles, and

Saharaouis") were unassimilable to France because Islamic religion, polygamy, and despotism had deformed the physical and moral organism: "The Arab people are in a state of moral and physical degradation . . . Theft and murder on the moral order, syphilis and mange in the material order."[53] Muslim polygamy overstimulated the "genito-sexual" system and created sex organs of monstrous proportion, distorted and burdened the circulatory system, and generated a hereditary and inherently Muslim ailment: syphilis.[54] Islam, "a simple, sterilizing and absolute submission," suppressed the nervous system and blocked the development of the brain's intelligence.[55] Islam deformed the "physical-moral economy"[56] and produced a "fatalist, superstitious, ignorant character," which was transmitted to progeny as the "Arab temperament." Since Frenchmen and Muslims had distinct physiologies, physiognomies, and pathologies, Bertherand argued that each race must have its own hospital and its own law code; France must govern each man in Algeria "as an individual and as a race."[57]

Bertherand could not prove that Algerians were sicker than Frenchmen, so he focused instead on proving the inferiority of their medicine. He prepared the voluminous and jumbled *Médecine et hygiène des arabes* (1855) to "prove" that Algerians had no true science, though he reveals the existence of sophisticated Muslim pharmacy and botany despite himself.[58] Bertherand derided Algerian medical knowledge as "empiric," "theoretical," improperly divided, wrongly classified, and unregulated by institutions of higher learning or law. *Atiba'* buried dead cholera victims "prematurely" and were reluctant to bleed patients from major arteries, which he claimed proved a faulty native understanding of anatomy.[59] Embarrassed by the limits of his own therapeutics in 1855, Bertherand could nevertheless show that Algerians did use magic to heal sickness: "The native fallen ill on Saturday writes verses on seven pieces of paper," with which he rubs his body for seven days with a mixture of oil, rue, anise, and sesame, in order "to calm the pathogenic rage" of the genie "Mimoune." Bertherand triumphantly concludes, "Imbued with the most deplorable superstition . . . attribut[ing] the cause of almost all phenomena to the constant action of malevolent supernatural beings, the Arabs have the most bizarre ideas of the origin of maladies."[60]

Evidence or not, politics in Algeria guaranteed the victory of race hygiene. In 1871–1872, the tribal leader Muhammad al-Muqrani and the Rahmaniyya *tariqa* led a general revolt against French rule, a "Kabyle uprising" that shocked French opinion much as the Sepoy Mutiny had outraged the British colonial establishment in India. French vengeance knew few bounds, and the inhabitants of eastern Algeria were presented a reparations bill of 36,500,000 francs, land confiscations, and the extension of colonial civilian government over all but the Territoires du Sud in the Pre-Sahara.[61] French physicians were instrumental in the process. Auguste Warnier inspired the 1873 law bearing his name, *la loi Warnier*, which accelerated the alienation of Algerian peasants from their lands.[62] At the 1881 Congrès de l'association française pour l'avancement des sciences, Émile's brother Alphonse Bertherand proclaimed the great victory of French *acclimatement* in Algeria, where "the blood, name, and the language of France will predominate forever."[63]

Émile-Louis Bertherand had attempted to separate Muslims from Frenchmen through the sciences themselves but lacked the conceptual vocabulary to achieve it. The social sciences of Auguste Comte, Ernest Renan, and Émile Durkheim would provide a language of the mind to separate Frenchmen from Muslims after 1860. In the Third Republic, the French civilizing mission would rest upon both a racial theory of the sciences and an idea of epistemology itself.

AN IDEA OF SCIENCE: COMTE AND COLONIALISM IN THE THIRD REPUBLIC

The architects of French imperialism in the Third Republic (1871–1940) claimed Auguste Comte as their inspiration. Jules Ferry (1832–1893), the prime minister of France (1880–1881, 1883–1885) and the engineer of French colonial rule in Madagascar, Indochina, and Tunisia, used Comte's *Catéchisme positiviste* (1852) to argue that "civilized" nations had the duty to bring positive science and rational law to non-Western peoples. A self-identified positivist, Ferry argued that positivism must oppose "Muslim fanaticism" everywhere in the world.[64] Pierre Laffitte, Comte's disciple and the leader of the Comité Positiviste, argued for a *grande politique arabe* and approved the imposition of a French protectorate in Tunisia in 1881.[65] On the eve of the Moroccan conquest, Deputy Eugène Étienne proclaimed to the French Senate that Comte's method would guarantee a rational colonial rule in Morocco: "Colonial experimentation has brought us to apply the doctrines formulated by Auguste Comte, for whom sociology is to politics what biology is to medicine. Let us be inspired by the *positivist spirit* in Morocco if we wish practical success. Let us begin where we finished elsewhere: by determining all that Moroccan society is in its ancient and contemporary evolution, to guide it more surely to its future: peaceful progress under the auspices of democratic France."[66] But Comte himself was an outspoken critic of French rule in Algeria, so convinced of its destructiveness that he suggested restoring Algeria to independence.[67] How then was Comte adopted as a guiding light by the French colonial lobby? Why did Jules Ferry, the École d'Alger, and the Comité du Maroc identify themselves as Comteans? Comte provided not jingoistic ideology but an idea of science, a conceptual framework through which the French colonial lobby could construct an imperial civilizing mission for Africa, Asia, and the Middle East.

In his *Cours de philosophie positive* (1830–1842), Comte imagined a causal relationship between science and society that generated human thought. The physical and moral were actually levels of a single system, one that obeyed natural law from the simplest to the most complex order of reality.[68] Comte believed that societies evolved through history to an awareness of this fact; thus, a society's approach to the physical world demonstrated its degree of cultural progress. In intellectual infancy, man attributes all causality to gods, then he observes reality abstractly, and finally he derives natural laws directly from the physical world. This maturation progresses chronologically through the sciences: first chemistry replaces alchemy, then astronomy astrology, until finally sociology replaces traditional religion and "metaphysical nonsense." Comte described the sciences themselves as hierarchically ordered, a mirror of the actual hierarchy of the universe. As number is the most basic element of the world, Comte's first science is mathematics. The other sciences follow in "chronological order," building upon the principles and realities of those that precede them. Sociology was the ultimate science, for it described human society as Comte's highest and most complex reality.[69] Comte's resultant *sociologie* was not merely the perfect way to know and manage society, it offered what Bruno Latour calls a "Constitution of the Universe," "defining humans and nonhumans, their properties and their relations," a global schema of nature and culture.[70]

Comte's sociology suggested a mission for France as the world apostle of positivism, a liberating and egalitarian science of true knowledge. Comte defined the "positive" as the real, the useful, the certain, the precise, and the constructive, a truth derived by scientific method from objective and verifiable "facts."[71] He believed that positivism would transcend the feuds between Islam and Catholicism to fuse Eastern and Western peoples into "an immense and eternal Being," for human thought would inevitably become homogeneous once all peoples shared a true and complete scientific knowing.[72] As an artifact of incomplete social progress, traditional religions would fall away. "In a word," Comte wrote, "Humanity definitively substitutes herself for God, without ever forgetting his provisional services."[73] Comte's disciple Jean Robinet argued that France must use her advanced sciences to demonstrate enlightenment and to persuade the peoples of the world to leave God for positivism.[74]

ERNEST RENAN, ISLAM, AND
A RACE THEORY OF THE SCIENCES

Orientalist scholar, philologist, historian, race theorist, and nationalist Ernest Renan used a theory of knowledge to constitute the Islamic world as a social, intellectual, and political Other. Though Edward Said has portrayed Renan as a racist who used science instrumentally, Renan's view of Islam evolved out of his larger project to realize scientific modernity in France.[75] To sweep away dogma and esotericism, he defined them as alien; faith and religion were essentially Semitic and Muslim, science and reason were Latin and secular. To argue his case, Renan deployed philology, the science of language, which he considered an "exact Comtean science of mental objects": "It is to the sciences of humanity what physics and chemistry are to the philosophic sciences of bodies."[76] Through philology, Renan built "Islamic society" into a historical module, an unchanging set of legal, social, political, economic, and cultural elements that traveled space and time, conquering new societies and absorbing them into the collective. Renan thus invented a durable French intellectual construct of Islam, one with wide currency among French colonial elites in Morocco and Algeria.

Renan described Islam as a historical construct of the "Semitic race," a social group originating in Arabia of which the Arab was the only true exemplar.[77] In his *Système comparé et histoire générale des langues sémitiques* (1848), Renan describes the Semite as "a phenomenon of arrested development [whose language is] . . . the first awakening of [man's] consciousness."[78] Because Arabic grammar had changed little from the Qur'an, Renan concluded that Semites were literalists, incapable of philosophy or speculative thought. Semitic monotheism was a rigid insistence on one God and a "unified" thought system that rejects drama, fiction, imagination, the plastic arts, commerce, public spirit, and civil life.[79] The Semitic mind generated a unique social order, polygamy, which blocks "the development of all we call 'society.'"[80] Semites also required absolute monarchy, or "monotheism on earth."[81] For Renan, Muhammad was an ordinary historical figure, "neither seer nor saint nor magician," whom

Semites built into dogma by codifying his mundane daily orders into religious scriptures (Qur'an, hadith).

Once created by Semites, "Islamism" became a historical actor, invading and conquering Aryans in Persia, Buddhists in Asia, and Berbers in Africa, everywhere enslaving minds and bodies: "Freedom is never more profoundly wounded than by a social organization in which dogma reigns absolutely over civil life."[82] After consolidating its world power by 1200, Islam "exterminated science down to the roots" and homogenized diverse races to Islam by crushing their minds with the "steel circle" of dogma.[83] Thus, Renan concludes, "What distinguishes the Muslim is a hatred of science, the conviction that research is useless, frivolous, impious: natural science, because it competes with God, and history, because it could revive the errors of the pre-Islamic period."[84]

Renan claimed science for the West alone, an extraordinary notion that required the wholesale reinvention of centuries of scientific history. In reality, Greek science first reached the Latin West and France via Arabic translations, but more importantly, the Arab physicians and philosophers were the first foundation of European medical and scientific learning.[85] European scholars modeled scholastic method on the Muslim madrasa, European medical schools composed their curricula from works by medieval Muslim physicians, and Aristotle was read through the commentaries of the Muslim Arab philosopher and physician Averroes (Ibn Rushd, d. 1198).[86] If France first learned her science from the Muslims, how could the Islamic mind be unscientific? Renan denied history by redefining it: "I am the first to recognize that we have nothing . . . to learn from Averroës, nor the Arabs, nor the Middle Ages."[87]

In *Averroès et l'averroïsme: Essai historique* (1861), Renan dismisses the entire Arab philosophic corpus as a bastardization of Greek thought; the Arab Peripatetics transmitted to Europe a "deformed and travestied form of original and sincere Greece," admixed by magic from Egypt and Syria.[88] The great Aristotelian Averroes produced a "Jansenism" that inspired true science only in France, a freethinking movement that led France astray from her rational Greek ancestor. Renan thus invented a fictive intellectual genealogy for France as the direct descendant of an equally fictitious rationalist Greece. He also thus reveals the necessary connection between his two identities, Renan the French nationalist and Renan the Orientalist. Renan could realize his secular France only by inventing the Muslim as an intellectual, racial, and scientific Other, a dumping ground for all that Renan rejected in French society: religious faith, dogma, tyranny, and "metaphysics."

Architects of colonial Islamic policy in North Africa were influenced by Renan. His concept of the Islamic world as a single civilization took shape as a chair of *sociologie et sociographie musulmane* at the Collège de France in 1902 and the founding of a comparative journal, the *Revue du Monde Musulman*.[89] His analytic categories informed the work of French ethnographers Louis Rinn, Octave Depont, and Xavier Coppolani and suggest why the ethnographer Lucien Rabourdin considered the self-mutilation, ecstatic dance, and fire-handling of the 'Isawa Sufi order to be political.[90] In the 'Isawa's *hadra* (trance prayer sessions), Rabourdin saw Renan's Islam made manifest, a dogma that obliterated individual reason and self-mastery: "Bound together by secret signs . . . bent under the yoke of a passive obedience to . . . their priests, [the 'Isawa] are all the more frightening as the exercises to which they deliver themselves up . . . lead them to disregard pain."[91]

Renan was the crucial pivot between French and Islamic political philosophies, for his views sparked response and debate across the Islamic world. Among his Muslim interlocutors was the pan-Islamic thinker Jamal al-Din al-Afghani, who formulated his ideas of Islamic modernity in direct response to Renan's controversial 1883 "Islamism and Science" lecture. In the Paris-based *Journal des Débats*, al-Afghani conceded the backwardness of Muslim countries, but blamed lazy religious scholars and despotic rulers rather than Islam; he insisted that Islam, unlike Christianity, was a religion of reason. Muslims were weak because they had forgotten true Islam, a rational faith of the ancestors (*al-salaf*). Once recovered, this original *salafi* Islam would provide a path to modernity and unify the fragmented, foreign-occupied, divided Muslim world into a single community.

Yet even as he rejected Renan's work, al-Afghani assimilated Renan's positive theory of knowledge. Al-Afghani insisted that Muslims would "march resolutely in the [Comtean] path of civilization after the manner of Western society," for all nations "have emerged from barbarism" on the "road of intellectual and scientific progress."[92] He envisioned reform (*islah*) not as traditional renewal (*tajdid*), but as a transformation of Islamic *shari'a* through rational sciences. Like Comte's positive philosophers, Muslim jurists educated in new sciences would integrate reason with Islamic law and raise the intellectual level of the people with a progressive *ijtihad* (legal interpretation). Al-Afghani rejected materialism (*zahiriyya*) in its European and Islamic guises, yet he unconsciously limited the transcendence of revelation by using it for this-world activity and the improvement of human society.[93]

Al-Afghani's *salafi* Islam thus mirrored the social utopia of Comtean positivism. As Comte sought to reconstruct a post-1789 France torn by violent politics through true science, so al-Afghani envisioned unifying a fractured Islamic world through a purified Islam into a harmonious *umma*. Indeed, the actual Comte anticipated al-Afghani, for he viewed Muslims as "ripe for positivist conversion because their faith was tolerant and simple, they were already focused on the needs of the community, and they had been preserved from the anarchic influences of metaphysicians and legists."[94]

ÉMILE DURKHEIM AND
THE SOCIAL PRODUCTION OF THOUGHT

Émile Durkheim made Comte's theoretical "science of society" an applied reality in the world of cultures, human bodies, and artifacts, and created empirical methodologies for deriving general laws of social process.[95] Durkheim provided a mechanics for Comte's evolutionary model. The "categories of understanding"—ideas of time, space, class, number, cause and substance—are neither a priori (Kant) nor the result of individual experience (Hume), but are collective representations arising from the social group: "Each civilization has its organized system of concepts which characterizes it."[96] These categories function to reproduce society, for "if men did not agree upon these essential ideas at every moment . . . all contact between their minds would be impossible, and with that, all life together."[97] In *The Elementary Forms of Thought and Religious Practice* (1912), Durkheim argued that religion is the first "system of ideas by means of which individuals represent to themselves the society of which they are members." Religion provided a total cosmology and a "first philosophy of nature," but it differentiated in complex society into the areas of law, morality, science, and democratic government.[98] Religion was thus the womb of science, but it inevitably gave way to natural law.[99] The primitive mind, bound by social affectivity, betrayed its presence through belief in magic and magical practices, rituals, legends, texts, and artifacts, all collectable by the ethnographic sociologist.

The École de Sociologie thus provided the theoretical basis for the peculiar juridical status of colonial peoples as "Republican subjects" and for the French policy of colonial association in Africa and Asia.[100] The primitive was considered incapable of republican citizenship because he could not think or act independently of the ritual mandates of religious society. *Sociologie* allowed France to dissect and categorize each colonized people according to its degree of evolution and to rule it according to its *menta-lité*. Colonial physicians appropriated this evolutionary scale to argue for the failure of universalism and the need for a medicine of association. As Dr. Georges Samné declared to the Colonial Congress in 1904, "Everyone knows that one does not treat an Annamite and a Congolese in the same way, for the pathology of Annam is as different from that of Congo as the Annamite language is from the Congolese language."[101]

Edmond Doutté (1867–1926) applied Durkheimian sociology to Morocco, a dramatic departure from the textual approach of his Orientalist predecessors.[102] The first Arabist editor of *L'Année Sociologique*, Doutté defined Islam as "the ensemble of techniques, institutions and beliefs common to a group of men during a certain time."[103] He collected religious texts, linguistic evidence, healing practices, rituals, and legends as social facts of equal value.[104] Doutté began his career as a colonial administrator in Algeria, studied with Auguste Moulieras and Henri Basset at the École Supérieure d'Alger, and became chair of the History of Muslim Civilization and the Berber Language at the Faculté des Lettres d'Alger in 1907.[105] The resident generals of Algeria, the Comité du Maroc, and the Ministry of Foreign Affairs sent Doutté on five scientific missions to Morocco between 1900 and 1909 to design a strategy for future French rule. He reported in the *Renseignements coloniaux*, in the *Bulletin de la Comité de l'Afrique Française*, in the monographs *Merrâkech* (1905) and *En Tribu: Missions au Maroc* (1914), and in secret intelligence to the Ministry of Foreign Affairs.[106] With *sociologie*, Doutté reversed the relationship between God and society. God did not create the world; it was society who created God, through its collective rituals and practices.[107]

In the Chamber of Deputies, Paul Doumer, Paul Deschanel, Eugène Étienne, and the governor-general of Algeria, Célestin Jonnart, acclaimed the future Moroccan conquest as a positive scientific project. Governor-General Jonnart called the physician "the true conqueror of native society," and Dr. Samné identified medical assistance as the "surest means of conquest." Modern physicians were Samné's Comtean "materialist priests" who would ensure that "each group keep[s] her natural place, France her civilizing superiority and Morocco her natural riches."[108] René Millet, resident general of Tunisia, lauded the "peaceful penetration" of Morocco through the exact sciences.[109] The École d'Alger and the Mission Scientifique du Maroc competed to control the French colonial strategy in Morocco, and the intellectual leaders of each group, Edmond Doutté and Alfred Le Chatelier, presented opposite methods. Le Chatelier argued for British-style indirect rule through the Moroccan sultanate, a *gouverne-*

ment chérifien.[110] Doutté recommended an overarching secular and technocratic state operating independently of local Islamic leaders.[111] Resident General Lyautey used both models to create the French protectorate in Morocco: indirect rule through a *sharifian* sultanate supported (controlled) by a parallel shadow state, the French military technocracy.

SUFI SAINTS AS *HOMMES-FÉTICHES*: EDMOND DOUTTÉ AND ALFRED LE CHATELIER

Alfred Le Chatelier, the first occupant of the chair of *sociologie et sociographie musulmane* at the Collège de France (1902), argued that the Islamic world reacted in two ways to the modern West. Complex societies like Turkey, Syria, and Egypt gradually abandoned Islamic faith in favor of nationalism, whereas "primitive" North African Muslims rejected modernity and mobilized in mystical Sufi brotherhoods like the Qadiriyya, the principal resistance to French invasion in Algeria.[112] Le Chatelier claimed that Sufism was Islam's rejection of civilization and resembled African primitivism: "There is no appreciable difference between the ecstatic *shaykh* who cures maladies and the negro sorcerer with his grisgris."[113] When Le Chatelier arrived in Morocco in 1890, he insisted that Moroccan Islam required its own intensive local study and thus created the Mission Scientifique du Maroc, its journal *Archives Marocaines*, and the monograph series *Villes et Tribus du Maroc*.[114]

Le Chatelier saw Morocco as a fragmented, feudal polity with a spirit of nationhood centered on the dynasty of Idris II, which he believed was destined to become a monarchy.[115] But Le Chatelier could not explain the Moroccan politics of 1900–1912 and the array of pretenders, saints, and *mahdis* who challenged the sultan for power. As Edmond Ferry reported from the field in 1905: "There is not one Morocco, but several Moroccos," each led by a holy person with *baraka*, "a kind of blessing or divine power":

> A single tie, the religious tie, unites these pieces of Morocco without creating a state . . . The sultan . . . is not recognized everywhere as the political leader, but Berbers, Arabs and Moors all accept him as religious leader. He is, according to an apt expression, a "crowned *sharif*," he is directly descended from the Prophet and his hereditary *baraka*—a kind of blessing or divine power—is the most powerful . . . The numerous religious brotherhoods are more powerful than the Sultan and [are] true directors of Muslim souls and sorts of theocratic states . . . The Sultan of Morocco

cannot do without the support of the *shurafa'* . . . Some of the latter even give [the sultan] a kind of public investiture, like the Sharif of Wazzan . . . Then, another competing *baraka* suddenly appears and imposes itself on public credulity through miracles or arms.[116]

It was the Durkheimian Edmond Doutté who provided a unified theory of Moroccan politics. *Baraka* was healing: "[To understand], study the marabouts in action, that is to say, their thaumaturgy."[117] Doutté saw Berbers as primitives who, unable to grasp an abstract monotheistic God, recast animist fetish-men as Islamic "saints" or marabouts (*murabitin*). North African Islam was thus actually animist healing. Observing that Muslim pilgrims to marabout shrines rubbed their sick bodies with stones and carefully placed them on a pile called a *kerkour*, Doutté used the work of the British anthropologist James Frazer to describe the *kerkour* as a "healing by magical transference."[118] The primitive attains relief from illness by rubbing the sick place with an object, thereby externalizing the sickness and trapping it outside his body. With the advent of Islam, Moroccans reinvented the *kerkour* as a sacred offering to a Muslim saint:

> We find ourselves in the general process of Islamization of the pagan beliefs and practices, or maraboutism . . . In long perilous journeys or mountain passes, when he wants to remove fatigue, effort, evil influences, to whom will he pray? Allah? The Supreme Being? Not yet, the brain of our Moroccan is not yet capable of abstract representation. It is to the saint who protects him and his country, to the marabout whose tomb he knows that he addresses himself, where he continues, though a Muslim, to accomplish the old animist rites. It's to him that he will pray and the pile of rocks of the Tizi n Miri Pass will become a *kerkour*.[119]

The marabout took the place of the healing stone by absorbing the tribe's maladies into his own body: "The bodies of the saints become receptacles of the ills of the community."[120] Thus the Muslim crowds vying to touch the *sharif* of Wazzan, to swallow his saliva, and to walk in his footprints were for Doutté sick persons seeking relief. Doutté noted that Moroccans called the trees, epileptic madmen, and shrine buildings they visited "marabouts," and thus marabout must signify "instrument of healing."[121]

Doutté approached Islam in North Africa as primitivism. In *Magie et religion dans l'Afrique du Nord* (1908), he argued that Moroccans inhabited a magical universe of demons, the emotional projections of the collective social mind.[122] Moroccans believed sickness to be a wicked spirit:

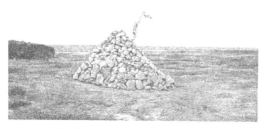

FIG. 25. — Kerkoûr de Sidi Dâher à Casablanca

FIGURE 2.2. *Kerkour,* the healing pile of stones, of "Sidi Daher," or Saint Tahir. (Edmond Doutté, *Merrâkech* [1905].)

"[The *jinn* says] I go to the woman who has conceived and I blow on her and make her miscarry,"[123] but the *jinn* could be countered with procedures that played upon imaginary magical sympathies. To cure an ulcer, one knotted the patient's blood, fingernail clippings, and hair into a cloth, which was placed in a riverbed; as the river washed the cloth, so the patient's body would be cured of sickness.[124] Magic by spirit intermediaries summoned the *jinn* and constrained them within frameworks of incantation, writing, geometry, or knots. Richard Keller has argued that the French viewed Islam as a space of madness, but Doutté's ethnography reveals this "madness" more precisely to be an inability to understand the physical world rationally.[125] Doutté concluded that North Africans were primitive minds incapable of science: "The doctor (*médecin*) is at base only a counter-sorcerer; the word T'ibb signifies magic as well as medicine: medicine is the daughter of magic. Even now, the doctor in North Africa is no more differentiated from the sorcerer than the malady from the djinn . . . the procedures to expel genies are beside therapeutic notes, rites of magic with the use of simples."[126]

He concludes that Islamic society has no medicine, public life, secular law, free thought, or public morality, because the Muslim's thoughts, words, and gestures are defined by a savage religion of "ritual, sacred, obligatory and immutable character."[127] Doutté acknowledged that Morocco had a political history, but for him, Moroccan politics was *maraboutisme*.[128] The *sharif* of Wazzan was an *homme-fétiche*, a fetish-man, a healing totem, rather than a political leader. Because the saint (marabout) was the product of primitive tribal society, Doutté concluded that saints could not be co-opted as intermediaries for a modern and centralized French colonial state in Morocco.[129]

Doutté thus revolutionized French approaches to Islam in Morocco.

Orientalists had studied Islam in theological texts but Doutté privileged lived social practice, which he called "the only Islamic reality." For Doutté, Islam was the *kerkour* pile of stones, not the Qur'an. He found validation in his every experience: if Moroccans avoided him, "savages are afraid of every novelty"; if they invited him to dinner, "savages use food to conciliate the stranger's magic power."[130] Doutté's sociology gave France a colonizing method for Morocco; if political authority were healing, then France could use medicine to prove French superiority to the Moroccan in the laboratory of his own body.[131] After Doutté selectively presented magical healing amulets to "prove" a primitive Muslim *mentalité* (see Fig. 2.4), French doctors adopted his attack on Muslim *atiba'*, viewing them as an affront to civilization, an impediment to liberty, and the antithesis of reason.[132] Doutté joined the metropolitan administrative-scientific complex after 1914 as secretary general of the Commission Interministerielle des Affaires Musulmanes; he occupied a chair at the École Coloniale and was a member of the Comité Parliamentaire de l'Action à l'Étranger, the Académie des Sciences Coloniales, and the Institut Ethnologique.[133]

Together, Doutté and Le Chatelier provided Lyautey with a strategy for Morocco. The men agreed that Morocco was a primitive tribal society whose *maraboutisme* blocked science, nationalism, and pan-Islamism, but Le Chatelier feared that modern economic development would pro-

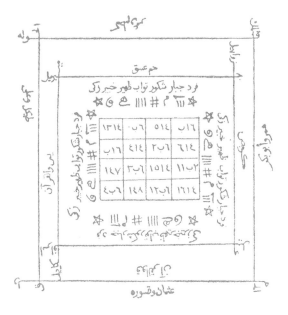

FIGURE 2.3. Muslim healing amulets deployed gematria and numerology to summon the *jinn* but confine them within Islamic boundaries. Here the call to the *jinn* (*daʿwa*) at the amulet's center is contained within a framework composed of the names of the four archangels, the four rightly guided caliphs, and God's Truth and Power. (Edmond Doutté, *Magie et religion dans l'Afrique du Nord* [1908].)

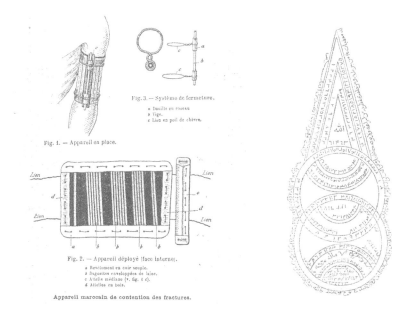

FIGURE 2.4. Doutté selectively presented examples of magic like Qur'anic amulets (*right*) to "prove" Moroccan primitivism, ignoring, for example, the bone-setting apparatus (*left*) that French military physicians collected in Morocco just one year after Doutté's *Magie et religion* was published. (Edmond Doutté, *Magie et religion en Afrique du Nord*; Deniau, Dercle, and Bachon, "Poste médicale et infirmaries indigènes au Maroc," *Archives de médecine et pharmacie militaires* [1909].)

duce "the bankers, businessmen and industrialists of a revivified [Oriental] Islam."[134] Doutté's Durkheimian analysis suggested how this modern revolutionary politics could be avoided: by preserving the primitive mindset of *baraka* and marabouts, the French ethnographic construct Spencer Segalla has named "the Moroccan Soul."[135] To study, manipulate, and preserve this Moroccan Soul, Lyautey institutionalized a Section Sociologique of native affairs under Le Chatelier's disciple, the sociologist Edouard Michaux-Bellaire.[136]

THE CIVILIZING SCIENCE IN MOROCCO:
LYAUTEY AND THE FRENCH DOCTOR

"In Morocco, between the medical corps and myself, there is only one spirit, one doctrine," wrote Lyautey, "to help Morocco evolve towards greater justice, well-being, and liberty under the guidance of France."[137]

Lyautey called medicine a "mission and an apostolate," and the physician "an agent of penetration, attraction and pacification."[138] Doctors were at the vanguard of Lyautey's armies and philosophy: Jourdran, his first director of the Service de la Santé et de l'Assistance Publique (later, the SHP), served with Lyautey in Madagascar and opened a medical school in Tananarive (Antananarivo).[139] From Algeria, Lyautey recruited Mauran, a *médecin de colonisation* who became a *médecin missionaire* in Morocco (1906) and the first director of native health.[140] Lyautey brought the *pied-noir* and future director of public health Jules Colombani from Algeria.[141] After accompanying Lyautey on his Shawiya campaign in 1907, Léon Cristiani became personal physician to the sultan's armies and founded the first French hospital in Fez for natives, the Hôpital Cocard.[142]

Lyautey drew from the Catholic corporatism of Adrien Albert Marie, comte de Mun (1841–1914), rather than the republican civilizing mission. He refused to teach Moroccans the exact sciences and opposed both the creation of a modern, European-style "Dar al-'Ulum" university or the introduction of modern science courses to the traditional Qarawiyyin university. He explicitly exempted native healers and midwives from all state regulation with a *dahir* of 1916. Yet Lyautey was a passionate believer in the power of medical science and doctors to "peacefully penetrate" Muslim society, at once improving material conditions for the natives, deploying a scientific gaze over the countryside, and attracting Moroccans to France by healing them in body and mind.

In contrast, the French doctors Lyautey recruited drew upon a medicine deeply entwined with republican values. The physicians Thévenin (1860), Seux (1870), and Ollive (1875) considered the Moroccan climate naturally healthy, and so concluded that epidemic disease must be caused by undisciplined populations and a failure of governance.[143] Castex, the physician of the French mission in Tangier, blamed the cholera epidemic of 1860 on the behavior of the city inhabitants: "[Imagine] all the miasmas that the most total human negligence can accumulate . . . The houses throw everything into the street where it decomposes freely; fish debris, domestic animals, etc."[144] Lucien Raynaud, a hygienist sent to Mogador by the Conseil Sanitaire of Tangier, attributed Moroccan epidemics of plague, typhus, and cholera to the sultan's government. Because the state failed to provide food in times of drought, he argued that the starving population resorted to eating cadavers, garbage, and insects in order to survive.[145] Hygienists insisted that the mark of civilization was a state that provided for the people's welfare.

French doctors in Morocco saw native healing as "empiric," a jumble of plants, religion, and superstition devoid of any governing scientific system. Mauran regretted that the grand science of the Islamic golden age had become "degraded to a base charlatanism, to the point that the marabout, the saint, the religious doctor, is . . . the 'sovereign guardian of public health,'" and "*kitaba*, astrology, incantation, exorcism, properties of gems, therapeutics of simples, and some notions of chemistry and antisepsy, even organotherapy are strangely mixed."[146] Raynaud illustrated the collapse of classical Galenism into magic in an interview with a Moroccan *tabib*: "There are, he told us, 4 temperaments, which are in relation with the 4 elements . . . To know the constitution of a patient, one must add the letters of his name and that of his mother, then divide by 7, one has the star under which he is placed and its day; and then dividing by four the patient will fall into the following classification: 1 fire, 2 earth, 3 air, 4 water."[147] The textual Moroccan Galenic tradition became a moribund scientific Orientalism conserved by the physician-turned-Orientalist Henri-Paul-Joseph Renaud, in his capacity as director of manuscripts at the Bibliothèque Générale de Rabat.

Doctors saw Islamic belief itself as a pathology of mind and society. Mauran wrote of the trance *hadra* of the Hamadsha Sufi order as "pathology, delirium and contagion" and political tyranny: "These exhibitions disgust me profoundly and I flee them . . . I accuse them of perpetuating fanaticism and ignorance, of capturing the soul of the people, preventing them from thinking, waking up, throwing off the yoke . . . which drags them down to the worst misery and servitude."[148] But French *sociologie* also informed how doctors saw the Muslim body, classified diseases, and collected biomedical data. Such a seamless incorporation of colonial racism to disease pathology illustrates the social production of biomedical knowing; as Jean Comaroff has written, it is "the [very] key to the social significance of knowledge itself."[149]

THE SYPHILITIC ARAB, OR THE ISLAMIC *MENTALITÉ* AND THE BIOMEDICAL BODY

In 1913, the director of the Tangier Institut Pasteur Pierre Remlinger wrote, "Venereal diseases . . . constitute the very essence of Moroccan pathology . . . Syphilis is the Moroccan malady par excellence."[150] In 1918, Georges Lacapère claimed that 100 percent of the residents of Fez were infected with syphilis.[151] In 1924, the *sous-directeur* of the health service, Jules Colombani, agreed: "Everyone knows syphilis is extremely common in the Moroccan population . . . around 80 percent."[152] How is it that doctors "saw," or made themselves to see, an epidemic that didn't exist? Pasteur's discoveries introduced a universal science that could theoretically transcend race, for man was evaluated as a set of microbiological factors rather than racial qualities.[153]

But the "syphilitic Moroccan" demonstrates the persistence and influence of *sociologie* despite the theoretical objectivity of bacteriology. In Algeria of 1855, Émile-Louis Bertherand claimed that Islam caused syphilis. In Morocco of 1912, doctors repeated his claim, despite the new Wassermann blood test (1906) for the *Treponema pallidum* spirochete and a network of Instituts Pasteur in North Africa.[154] Guided by sociology, doctors "found" Muslim syphilis in statistics, clinical observation, and medical photography. As Meghan Vaughan has argued, "Biomedical knowledge on Africa was both itself socially constructed . . . and 'social constructionist.'"[155]

Arab syphilis was an old trope in French military, travel, and medical accounts of North Africa, from the "blooming chancres" that fascinated Gustave Flaubert in the anuses of Egyptian soldiers at Qasr al-'Aini hospital to the eyeless death-heads whom doctors encountered in the Moroccan countryside.[156] Colonial syphilologists in France and Britain theorized that deviant native sexual behavior caused extremely high rates of syphilis infection.[157] In Morocco, Remlinger of the Institut Pasteur argued that the polygamous family was itself perverse, characterized by an indiscriminate, frenzied, bestial sexuality. He imagined Muslim women engaging in lesbian tribadism in the harems and then prostituting themselves in the streets; their husbands "copulated with multiple wives" and then engaged in homosexual sex at the public baths.[158] The *sociologue* Edmond Doutté claimed that female marabouts "prostitute themselves regularly and continuously . . . A true *baraka* appears attached to prostitution."[159]

The architect of antisyphilis campaigns in Morocco was Georges Lacapère of the Paris Saint-Lazare Hospital, a disciple of Alfred Fournier (1832–1914), who viewed syphilis as a scientific rather than a moral problem.[160] For Lacapère, Muslims were syphilitic because they were ignorant, because Islamic law did not regulate society; barbers were not prevented from circumcising boys with dirty razors, syphilitic mothers were nursing their newborn infants, and prostitutes were allowed to roam the streets.[161] For Lacapère, Arab syphilis demanded a regulation and medicalization of Islamic society by a hygienic protectorate state.

How could medical data prove an epidemic that did not exist? French doctors from 1900 to 1912 compiled morbidity data from tiny, high-risk groups of soldiers and prostitutes, then generalized their findings to the entire population. In Mazagan, Remlinger found 150 of 170 native soldiers syphilitic, 230 of 275 soldiers in Mogador, and 428 of 500 soldiers in Tangier.[162] Syphilis also produces skin lesions that are easily confused with many other skin diseases, such as cutaneous tuberculosis (scrofula), favus, lupus, and yaws; for this reason syphilology was (and is) a branch of dermatology.[163] Yet in 1917–1918, the military physician Laurent Leredde instructed his doctors to diagnose syphilis sores by sight alone, which he admitted had great potential for error.[164] Even when the Wassermann blood test for syphilis was used, Lacapère observed that the test yielded false positive results in the presence of malaria, tuberculosis, and scarlet fever.[165] Conversing with native patients did not contradict the syphilis diagnosis, for French-Arabic medical dictionaries translated vague dialectical Arabic expressions such as *mard al-kabir* (the great illness), *al-bird* (the cold), and *mard al-fassad* (the rotting disease) as "syphilis."[166]

Data contradicting the syphilis diagnosis were explained away. Doctors noticed that North African Muslim "syphilis" patients did not suffer the classic neurological symptoms of tertiary syphilis like tabes dorsalis (nerve degeneration), insanity, and paralysis.[167] But rather than question the diagnosis, Lacapère asserted that "syphilis does not like the Arab brain," because Muslim brains were too rudimentary, "never developed by intellectual work."[168] Neurological syphilis was thought to afflict only the civilized and culturally evolved, whereas "primitives" suffered purely physical and cutaneous symptoms.[169]

French colonial syphilologists thus translated the civilizing mission to pathology. Dr. Edouard Jeanselme claimed in his *Histoire de la syphilis* (1931) that natives developed "exotic syphilis"[170] because "the races of color live a style of life in which [mental] activity is reduced to a minimum."[171] But natives who received a modern French education and wore European clothing could develop "civilized" syphilis; doctors attributed the paralysis of a Tunisian Muslim man to his French secondary-school diploma and sartorial penchant for suit and tie.[172] In Morocco, native Jews attended French-language Alliance Israélite Universelle schools and were believed to suffer neurological syphilis, whereas Muslims were "completely uncivilized, not sharing the habits of European life."[173] The high incidence of neurological symptoms among the "evolved" was a likely result of French medications. Doctors treated syphilis with compounds of mercury (salvarsan) and arsenic (novarsénobenzol), assuming that such toxins were excreted by the kidneys. In reality, heavy metals settle in body fat, especially the fat cells sheathing the nerves, eventually causing paralysis and insanity.[174] When "modern" European medications were introduced in China and the Dutch East Indies, European doctors noted a sudden, dramatic increase in "civilized" neurological syphilis among natives.[175]

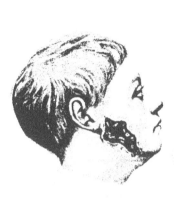 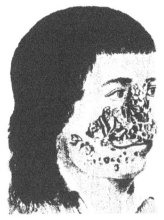

Figure 12.1: Scrofuloderma (chronic scrofulous ulceration), lithograph from Radcliffe Crocker's *Atlas of the Diseases of the Skin* (1903).

Figure 12.2: Lupus vulgaris, Plate LXVII from Bateman's *Delineations of Cutaneous Diseases* (1817).

FIGURE 2.5. Cutaneous tuberculosis (scrofula), lupus, yaws, and other skin diseases produce lesions that were often confused with those caused by syphilis. (Crissey and Paris, *The Dermatology and Syphilology of the Nineteenth Century* [1981].)

The clinic is an imaginative space in which doctors collect symptoms from hundreds of patients to create a "biography of disease," as Michel Foucault has argued.[176] Moroccan syphilis demonstrates that colonial clinics also drew upon racial stereotypes, native *sociologie*, and historical cliché to compose disease biographies. In 1916, the physicians Lacapère and Leredde founded a native syphilis clinic in the Lamtiyyin neighborhood in Fez, where they registered eight thousand "syphilis cases." From experiences at the clinic, Drs. Decrop and Salle created a photographic syphilis atlas (1921), and Lacapère composed his magisterial *La Syphilis Arabe: Maroc, Algérie, Tunisie* (1923). These texts invented "Moroccan syphilis" from the diverse rashes, sores, and tumors of the Lamtiyyin clinic's Muslim patients.[177] As we have seen, the lesions caused by tuberculosis, yaws, and other diseases were often falsely identified as signs of syphilis. Lacapère created a visual "history" of Arab syphilis by assembling photos of different patients into a purportedly chronological disease biography, a scientific creation that "demonstrated" the progression of the disease over time (see Figs. 2.5 and 2.6).

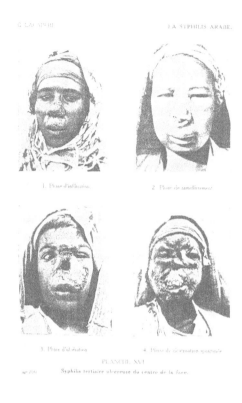

FIGURE 2.6. Lacapère assembled several patients from the Fez clinic into a disease "biography" of syphilis progression, thus inventing Arab syphilis from the diverse rashes of actual bodies. (Georges Lacapère, *La Syphilis Arabe* [1923].)

Syphilis in Morocco illuminates the connections between colonial knowing, the clinic, and pathology-as-knowledge. Ludwig Fleck and Thomas Kuhn argue that scientists know the world through received ideas, a "thought community" that defines the legitimate objects of scientific study.[178] Colonial *sociologie* conditioned what doctors knew; Muslims were "known" to be perverse, a "fact" that physicians confirmed with medical photography. In the French medical journal *Maroc médical*, Muslim physiology is a house of horrors—the death's head rotted by syphilis, the enormous scrotum of elephantiasis, hideous tumors that deform the face and eyes. Clinical data interlocked to assert, repeat, and re-inscribe syphilis onto the Moroccan body, a medical discursive edifice analogous to Edward Said's "Orientalism." The Muslim literally wore his barbarism on his body, a body rendered eloquent by French medical technology to speak its suffering, a pathological condition inflicted by the [irrational] Muslim *mentalité*.

For French doctors and republican science, the documented existence of Moroccan syphilis provided a moral victory over Islam. Muslim syphilis "proved" that Islam threatened the human body and the survival of the Moroccan population; doctors "demonstrated" how Islam killed infants in the womb and condemned children to a life of intellectual and physical deformity as hereditary syphilitics (see Fig. 2.7).[179] Syphilis provided justification for the entry of French physicians into the Muslim home and made a mockery of Muslim morality. Decrop and Salle bragged that the most veiled women "allow themselves to be examined completely . . . We achieved the nude photos without difficulty."[180] Medical Orientalism laid claim to the real and the positive, for "North African pathology" was developed in a hands-on interaction with native bodies.[181] But as Fleck argues, "Scientific facts are not . . . so much discovered as invented in a prolonged social process."[182] Thus was a French republican positivist war against Islam engaged, at the biological and even microbiological levels.

THE FRENCH CIVILIZING MISSION in North Africa from 1830 to 1900 moved from a radical assimilation policy in Algeria (1830–1870) to a policy of association with natives in the Moroccan protectorate (1912–1956). Superficially, French association policy resembled British indirect rule in India, but each colonial strategy sprang from different premises. British colonial policy separated the races through biology; human difference was a matter of "blood and color," elaborated in Darwinian theory and physical anthropology. French colonialism conceptualized difference in the mind; the native could evolve to a state of civilization if he learned to

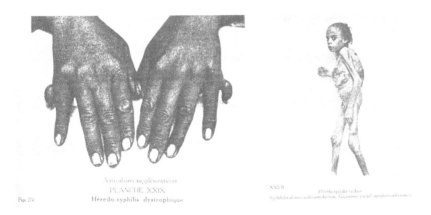

FIGURE 2.7. Lacapère also used the Fez clinic to document Muslim "hereditary syphilis." He used an array of birth defects, nutritional disorders, and even a genetic abnormality like vestigial fingers to "document" the ubiquity of syphilis among Muslims. (Lacapère, *La Syphilis Arabe* [1923].)

think like a Frenchman. But Auguste Comte, Ernest Renan, and Émile Durkheim argued that individual human thought was a collective social product; as a consequence, direct assimilation of natives to France would be doomed to inevitable failure. Colonial generals Joseph-Simon Gallieni and Lyautey confirmed the destructive effects of direct French rule in Madagascar, Indochina, and Algeria and advocated a policy of association. The colonialism of the Third Republic deployed an idea of science—an aggressive positivism—to civilize, classify, and administer the diverse peoples of the empire and to evolve them gently toward a universal secular modernity.

French hygiene theories about North Africans were intertwined with the emerging French sociology of Islam. The hygienist Périer saw man as a product of his environment and envisioned a blending of Frenchmen with Algerians. But after positivists located human difference in historically-constructed mental races (Renan) and used native healing practice as evidence of socially-constructed worldviews (Durkheim), assimilation was rejected in the French Colonial Congresses of 1904–1907.[183] French doctors' views of native medicine evolved in parallel. In 1865, French physicians proposed using *atiba'* as agents for the French colonial health service; in 1905, the same native *atiba'* were rejected as magicians with an antiscientific Muslim *mentalité*. In Morocco, French doctors described distinctively "Muslim" pathologies—the physical manifestation of Islam on the biological body.

The French sociology of Islam also created a fundamental tension within the French protectorate in Morocco. To govern Morocco effectively, Lyautey wished both to preserve its primitive Islamic *mentalité* and to engineer a peaceful coexistence between Muslim and French civilizations scientifically. To this end, he created a Section Sociologique of native affairs to catalogue each Moroccan tribe and respect its local saints, lineages, language, and customs.[184] But to extract wealth from Morocco, the country would be obliged to modernize and industrialize, and the sociologist Edmond Doutté warned that industrialization would destabilize both the Moroccan family and the Islamic religion.

Not so in the Islamic world, where Muslim *salafi* intellectuals adopted the French positivist languages of civilization, modernity, and progress in order to purify the religion and reform society. *Salafis* called themselves Islamic Comteans; al-Afghani's student and collaborator Muhammad 'Abduh saw Islamic law (*shari'a*) as evolving with the "collective knowledge of a people" toward an enlightened social order.[185] 'Abduh derived general laws of social process from the Qur'an, a project pursued by sub-

sequent Islamic thinkers from Sayyid Qutb (1906–1966) to ʿAli Shariʿati
(1933–1977).[186]

But in adopting the terms of modernity from French positivism, *salafi*
intellectuals also absorbed its positive theory of knowledge. Muslim *salafis*
condemned esoteric (*batini*) Sufi knowing as heretical and alien to Islam, a
cause of social decay, doctrinal schism, and despotism. As ʿAbduh wrote:
"[Among the causes] of social illnesses of the Orient . . . are the beliefs
and opinions introduced into Islam by different groups like the Sufis . . .
The [Islamic] reformation will extract these beliefs from the nation."[187]
The Moroccans who imported Islamic modernism from Cairo to Fez thus
brought with them a *salafi* epistemological war on Sufism, one that originated not with Islam, but with France and the French civilizing mission.

THE MANY DEATHS OF DR. ÉMILE MAUCHAMP: CONTESTED SOVEREIGNTIES AND BODY POLITICS AT THE COURT OF THE SULTANS, 1877–1912

ON MARCH 19, 1907, French physician Émile Mauchamp was beaten to death outside his clinic in the city of Marrakesh. This spectacular murder served as the official pretext for a French military invasion of the city of Oujda in 1907 and the creation of a French protectorate in Morocco in 1912. The French ambassador to Morocco, Henri Regnault, eulogized the doctor as a martyr to France's civilizing mission, "the evolution of peoples is never accomplished without sacrifices and without victims."[1] Mauchamp's biographer Jules Bois suggested that antiscientific Islamic "sorcery" was responsible: "The sorcerers jealously conserve corrupted and corrupting traditions . . . Ulémas and talebs are the great enemies of our intervention . . . It is not the sultan with his ministers who in reality governs, directs and exploits Morocco: it is the sorcerers who profit from the credulity, the timidity, the darkness . . . of these people."[2]

But in an entry from his private diary dated November 8, 1905, Mauchamp mused, "The rumor circulates that I am not a doctor but a secret envoy of the French government sent to make maps, do topography and spy to prepare for French invasion."[3] As Luise White has suggested, medical rumor can reveal a deeper history of social experience than high politics.[4] Many Europeans were attacked in Morocco after the Algeciras Conference of 1906, but an international political crisis crystallized around the body, not the person, of a French doctor, because the human body intersected with Moroccan politics in 1907.

Émile Mauchamp's corpse offers a window into the political culture of precolonial Morocco, where biological bodies were linked to the integrity of the body politic. Rumor offers historians "a way to see the world the way the storytellers did," and Moroccans told of a poisoning French doctor in order to describe invisible forces assailing post-1860 Morocco.[5] The doctor came to personify internal and external threats to the body politic and was made to suffer "many deaths," for European commercial encroachment, rural rebellion, famine, civil war, and a disintegrating Moroccan state.[6] Mauchamp's murder was a political event, an act of popular Moroccan defiance and rage at the sultan's impotence before the European powers. The suspects to Mauchamp's murder were the forces fighting for political legitimacy in 1907: Sultan 'Abd al-'Aziz, his brother 'Abd al-Hafiz, the jihadist Ma' al-'Aynayn, and the regional overlords of Marrakesh, the Glawa. Through the body, we explore Moroccan experiences of foreign invasion, the state's collapse, and a reconstitution of the Islamic sultanate under French rule.

THE FRENCH DOCTOR AT THE COURT OF THE SULTANS

In contrast to the Ottoman Empire, which imported European experts to reorganize its military and create institutions of higher learning,[7] nineteenth-century Morocco has been seen by historians as closed to European penetration. The sultan Mawlay Sulayman (1793–1822) disbanded the Moroccan fleet and stopped maritime trade on Moroccan ships in 1817. Ambassadors sent by Mawlay 'Abd ar-Rahman (1822–1859) to London and Paris recognized European technological superiority but advised the sultan to minimize Morocco's contact with Europe.[8] The sultan Mawlay Hasan (1873–1894) accepted European military training missions under foreign pressure, but these missions have not been considered significant.[9] Edmund Burke argues that the tardy modernization efforts of Sultan 'Abd al-'Aziz in 1900 failed because the 'ulama' opposed the introduction of European experts and their technology.[10] Nineteenth-century European diplomats described the Moroccan court as closed, a place where "doctors of law" frowned on all but commercial interactions with Christians.[11] But in fact, the Moroccan sultans, the 'ulama', and the rural populations were keenly interested in Western science from the beginning of the nineteenth century and actively sought to acquire it. But as they adopted new technologies for their own ends, Moroccans invested French science with local social meanings.

The Moroccan sultans invited French and English physicians to court from the sixteenth century, when the Sa'adiyyan sultan Mawlay 'Abd al-Malik engaged the Frenchman Guillaume Bérard as his personal physician.[12] "Maritime jihad," or piracy against European ships, provided the greatest source of European doctors, engineers, and military experts in Morocco. Piracy has been recognized as labor exchange—Sultan Mawlay Isma'il (1672–1727) used Christian slaves to build his Meknes palaces, and Louis XIV powered his galleys with Moroccan slaves, but slavery also provided access to foreign scientific expertise.[13] European doctors served the Moroccan court as slaves, were sent to minister to European slaves in Morocco, or converted to Islam and joined the Moroccan army as renegades, or *renegados*.[14] France, Spain, and England sent doctor-clerics (Franciscans, Trinitarians, Mercedarians, Dominicans, or Protestant missionaries) to care for their enslaved countrymen. In 1691, the Spanish crown founded a royal hospital and friary for the Spanish captives of Meknes, which the sultan placed under his protection.[15]

The sultans also had access to European technical knowledge through renegades—European officers captured at sea, escapees from European penal colonies, or deserters from the French army in Algeria who converted to Islam, took Moroccan wives, and assumed a rank in the sultan's army.[16] In 1825, the Piedmontais renegade Ahmad ibn Sulayman was chief of artillery, since he alone knew how to operate and repair the gun-carriages purchased in Europe. In 1810, a renegade Portuguese surgeon accompanied the sultan on campaign to treat the wounded and compose drugs for the officers and rich soldiers.[17] The French engineer Théodore Cornut designed the Moroccan port city of Mogador (modern Essaouira) in 1764, with straight streets, European-style windows, a sewer system, and a covered aqueduct with clean drinking water.[18] The English renegade Isma'il Ingliz ("English Ismael") served as tutor to the adolescent Mawlay Hasan. Under his direction, Hasan organized an infantry battalion of Susi tribesmen in the Western style and developed the infantry as a branch of the Moroccan army.[19] With the end of piracy came an end to the supply of European technical personnel, but as late as 1877 the French *mission militaire* found a French *polytechnicien* canalizing the River Fez, the Baron de Saint-Julien serving as personal physician to the grand vizier, and a renegade Spaniard directing a royal brass band that could play "God Save the Queen" and other military airs.[20]

European travelers were another source of information about the new science. In 1803, Sultan Mawlay Sulayman received "'Ali bey al-'Abassi," the assumed name of the Catalan adventurer Domingo Badia y Leblich, who disguised himself as a Turkish savant.[21] As Badia claimed to have studied in London and Paris, the sultan questioned him about modern European education. Whether the Moroccans were fooled by his disguise is debatable, for the sultan delighted in having Badia read Arabic and gently correcting his mistakes.[22] The first Friday sermon included pointed remarks from the imam that "it was a great sin to cultivate any commerce with the Christians, or to sell or give them any sort of food or nourishment."[23] The sultan posed many questions about the measurement of temperature, astronomical observation, and electricity:

> I ordered my electrical machine and a camera obscura to be brought in. I presented these to him as objects of mere amusement, which had no scientific application . . . He afterwards amused himself with seeing the electric jar discharged, and had it often repeated; but what surprised him most was the experiment of the electrical shock, which I was obliged to repeat a great many times, all of us holding ourselves by the hands in order to form the human chain. He asked me many and various explications of these machines, and also of the influence of electricity.[24]

After the Moroccan army suffered stunning defeats in the Battle of Isly with France (1844) and the Tetouan War against Spain (1860), Sultan Mawlay Hasan (1873–1894) recognized the urgent need for state-directed military reform and the acquisition of European technology and science.[25] Mawlay Hasan sent Moroccan students to study artillery in Belgium, England, France, and Spain, where some attained the rank of *maître-ouvrier* and returned to assume direction of the arsenal in Fez.[26] The Moroccan physician 'Abd as-Salam al-'Alami was sent to study European medicine at the Qasr al-'Aini medical school in Egypt founded by the Frenchman Bartholomé Clot,[27] and Muhammad Gabbas returned from the School of Royal Engineers in Great Britain in 1880 to become minister of war and then minister of foreign affairs. Mawlay Hasan cooperated with the Spanish government to train Moroccan military physicians in European medicine at the Spanish hospital in Tangier.[28] His successor, Sultan 'Abd al-'Aziz, used Arab graduates of the French medical school in Algiers as military doctors.[29] In 1861, the Moroccan state spent 62,747 francs on imported pharmaceutical drugs from France; this was more than the value of all Moroccan exports to France combined.[30]

Under pressure from the European powers, Mawlay Hasan accepted official missions from European governments to train his military after 1870. The sultan knew that these European experts were government spies, topographers, and commercial agents, but he desperately needed trained personnel—he had resorted to using religious students to manufacture cartridges, maneuver artillery, and keep records. To prevent any one European power from knowing the full capacity of his military, he divided the missions between its different branches—the French trained the artillery, the English trained the infantry on Gibraltar, and the Italians set up foundries for the arsenal in Fez at a portal known as "Bab al-Makina," or Portal of the Machine.[31] The military missions were financially and politically costly for Mawlay Hasan—the French artillery mission alone cost 60,000 francs per year and 100,000 francs more when tribesmen killed a French officer in 1887.[32]

In an attempt to extract scientific knowledge without paying the political price, Mawlay Hasan incorporated individual "men of science" into his entourage and kept the rest of the 1877 French mission at a distance. He took the physician Fernand Linarès with him to the palace, and had the artillery expert Jules Erckmann lead a group of Moroccan students to the École de Génie in Montpellier for engineering training.[33] Erckmann also served as palace astronomer, directing the *muwaqqitin* (mosque functionaries who determined exact prayer times) in the use of the sultan's astronomical instruments, which included the English Quarter, sextants, theodolites, and a glass mounted on the equatorial.[34] Unlike the renegades, these *mission* experts extended the reach of the French military into Moroccan society and laid the groundwork for the French invasion of 1912. The artillery expert Nestor Prosper Larras was an adept cartographer and secretly conducted topographical surveys while at court; his maps were used to execute the French invasions of Casablanca in 1907 and Fez in 1912.[35]

Through the person of Dr. Linarès, French medicine became the tool of European espionage par excellence. He acquired great influence at court and became the sultan's personal physician, accompanying him on the famous *mahalla* (traveling court) of 1893.[36] After gaining the sultan's confidence, Linarès deftly promoted French interests, acting on constant instructions from the French legation in Tangier. Linarès was able to block efforts by the British and the Germans to introduce the telegraph, a state bank, and the post office, reserving these strategic interests for France.[37] On the diplomatic front, Linarès single-handedly mediated between Paris, Madrid, and the *makhzan* in the Melilla crisis of 1893, averting war between Morocco and Spain. His detailed accounts of everyday court intrigue, many of them in numeric code, helped the French to monitor contacts between Morocco and Turkey. After Sultan Mawlay Hasan died in 1894, Linarès was the first European representative received by the new sultan, ʿAbd al-ʿAziz.

So successful was Linarès that after his departure from Morocco in 1902, the French organized a corps of doctor-agents (*médecins missionaires*) attached to the Ministry of Foreign Affairs, who were to gather local intelligence and win the natives' confidence.[38] Beginning in 1904, the French created dispensaries for these scientific "missionaries" along the Moroccan coast (in Casablanca, Mazagan, Mogador, Larache, Rabat, Safi) and in Marrakesh and Fez. Dr. Mauchamp was the *médecin-missionaire* for the clinic in Marrakesh. Other European powers soon besieged the sultan with their own doctor-agents, offering medical and military advice. French doctors did not see themselves as spies; they fulfilled intelligence duties in order to pursue medical goals. Indeed, the Ministry of Foreign Affairs forced Linarès into retirement for what it considered his excessive sympathy for Moroccans.

After 1900, the French made of medicine, science, and technology Daniel Headrick's "tentacles of progress," ensnaring Morocco in a web of debt and technological dependence. The French Algerian *député* Eugène Étienne and his Comité du Maroc organized the Mission Scientifique du Maroc in 1905, to interest metropolitan investors in the natural resources of Morocco and to persuade the Chamber of Deputies to invade and colonize.[39] The French entrepreneur Henri Popp raised 600,000 francs for his Moroccan Telegraph Company in September of 1907 and installed stations in Casablanca and Tangier without the sultan's permission. After the French occupied the Shawiya in 1907, they offered to withdraw on condition that the sultan buy the telegraph, railroads, and other technologies installed by the army of occupation and hire Frenchmen to supervise.[40] The *makhzan* bought Popp's four telegraph stations for 560,000 francs and named Popp the director of the new Moroccan Telegraph in 1908.[41] The French technical personnel of precolonial penetration thus transitioned to the functionaries of the French protectorate in 1912.

THE FOREIGN IMPORTED BOX OF FIRE: SCHOLARS AND TRIBES DEBATE TECHNOLOGY

Many Moroccan *'ulama'* condemned the sultans' interest in European science, which they saw as a road to debt, foreign influence, and an inappropriate strengthening of *makhzan* state power. The Qarawiyyin jurist Ja'far ibn Idris al-Kattani (d. 1905) denounced foreign inventions in his *Blessed Composition in Judgment of Soap of the East and Candle "the Bougie" and the Foreign Imported Box of Fire, These Things from the Countries of the Unbelievers, God Curse Them . . .*[42] Scholars attacked the hated protégé system, which placed international commerce and merchants under the jurisdiction of European law courts, and they criticized the sultans' modern reforms (*nizam*): a European-style standing army, a modern bureaucracy, and a new tax system.[43] A smaller group of scholars saw a reformed state as the only guarantee for Morocco's survival; a regime apologist chided his countrymen: "How strange, the Moroccans! The enemy is at their door, he has already planted his claws in their flesh, and they still hesitate to sacrifice . . . to reinforce their army and permit it to repel them."[44]

Between 1900 and 1904, the Moroccan *'ulama'* saw the country go into economic free-fall, losing its treasury surplus and going 100 million francs into debt. The young sultan 'Abd al-'Aziz, with his taste for extravagant European inventions (a bicycle, a solid gold camera, fireworks), did not inspire confidence. 'Abd al-'Aziz's ambitious program of reform, including roads, bridges, the telegraph, and modernization of the ports, was undermined by its inept application. Heavy taxation for a hypothetical *jihad* that never arrived and notoriously corrupt Moroccan ministers who colluded with European interests to pocket public funds helped to unify the scholars in opposition. When Sultan 'Abd al-'Aziz requested a legal opinion (*fatwa*) on "the cause of our present decadence," he received a resounding rejection of European advisors: "The foreigners are the original cause of our misfortunes. It is to them that our decadence, our anarchy, our internal strife, the loss of our independence and our ruin must be imputed . . . Of what utility are they? What new sciences have they taught us?"[45] On December 22, 1904, a delegation of *'ulama'* led by Ja'far ibn Idris al-Kattani demanded the expulsion of French military advisors and the firing of two viziers seen as agents of France.

However, the *'ulama'* did not object to European technology itself or declare it contrary to Islam. A member of the same al-Kattani family secretly visited the French in Tangier for a demonstration of the telegraph and telephone.[46] European technology was an element of religious observance in everyday life; European clocks kept prayer times for the Fez mosques from 1803.[47] The *'ulama'* did not oppose technological reform itself and indeed proposed inviting Egyptian or Ottoman experts to direct reforms in place of the Europeans. 'Abd al-'Aziz suspended the French military mission and dispatched the minister Muhammad al-Muqri to the Orient.

Rural tribesmen also appropriated French medicine and technology despite hostility to foreigners and the *makhzan*. Rural folk did not have access to the accounts of elite travelers like as-Saffar,[48] but pilgrims to Mecca saw the military and technological reforms in Algeria, Tunisia, and Egypt on the journey across North Africa. In 1843, the French sent the military physician Dr. Candé to the Middle Atlas Mountains to treat a Berber Banu Snassen tribal leader who had aided the French against Amir 'Abd al-Qadir in Algeria. Among the tribesmen, Candé found European technologies the subject of lively popular discussion, particularly for those who had made the pilgrimage: "They were enchanted by the relations they had had with the French in Cairo . . . one of them had spent three months in Tunis, and recounted with enthusiasm . . . the Bey circulating in a carriage which the king of France had given him, a troupe of musicians who played together . . . the troops maneuvering in the European style."[49] But the Banu Snassen were well aware of the relationship between French science and her military. When Candé took a notebook from his pocket, the nephew of the chief remarked, "That's how the French are. When they go to a country, they take the description of the localities and map the cities so they can take them later."[50]

Moroccans were also accustomed to French medicine before Mauchamp arrived in 1905, because Muslim pilgrims endured quarantine on the hajj, imposed on Moroccan ships by the Conseil Sanitaire (hygiene council) in Tangier after 1840. In principle, the council protected the safety and health of Moroccans, but its second raison d'être was to facilitate the export of goods to Marseille and hide Moroccan epidemics from French metropolitan health authorities.[51] The council argued that plague and cholera outbreaks were due entirely to pilgrims returning from Mecca; thus, putting them in quarantine would suffice to protect Mediterranean shipping.[52] The city of Tangier provided Moroccans with more benevolent examples of Western medicine; Tangier enjoyed one French, one Spanish, and two English hospitals by 1902.[53] The native Jewish community in Tangier was so impressed with European medicine that a Jew named Benshimol founded a French hospital for Moroccan Jews with his private fortune.[54]

Even the Shawiya and Marrakesh tribes, who waged jihad against the French invaders in 1907, asked their enemies for medical assistance. Shortly after the French occupied the Shawiya in 1907, the M'Zab and 'Ash'ash tribal councils approached the French military post to request native infirmaries for their populations, which they offered to support at their own expense.[55] In the nine French dispensaries founded in the Shawiya, the Muslim clientele climbed to three hundred consults per day by September 1908.[56] In 1905, when the dissident Zenaga tribesmen captured a French explorer, the marquis de Segonzac, they seized his pharmaceutical supplies and required him to treat the sick. As they released him into the custody of the Glawa, the Zenaga asked their former prisoner to send them Frenchmen for civil engineering.[57] "Medicine," wrote Dr. Trolard on August 29, 1907, "is a letter of safe-conduct in Morocco."[58]

In his (posthumous) work *La Sorcellerie au Maroc*, Mauchamp wrote of French medicine as civilization and Moroccan healing as barbarism, but Muslim healers saw no conflict and borrowed freely from European techniques, equipment, and medical training. In 1865, an Algerian "syphilis specialist" approached the French physician H. Cenac to request an *ijaza*, a certificate of competence. Nancy Gallagher has argued that European signatures on *ijaza* illustrate European hegemony, but one may also see them as a consequence of the fluidity between French and Islamic medical traditions.[59] The Algerian *tabib* already "enjoyed a great reputation among the Ouled Sellem tribe" and possessed considerable lands, but "all Arab doctors are specialists and seek to perfect their art by all means in their power."[60] In their interview, Cenac was astonished by the similarity between the "Muslim" description of syphilis and its clinical study at the Paris Hospital:

> CENAC: Every individual who has sores thus has the disease?
> TABIB: No, there are sores and sores. If they eat at the flesh, it is mange. There are also sores from the heat. Those of syphilis are grouped in a circle by place, all circular ulcers or union of circular ulcers have the same cause. When the bones are swollen in certain spots, in the elbows, the legs, the cranium . . . this is syphilis.[61]

The enthusiasm of Moroccan healers for French medicine caused embarrassment once the protectorate was established. The Moroccan Muhammad ibn Salim Balkhayat, who began his dental practice in 1892, scandalized French doctors with his modern European equipment. One doctor exclaimed, "He even bought his apparatus in Casablanca!"[62] A *dahir* (royal edict) of 1916 applied strict standards to European pharmacists, physicians, and midwives, but had no provision for natives who learned "modern" French medicine informally: "This is not a case of bone-setters practicing traditionally in the Moroccan crowds, but Muslim or Jewish natives having more or less frequented the medical milieu . . . the native Mahboub, former doctor of Abd el Krim [al-Khattabi], has in the medina a veritable medical cabinet, with instruments, examining table . . . his prescriptions are filled in the pharmacies, notably that at K'tarine in the medina."[63]

VACCINATION AND A POLITICS OF
THE BODY IN MOROCCO, 1860–1907

As they assimilated French medical technologies for cure, Moroccans used them to debate the erosion of state, territory, and sovereignty in Morocco. As Luise White has argued, "New technologies and procedures did not have meaning because they were new or powerful, but because of how they articulated ideas about bodies and their place in the world."[64] Morocco began to disintegrate politically after 1860, torn between European commercial encroachment, reparations, protégés, loans, Sultan Mawlay Hasan's efforts to extend the centralized state, and, after 1900, pretenders to the throne, open tribal revolt, and civil war.[65] Rumors about foreign medical technologies provide a history of perception behind rural revolt and revolution.

To evaluate the Mauchamp rumors, we should first consider the social meanings of smallpox vaccination in Morocco. Moroccans were not opposed to smallpox vaccination in principle, and indeed practiced variolation, a traditional form of inoculation. According to an account by the French traveler Léon Godard in 1860: "The mountain Berbers know inoculation against smallpox from time immemorial, and they practice it."[66] The historical forerunner to vaccination, variolation operates according to the same principle, stimulating the body to produce natural antibodies.[67] Whereas the Jennerian vaccine is a serum of cowpox harvested from infected cattle, Moroccan variolators took pus directly from a person ill with smallpox and introduced it to a small incision on the healthy body: "When smallpox (djidri) is discovered, the parents of the child to be inoculated buy one or two sores through a small gift to the young infected person. These are cut and the contents are rubbed against an incision in the region that separates the thumb from the root of the index finger on the person to be protected."[68]

Moroccan populations thus had no objection to the concept of vaccine itself, but they did object to *the use of needles to create marks on the body*. In Morocco, marks on the body, particularly tattoos, had military, religious, or tribal significance. All members of the corporation of riflemen attached to the Nasiriyya Sufi brotherhood were identified by a tattoo on the shoulder.[69] Native Jewish women carried off by rural tribes in the sacks of the mellahs of Fez and Casablanca were then tattooed with the *siyala*, the facial tattoo of Berber women.[70] Perhaps most troubling to Moroccans, soldiers of the sultan's *jaysh* troops were identified by a tattoo between the thumb and forefinger to prevent desertion.[71] Mawlay Hasan's military reforms put increased pressure on the general population to provide conscripts.[72] The people of Fez rose in the tanners' revolt of 1873 to prevent military recruitment of their children; Mawlay Hasan's army included boys as young as ten.[73] Because tattoos could transform social identity, Moroccans suspected any procedure that could permanently mark the body.

Vaccination was associated in the popular imagination with the *makhzan*; those who accepted French vaccine were closely affiliated with the sultan's court. In Safi, a coastal city near Marrakesh, Dr. Trolard remarked in 1907 that vaccination was "admitted in the city by notables and universally requested by the Jews, [but] it is absolutely rejected by natives of the countryside [the Rahamna and Haha tribes]."[74] Trolard's Muslim clientele consisted of governmental administrators, soldiers, and functionaries of the state. Likewise, Moroccan Jews served as the sultan's commercial agents in international trade; the Jew was the *tujjar al-Sultan*.[75] Those who rejected vaccination were rural tribesmen hostile to the *makhzan*; this distinction was observed by French doctors in the cities of Oujda (1844), Mogador (1875), and Safi (1907). Rahamna and Haha tribesmen walked days to be treated in the Safi clinic, yet they refused vaccination. Soon after, the Rahamna were in open revolt; they switched their allegiance from Sultan 'Abd al-'Aziz to his brother, 'Abd al-Hafiz.[76]

Thus, Mauchamp's vaccination sparked rumors not because Moroccans feared or misunderstood the procedure, but because of how the vaccine was administered and for whom. Needles could penetrate the body to transform identity and the vaccinators were French doctors, associated with the court. Rural patients both crowded French dispensaries and accused French doctors of poisoning them.[77] In Mogador in 1909, a crowd tried to murder Dr. Dinguisly, then approached his colleague Henri de Leyris de Campredon for vaccine, "assuring us that smallpox is in the city."[78] The people of Morocco did not reject Western medicine, contrary to the claims of the French colonial lobby. But in 1907, French medical technologies were implicated in systems of social meaning, articulating the invasion of bodies and bodies politic.

THE MANY DEATHS OF DR. ÉMILE MAUCHAMP, 1905–1907

Of interest here is not Dr. Mauchamp's biography or his actual death but his "many deaths," the rumors surrounding him in life and the treatment of his corpse after death.[79] Although Mauchamp's spectacular demise in 1907 was the cause célèbre of French colonial interests and the pretext for invasion, Mauchamp himself was a minor figure. Unlike Dr. Linarès, who influenced Moroccan foreign policy, Mauchamp unsuccessfully courted 'Abd al-Hafiz and the Glawa, offended the *makhzan*, and snubbed his French colleagues.[80] His medical dispensary was one of seventeen in Morocco and other clinics boasted triple his clientele.[81] So why did the death of this minor actor involve the sultan, his brother 'Abd al-Hafiz, and the government of France in an international crisis? Mauchamp became a vehicle for the articulation of a post-Algeciras (1906) crisis of Moroccan political legitimacy. Through the body of a French doctor, the people of Morocco indicted the rule of Sultan ʿAbd al-ʿAziz and demanded an end to foreign encroachment in Morocco.

The murder may have been instigated by the sultan, his brother ʿAbd al-Hafiz, European agents, Maʾ al-ʿAynayn, or local officials. Nooman Kouri, the French consul in Mogador, concluded in his 1910 investigation that ʿAbd al-Hafiz had staged the incident in order to destabilize his brother's regime.[82] One Moroccan witness testified that the crowd assembled on the order of the sultan,[83] and the *makhzan* did provide financial support for jihad against France in Mauritania.[84] There were other suspects. Supporters of Maʾ al-ʿAynayn, the Saharan jihadist, confronted but failed to kill Mauchamp on September 24, 1906. Mauchamp also disputed with his landlord, the Marrakesh pasha Warzazi, the German renegade and double-agent Judah Holzmann, and the British vice-consul, Alan Lennox. Politics further complicate the facts: the French used the murder to justify invading Oujda,[85] and some Moroccan witnesses changed their testimony between 1907 and 1910.[86] However, if someone did assemble the crowd, he only unleashed a popular rage that already centered on Émile Mauchamp.

From the moment Mauchamp arrived in Marrakesh, he was the subject of multiple rumors. In 1905, he heard a story that he was not a doctor at all, but a spy sent to make maps and prepare for a French invasion.[87] In January of 1906, Mauchamp noticed that his former Muslim patients were avoiding him; sent to investigate, his servant returned with the following rumor:

> [Mauchamp] belongs to a kind of French Christian freemasonry sworn
> to destroy the Muslims of Morocco. Savant and capable doctors like
> Dr. Mauchamp are chosen and sent among Moroccan populations. There,
> the doctors care for Arabs with the appearance of a great benevolence,
> curing them . . . gaining the confidence of all . . . but they have adminis-
> tered a subtle poison which only acts two, three or four years later, and
> [the patients] will surely die. When these doctors return to France, they
> consider it a great accomplishment to have killed two or three hundred."[88]

Shortly before Mauchamp's death, the sultan heard that the French geologist Louis Gentil was smuggling telegraph equipment into Morocco and contacted his governor: "It has come to our noble attention that a Frenchman named Gentil has gone to Marrakesh with a wireless telegraph apparatus with the intention of installing it in that city . . . If you have established that he has arrived in Marrakesh with the apparatus in question, you will keep him under surveillance by secret agents and take all measures needed to prevent him from installing it."[89]

A rumor circulated four days before the attack that Mauchamp planned to plant the French flag on his roof and signal waiting French troops to invade Marrakesh.[90] The morning of the murder, the pasha's agents warned Mauchamp to remove a suspicious antenna from his roof, which was drawing a hostile crowd. When the doctor walked out of his clinic to remove it, the crowd killed him.

Certainly, the rumors surrounding Mauchamp reflected historical realities. Mauchamp may not have been a freemason, but he was an agent of the Ministry of Foreign Affairs and French doctors did gather intelligence. All members of the 1877 French artillery mission engaged in espionage, and the 1905 Mission du Maroc and French scientific explorers did prepare the 1907 and 1912 invasions. As for the wireless telegraph, a Frenchman *was* installing telegraph stations on the west coast of Morocco. But it was the entrepreneur Henri Popp, not Gentil or Mauchamp. Moroccans were right to believe that French technologies were paving the way to invasion, for the French army executed the 1907 invasions of Oujda and Casablanca from Oran by wireless telegraph.[91]

However, the rumors also shed light on the Hafiziyya movement as a people's revolution. 'Abd al-Hafiz, brother of the sultan, conspired with the powerful Marrakesh *qaid* Madani al-Glawi to take the throne in 1904. But the "Hafiziyya" only became popular after Sultan 'Abd al-'Aziz signed the Act of Algeciras on June 18, 1906. The act, which gave France broad political powers to intervene in Morocco and made the Banque de Paris et des Pays-Bas the director of Moroccan finances, "consummated the break between the sultan and those Moroccans who favored continued resistance to France."[92] 'Abd al-Hafiz gained the support of the powerful Marrakesh *qaids* Madani al-Glawi and 'Abd al-Malik al-Mtuggui and the *'ulama'* of Marrakesh, who declared 'Abd al-Hafiz sultan on August 16, 1907. The French invasion of the Shawiya in 1907 radicalized the Hauz tribes, who lent their support to 'Abd al-Hafiz and then compelled him to send 3,000 men to fight the French on September 16, 1907.[93] The Hauz tribesmen were the core of the anti-French jihad. The question is how and when they developed this political consciousness.

The Mauchamp rumors describe an organized conspiracy of doctors who inject Christianity, foreign government, and secularism through the needle, a poisoning that will destroy Morocco internally. The French army will invade using information carried by invisible technologies—vaccines, the wireless telegraph, the topographical survey.[94] Rumor describes French "cure" as a slow poison, an apt metaphor for the French administration of ports and the French loans that devalued Moroccan currency and produced food shortages and famine. In 1906 Marrakesh, a third of the population nourished itself on boiled locusts, a typhus epidemic claimed 1,500 victims, and "twelve people die daily of hunger in the mellah."[95] But it is curious that of twenty-five Europeans living in Marrakesh in 1907, rumor should identify the boorish Mauchamp as the architect of foreign threat.

By accusing a French doctor, the rumors indirectly accused Sultan 'Abd al-'Aziz and his modern reforms of eroding Moroccan sovereignty. As we have seen, French doctors were the sultans' agents and Moroccans who accepted vaccination were close to the court. Rumors of a poisoning doctor blame 'Abd al-'Aziz for introducing Europeans and their sciences, forces that have gone out of control to menace Moroccan integrity itself. The murder of Mauchamp was a critique of Sultan 'Abd al-'Aziz, who understood it as such and condemned the murder in an open letter read in mosques throughout the country.[96] The Mauchamp rumors expressed a popular political will that became murder, revolt, and jihad. The crowds first killed Mauchamp, then declared 'Abd al-Hafiz the sultan, then pushed their new sultan to fight the French invaders. Popular politics begun as rumor took juridical shape in the contract of rule (bay'a) presented to 'Abd al-Hafiz in 1908.

From a variety of Moroccan eyewitnesses, we know that an armed crowd of men, women, and children led by the *muqaddimin* of the quarter waited outside Mauchamp's clinic in 'Arsa Mawlay Musa street and attacked when he emerged, clubbing and stabbing him over twenty-five times.[97] The crowd stripped the corpse naked, tied a rope around its neck, and dragged it to an empty lot. As they debated whether to burn it with kerosene, *khalifa* (royal) troops arrived to confiscate the body and return it to Mauchamp's dispensary. The crowd threw rocks at the mounted soldiers as they took the corpse, shouting, "Cursed be the father of Haj Abd as-Salam (Pasha Warzazi) the Christian."[98] The pasha Warzazi arrested ten Moroccans, all residents of the quarter and migrants from tribes outside Marrakesh: three Masfiwa, two Zamran, an Ought, a Dra, a Susi, and a deaf-mute person of unknown origin. The men worked in the Marrakesh market as vegetable, bread, and water sellers, grain measurers ('abar), and carpenters.[99]

We cannot know if these were the actual assailants, but their residence in Marrakesh shows the engagement of rural tribes in Morocco-level politics.[100] *Makhzan* sources identify the assailants as "Rahamna," a reference to the tribal confederation organized by the Rahamna tribe.[101] The origins of the accused murderers suggest the membership of the Rahamna organization—the Masfiwa, Zamran, Ouzgita, Dra (and Sagharna) tribes.[102] In May of 1907, the Rahamna group demanded that the prisoners not be handed over to the French, that Europeans leave Marrakesh, and that Jews uncover their heads and go barefoot in the city.[103] In August of 1907, the Marrakesh *'ulama'* judged Sultan 'Abd al-'Aziz to be "morally deceased" and the Rahamna tribes swore fealty to his brother in a *bay'a* of 1907. The tribes acted contrary to their own local interests, for their enemies, the rapacious Glawa governors (*qaids*), were 'Abd al-Hafiz's allies.[104] But in 1907, the tribes put the defense of Morocco above their own private interests and pressured the new sultan to honor his duty and wage jihad on the French.

When the Hafiziyya movement spread to Fez, the city echoed the Rahamna demands. On December 30, 1907, a mob of tribesmen and urban dwellers thronged the Fez streets declaring themselves independent of both the sultan and the *'ulama'*. Forty thousand people are said to have crowded the Qarawiyyin mosque, demanding that the *'ulama'* write a *fatwa* to declare 'Abd al-'Aziz an illegitimate ruler. On January 3, 1908, tribal chiefs, notables, the *'ulama'*, and the crowd proclaimed 'Abd al-Hafiz sultan. However, the 1908 Fez *bay'a* presented the new sultan with a list of conditions, including the suspension of the Algeciras Act, the restoration of Morocco's territorial integrity, the expulsion of the French, and the restoration of Islamic institutions, taxes, and privileges.[105] The *bay'a* was less a vote for 'Abd al-Hafiz than a definition of legitimate Moroccan political authority by the people and the *'ulama'*.

The line from the Mauchamp rumors to the 1908 Fez *bay'a* suggests that the public used Mauchamp to conceive a Moroccan polity larger than local interests. Rumors spread ideas and mobilized crowds in the streets of Fez and Marrakesh. The Mauchamp rumors identified the community under threat as the *umma* of Morocco, not local tribes or cities, and the people collectively demanded action from the sultan. The corpse of Dr. Mauchamp, like the Fez *bay'a*, is a text upon which to read these popular political sensibilities.

A TALE OF TWO BODIES: THE SULTAN OF MOROCCO AND DR. ÉMILE MAUCHAMP

In pre-protectorate Moroccan royal processions, court-led Muslim festivals, and diplomatic rituals, the sultan's body was displayed as the sym-

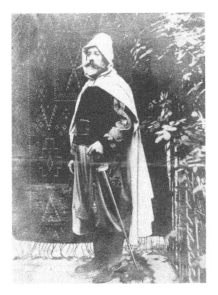

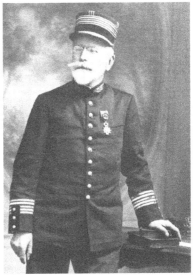

FIGURE 3.1. Dr. Fernand Linarès dressed in Moroccan military attire, symbolizing his incorporation into the Moroccan sultan's court. (Collection Ministère de la Défense—SHD—Armée de Terre, France.)

FIGURE 3.2. Fernand Linarès in French military dress. (Archives Historique du Service de Santé Militaire et Musée du Val-de-Grâce, Paris, Linarès personnel file.)

bolic center of the Moroccan state. In a *hadiyya*, or "gift" ceremony, tribal delegations presented the sultan with gold, carpets, and livestock, performing their deference to royal authority and filling the royal coffers.[106] The sultan traveled six months of the year through the country on *mahalla*, or "mobile court," from which he meted out justice, punished wayward provinces, and performed pilgrimage at the tombs of the saints.[107] The person of the sultan himself was a source of *baraka*, and his cannon offered a space of asylum (*hurm*).[108] So essential was the sultan's body to state cohesion that Sultan Mawlay Hasan's death while on *mahalla* campaign in 1894 was concealed until the court was safely returned to Fez.

The relations between the Moroccan sultans and Europeans were also enacted through corporeal symbolism. When the French consul Louis de Chenier angered Sultan Muhammad ibn 'Abdallah (1767–1784), he was "led around the city of Rabat on a donkey, his face turned toward the tail, which he was obliged to hold in his hand."[109] Sultan Mawlay Hasan insisted that members of the French military mission of 1877 wear Moroccan uniforms. This "disguise" was symbolic submission to the sultanate and a physical incorporation of French experts to the Moroccan court. When Dr. Linarès accompanied Sultan Mawlay Hasan on *mahalla*

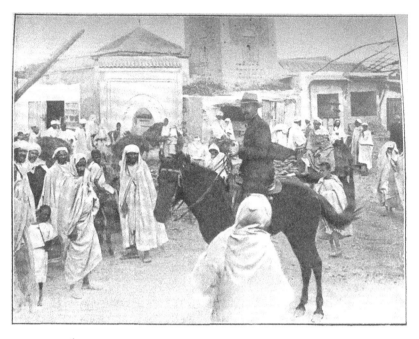

FIGURE 3.3. Émile Mauchamp shortly before his murder. Mauchamp asserted his foreignness and defied Moroccan authority by appearing in French costume on horseback. (Émile Mauchamp, *La Sorcellerie au Maroc* [1911].)

in 1893, a member of the crowd exclaimed, "There is a Christian among you!" Linarès responded to the heckler in Arabic, which affirmed the sultan's official fiction and drew appreciative laughter from the crowd.[110]

But as the Moroccan state weakened and social crisis grew, the symbolic order of Sultan 'Abd al-'Aziz began to unravel. After 1900, the Marrakesh population attacked the sultan's commercial agents, native Jews, forcing them to remove their shoes outside the mellah.[111] The French military mission became less willing to affirm royal authority at court ceremonies. In 1899, artillery expert and commander of the French military mission Burckhardt declined to appear at the *hadiyya* ceremony and refused to follow orders given by his Moroccan superior.[112] Dr. Mauchamp refused to dress in Moroccan clothes or speak Arabic. He declared, "I am here . . . as a French doctor, to make France known and loved; the natives must recognize me as a Frenchman."[113] With his fedora, tailored suits, and French language, the arrogant Mauchamp was a final affront to Moroccan authority.

On March 19, 1907, a crowd of men, women, and children took to the streets and beat Mauchamp to death, looted his house, then attacked the homes of Dr. Assiegeait and the British consular agent Lennox. Hours later, Professor Louis Gentil, his compatriot M. Lassalas, and a Moroccan agent of the French consulate discovered Mauchamp's corpse laid out on the floor of his dispensary. The corpse was not naked, as the soldiers must have found it. Nor was it wrapped in a white shroud, the custom for Muslim burial. Rather, someone had taken exquisite care to dress the corpse in a Moroccan man's white *qamis* and *jallaba*, place a turban on its crushed head, and lay the body on freshly cut grass.[114] Mauchamp lay dressed as a living Moroccan Muslim man.[115] The anonymous authors of this mock funeral used Mauchamp's corpse as a political commentary, to demand a restoration of Moroccan authority over agents foreign and domestic and over the human body itself.

Instead, the Moroccan sultanate collapsed. As sultan, 'Abd al-Hafiz found himself in the untenable position of his brother, forced to uphold the Treaty of Algeciras, reinstate the French *mission militaire*, and contract new foreign loans. He tried to consolidate his power by attacking constitutionalists and the Sufi Muhammad ibn 'Abd al-Kabir al-Kattani, but was assailed by revolt and five pretenders to the throne: his brother Mawlay Muhammad (1908), his brother 'Abd al-Kabir (1909), 'Abd al-Rahman al-Sulayman (1911), Zayn al-'Abadin b. Hasan (1911),[116] and the son of Ma' al-'Aynayn, Ahmad al-Hiba. 'Abd al-Hafiz's own (Shararda) troops turned against him, plotting first to kidnap him, then joining the rebel tribes blockading him inside Fez in 1911.[117]

The besieged man in Fez asked the French for help and signed the Moroccan state over to France on March 30, 1912. The sultan's troops flooded out of their Fez fort (*qasba al-shararda*) on April 17, killing their French instructors and leading the city in rebellion against the treaty.[118] The French army bombarded Fez mosques, crushed the revolt, and disbanded the sultan's army.[119] Sultan 'Abd al-Hafiz abdicated on August 11, 1912, to become a protégé of France. As he embarked on a ship bound for Europe, he broke the royal parasol, signifying the death of the sultanate. As the Moroccan historian Abdallah Laroui has observed: "Thus ended the Hafizian 'revolution,' with the spectacle of a sultan who begged the foreigner to accord him individual protection . . . the symbolic character of the sultanate was almost completely erased."[120]

A COLONIAL REBIRTH: THE SULTAN AS MOROCCAN SOVEREIGNTY EMBODIED

But to rule Morocco, the French needed a native Islamic authority at once useful, centralized, and legitimate, a royal embodiment of *baraka*.[121] Thus the 1912 Treaty of Fez constructed the sultan as a sovereign, so that he could delegate the Moroccan state to France.[122] France would determine "useful reforms" to protect Moroccan territory, finances, and religious institutions, which His Sharifian Majesty was obliged to legitimate as his own edicts (*dahir*). The representative of France, the *résident général*, thus executed French policies as Moroccan royal edicts, the sultan's "will." Despite this elegant fiction, popular revolt continued after Resident General Lyautey appointed Mawlay Yusuf (1912–1927) to be the new sultan. The rebellious city of Marrakesh proclaimed Ahmad al-Hiba sultan on August 18, 1912.[123] France needed legitimacy for Mawlay Yusuf in order to consolidate, subdue, and protect her Moroccan conquest against internal and external challenge.

Under French rule, the sharifian sultan was reborn as a Moroccan sovereign with "two bodies," "a Body natural and a Body politic."[124] Lyautey affirmed Moroccan sovereignty in the sultan's person on May 25, 1912: "I am committed to His Majesty the Sultan, sovereign of this country"; on December 1, 1916, "Not only because we are tied by the treaty of protectorate to the conservation of His sovereign power, but precisely because in the eyes of all Moroccans, [it] is the supreme guarantee of all the rest"; on November 24, 1919, "The principle of protectorate . . . is that Morocco is an autonomous state, of which France has assured the protection, but which remains under the sovereignty of the Sultan"; on December 7, 1919, "I personally renew to Your Majesty the formal assurances from the Government of the Republic to You that the regime of protectorate, guaranteed by treaties, founded on the sovereignty of Your Majesty . . . will assure its material and social development, its security and its strength."[125]

Lyautey devoted himself to restoring the sultan's public body, "his traditional aspect and his integrity (*intégrité*)," "with ancient Moroccan ritual."[126] In a first, carefully staged royal visit to Fez on September 30, 1916, the legal fiction of protectorate was performed for an enormous and silent crowd. Mawlay Yusuf breathed life into the moribund sultanate by receiving *hadiyya* under the royal parasol, leading public prayer at 'Aid al-Adha (feast of the sacrifice), and making a pilgrimage to the Mawlay Idris shrine. Lyautey and his officers performed French submission to Moroccan sovereignty by walking on foot before the sultan's horse. Lyautey deferred to the sultan with elaborate verbal expressions of humility: "Here the source of all authority is with Sidna (Our Lord) . . . Though representing the French government, I am honored to be the first servant of Sidna."[127] In a private letter, Lyautey toasted Mawlay Yusuf as his "greatest success," saying, "The attractive force of a restored sultanate gives all profit to our pacifying effort."[128]

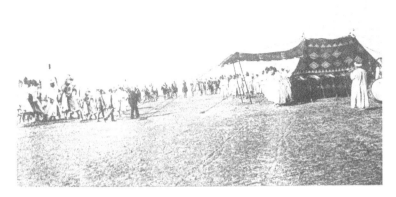

FIGURE 3.4. Sultan Mawlay Yusuf performed a new royal body to which French officers were the obedient hands and feet. (Reveillaud and Bel, *Maroc pittoresque* [1919].)

But Mawlay Yusuf was not a sultan restored, he was a sovereignty re-embodied, intended by Lyautey to "incarnate all of the tradition."[129] In preconquest Morocco, the ʿAlawi sultans invented a public royal ram sacrifice at ʿAid al-Adha to claim a prophetic inheritance, reenacting Abraham's sacrifice and the Prophet Muhammad's sacrifice in 624.[130] The protectorate appropriated, enhanced, and staged such royal celebrations to display the sultan's newly-defined sovereign body.[131] In court ritual, the sultan and French officers performed a royal Moroccan body and *makhzan* state to which French officials enacted the obedient hands and feet. Under French rule, the ʿAlawi monarchy achieved a symbolic power it had never previously enjoyed; the sultanate became the "means by which God could see the collectivity's faith and grant His favor."[132]

Makhzan court ceremonies, like the sultanate itself, were transformed by French rule. In the traditional *hadiyya* ceremony, the tribal leader symbolically submitted to the sultan by petitioning him with gifts: a daughter (alliance), cattle, grain, food (recognition), poetry (thanks), or animal sacrifice (begging the sultan's pardon). The sultan responded with counter-gifts of ceremonial clothes and food for the tribe's leader.[133] When the tribes rejected Mawlay Yusuf as the new sultan, a disastrous 1913 Feast of the Sacrifice celebration made visible his weakness; a "few dozen miserable tribesmen" brought six horses "too pathetic to offer."[134] To rescue the sultan's prestige, Lyautey orchestrated a magnificent 1915 Prophet Muhammad's birthday (*mawlid*), with paid prayer reciters, flag bearers, and thousands of splendidly appointed tribesmen, all coerced to pay homage with gifts bought by the French Résidence.[135] Since the Protectorate had purchased the sultan's counter-gifts, the gift exchange itself disappeared. *Hadiyya* became a public act of submission to the protectorate state and a time for tribes to curry favor with the resident general.

The French quelled rural revolt by courting the saints and Sufi brotherhoods, who responded as in Algeria with revolt, bet-hedging, and accommodation.[136] Because the French viewed the *sharif* of Wazzan as a "prince" with an "independent fiefdom," and since Wazzani *shurafaʾ* were historically mediators between sultans and the tribes, the *sharif* of Wazzan ʿAbd al-Salam was made a French protégé.[137] For Sufi brotherhoods like the (formerly anti-French) Kattaniyya, the protectorate became a shield against the theological attacks of *salafi*-oriented *ʿulamaʾ* like Abu Shuʿayb al-Dukkali. The brotherhoods performed their traditional mediating role on behalf of the new state; at Lyautey's request, ʿAbd al-Hay al-Kattani wrote to the tribes under his influence, the Bani Mtir, Bani Mgild, and Aït Yusi.[138] "I know with certainty," wrote al-Kattani to Lyautey in 1914, "that with France victorious, it is the triumph of science over ignorance . . . the guarantee of Morocco's security against internal and external disorder."[139]

Rumors reveal the social trauma of foreign conquest and the resulting crisis of Moroccan sainthood. In 1913, the Sufi Mahmud ibn Ahmad al-Tijani traveled from Algeria to Fez to collect tribute from his Sufi lodges. On the road, Ghiyata tribesmen glared at the traveling saint: "Everywhere it is repeated that the saint comes from France, that he carries cannons and artillery in his baggage, that the general is hidden in his trunk, that as soon as he arrives in Taza, he will install the cannons in a battery on a high terrace and bombard the villages of the Ghiata, while a column leaving from Moulouya will march on Taza. It is also said that Cherif Tijani did not leave a son and this is a Frenchman, for he wears gloves and an Algerian costume."[140] In fact, the Tijaniyya Sufi order did reach an entente with the French in Algeria,[141] and Europeans did adopt Moroccan disguise for exploration in Morocco: Charles de Foucauld dressed as a Moroccan Jew for his *Reconnaissance au Maroc*, the geologist Louis Gentil passed as a *majnun* to explore the Atlas Mountains, and the marquis de Segonzac posed as the mule driver to a minor sharifian personage in order to conduct five geographic explorations in southern Morocco (1899–1904). However, the rumor reveals how the Ghiyata experienced foreign technologies and saintly opportunists from 1900 to 1912.

The disguised figure evokes "Abu Himara," the messianic pretender and former court functionary Jilali ibn Idris al-Zarhuni, who represented himself to the Ghiyata as a miracle-working saint and the elder brother of the sultan.[142] In 1902–1903, he led a tribal coalition against ʿAbd al-ʿAziz, to which the sultan responded with cannon bombardment in 1903. Abu Himara retreated north of Moulouya and set up his own *makhzan* state. But the Ghiyata turned against Abu Himara when he failed to lead jihad; indeed, he sold mining and railroad rights on their tribal lands to Spanish and French companies to his own profit. Abu Himara was captured and spectacularly executed by Sultan ʿAbd al-Hafiz in 1909.[143]

The Ghiyata rumor describes a contaminated Islamic saint subverted by France. The Sufi saint is a gateway to French invasion, "the general is hidden in the trunk," and the French have stolen the saint's body, "Cherif Tijani did not leave a son, and this is a Frenchman." Sainthood has become a hollow shell, an Islamic vehicle for a power-hungry traitor who arms himself with foreign cannon. A series of messianic saintly tribal revolts against French occupation after 1912 failed: the angels did not ride into battle with Muslims at Bu ʿUthman on September 6, 1912; a cataclysm did not swallow French soldiers at the Kerkour of Tafassasset in 1922; and even General de Loustal could not bear to continue firing into the unarmed body of the *murabit* Sidi al-Wali in 1930. Ross Dunn notes the "unqualified failure" of mahdism and militant Sufism to unite large-scale rural resistance to French rule.[144] The Ghiyata rumors betray a disillusionment with saints—and the death of political sainthood itself.

THE FRENCH CONFRONT *BARAKA*: COLONIZING STRATEGIES AT COCARD HOSPITAL

And not a single person went to [the French hospital] . . . The French said, who is curing the people here? They said in Dar Dmana [House of Guarantee]. A *grande maison*, very old, belonging to the Wazzan. Those Wazzan, the people had *niya* in them. *Niya*. It means, I have *confiance* in you. You, I have *confiance*. If I were sick, and you want to treat me, whatever you give me, I will eat it, and God will bring easiness. When I come to you, I tell you I am sick. At that time, there was the sickness of urine (*marad at-tayr*). Now they call it *le cancer*. At that time, we didn't know *le cancer*. *Le cancer* just now came. We called it *tayr*. *Tayr*, how do we treat it? There were those who treated it just with the urine of children. They make *un petit pansement* like that, they do a little bit like that . . . Over there, the *shurafaʾ* of Wazzan, they are the ones who cured people (*yadawwi an-nas*). Just a little piece of *compress* like that . . . the person folds it up like that, they put a little *pommade* in it, [the child's urine] a month, fifteen days. In that place where there is that hole, which loses pus . . . that closes that thing for him. It doesn't remain.[145]

The *baraka* of healing was more elusive to colonial co-optation, not least because French doctors and sociologists viewed it as humbug.[146] Alfred Bel said with regret, "[Sick natives] take a bit of earth . . . impregnated with urine from this saintly man [al-Wazzani] . . . and carefully fill a wound that the French doctor didn't cure quickly enough."[147] Edmond Doutté derided the *sharif* of Wazzan as an alcoholic hypocrite who married a British governess and consumed aperitifs at Parisian boulevard cafés.[148] Doutté dismissed the *majnun* as simply insane: "The mad, in effect, the idiots, and those who pretend to be insane (because there is reason to believe there are many fakers), are surrounded by popular veneration."[149]

But Dr. Léon Cristiani adapted French medicine to the idioms of saintly healing. Cristiani arrived in Morocco as surgeon-general to the sultan's army and created a new hospital in the *qasba* of the Shararda,[150] the fortress for the native troops who led the bloody 1912 Fez uprising. But Cristiani fearlessly resided in the *qasba* with his wife and children. He saw himself as the "*shaykh* of a *zawiya* of which the sick are the faithful— he must live near them if not among them," and he described medicine as a personal relationship, "the man of the countryside comes to accept one face, one person; he does not want to leave his family to fall into the hands of a stranger."[151] Cristiani personally saw more than a hundred patients daily without the benefit of X-ray, laboratory, or laundry.

Cristiani presented the French hospital to Muslims as a space of healing by reproducing architectural elements from saint shrines. In its green-tiled roof, internal courtyards, and court fountains, Cocard Hospital incorporated design elements from shrines and mosques. Cristiani even had an elaborate artificial "saint's shrine" built into the hospital wall at Cocard, with a fake saintly "grave" and a niche where visitors could light candles. The Cocard Hospital grounds seamlessly incorporated the "second tomb" of Sidi Qasim, *wali* of the Shararda, which provided hospital patients with two Muslim saints to visit.[152]

Other French dispensaries in Fez were also located next to the shrines of popular saints, like "Sidi Bou Jida." Abu Jayyida ibn Ahmad al-Yazghi (d. 978), a Maliki jurist buried at the Bani Musafir portal, was famous for protecting Fez against the invading armies of the Fatimids in 960 and the Umayyad regent (978–1002); women especially visited him to ask for help.[153] The French built a dispensary a few meters from Sidi Bou Jida's shrine to draw *baraka* as well as patients from the saint.[154]

The Muslim patient population at Cocard Hospital reflects the success of Cristiani's strategies. At first (1913–1916), Cocard was a mobile field hospital in the *qasba* and the patient intake registers reflect a military

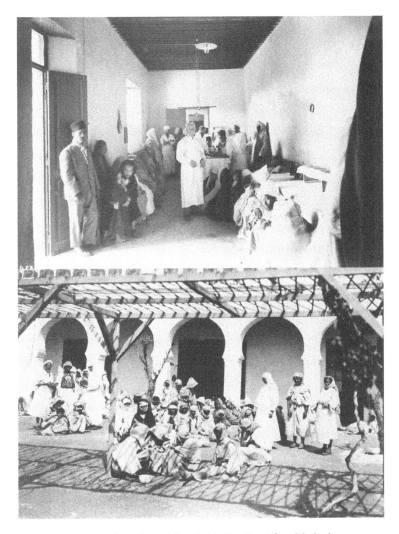

FIGURE 3.5. Scenes from Cocard Hospital in Fez. *Top*: Léon Cristiani, *médecin-chef* of the hospital. *Bottom*: In the courtyard, rural tribespeople await treatment, attended by the nurses, who are Franciscan nuns. (Archives of the Bibliothèque Nationale du Royaume du Maroc.)

clientele: Hayaniyya, Shararda, and Awlad Jama' soldiers with trauma wounds evacuated from the eastern front.[155] In 1916, Cocard saw 1,500 patients per month, fewer than native hospitals in other cities.[156] After 1916, tribes around Fez began to enter the hospital, largely because the large public livestock market on Thursdays (*suq al-khamis*) was held just

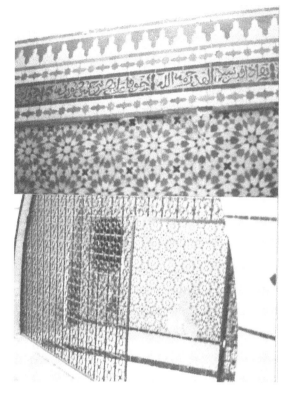

FIGURE 3.6. The "saint grave" built by the French in the wall of Cocard Hospital. This fabricated saint recapitulates the architectural and artistic forms of *wali* shrines. (Author photograph.)

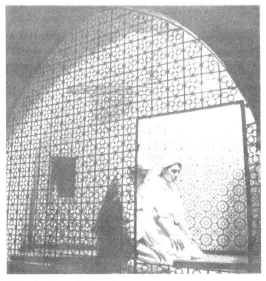

La prière des infirmières à l'hôpital Cocard

FIGURE 3.7. Colonial-era image of the "saint grave" in Cocard Hospital, staged with Moroccan female nurses praying; one is kneeling on the "grave." (Edmond Secret, *Les Sept printemps de Fès* [1990].)

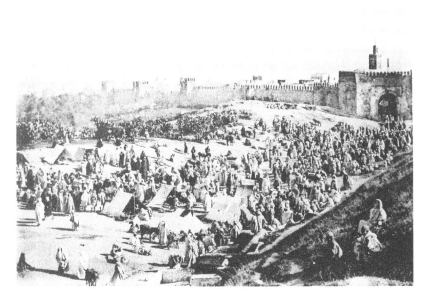

FIGURE 3.8. Thursday *suq* (market) was held outside the *qasba* of the Shararda/ Cocard Hospital in Fez. Patients could shop for cures, first consulting traditional healers under the tents and then entering the hospital for a second treatment. (Reveillaud and Bel, *Maroc pittoresque* [1919].)

outside the hospital walls. Elderly residents of Fez now recall that Fez city inhabitants were the last to accept Cocard Hospital, but they came for treatment because of the personal reputation of Léon Cristiani:

> At that time when the French came, and they opened the hospitals, they opened *spitar* [Hospital] Cocard, not a single person went to it. The people don't come. The people didn't used to go to *spitarat* . . . There are some families, it is among their customs, they don't come out of their houses . . . There was at the head of it Doctor Cristiani. Cristiani was in 1929 or 30 or 40. He used to walk ʿarj, like this [limping]. The people entered the hospital.[157]

> There were those who went to [Cristiani], who live up . . . in the Talaʿ up there, Kabira with Fez Jdid, with what, they call al-Qisba, Bu Julud and the Qasba of an-Nawar . . . If there were people who were poor, from a poor family, and you explain the way to him, he comes to you. He comes with his nurses, with his suitcase in his hand, and he went in to see you. Where is so-and-so, man or woman, he goes in and he sees and he examines.[158]

By 1926, the patient population of Cocard Hospital had expanded ten-fold, to 10,214 consultations in the month of December alone.[159]

Cristiani finally entered the therapeutic universe of Fez, for contemporary oral memory attributes to him a saintly Moroccan wife and nursing staff. A Moroccan physician at the modern ʿUmar Idrisi Hospital told me that Cristiani was married to a Wazzani woman and that her relatives became the hospital nurses.[160] Patients at Funduq al-Yuhudy clinic remember Cristiani as married to a saintly ʿAlawi *sharifa*: "Ah Cristiani! He was very good, a very good man, he cures (*kayadawwy*), he would listen to your chest with only a towel on, and tell you everything, tell you go on in the way of God. He was married to a *sharifa* ʿAlawi, that was his wife. He did it all and without money, for free."[161] In reality, Cristiani's wife was French and the nurses of Cocard Hospital were native soldiers and Franciscan nuns.[162] But Cristiani's strategic adaptation to saintly healing garnered him a measure of acceptance and even saintly authority. Fassis imagined that a saintly *sharifian* family, the Wazzani (saintly head of a Sufi order) or ʿAlawi (the royal dynasty), were curing the people with him at Cocard Hospital.

FRENCH MEDICINE DID NOT PROVOKE a "clash of civilizations" in Morocco, contrary to the claims of the French colonial lobby. An opposition between Islamic society and Western science is a frequent theme in antimodernist Islamic thought, Middle East studies, and colonial studies. The historians Daniel Headrick and Michael Adas have argued that Western technologies—the railroad, guns, the telegraph, quinine—inevitably led to Europe's victory over the non-West.[163] Postcolonial theorists have often assumed that the very introduction of Western science created Foucauldian systems of social control.[164] But from the sixteenth century, Moroccan sultans used Western science to enhance their own power. The sultans captured Europeans in Mediterranean piracy and used them to gain access to new medicine, civil engineering, and military training. By appropriating individuals, the sultans separated scientific knowledge from the institutions that create it and avoided interference by European states.[165] The relative autonomy of Moroccan scientific borrowing changed when Sultan Mawlay Hasan was obliged to accept official governmental military missions after 1877, whose members cemented tribal alliances, mapped cities, and laid the technological infrastructure for a French invasion. French medical knowledge itself was not necessarily anti-Islamic, colonizing, or an instrument of "bio-power."

Medicine in Morocco in 1877–1912 suggests the ambivalent relationship between exact sciences and colonial conquest. French doctors were deployed as agents of reconnaissance, but medical technologies, instruments, and drugs could also be detached and re-assimilated by *atiba'* to their own practices. Vaccination in Morocco shows the limitation of scholarly approaches that essentialize "Islamic" and "Western" medicines, for "Islamic" variolation is both similar to "European" vaccine and its forerunner.[166] Yet European exact sciences did become inextricably linked to European states over the nineteenth century, ultimately facilitating the French conquest of Morocco.

The real death 1907–1913 was of precolonial Moroccan sainthood and the idea of a Muslim community protected by saints against the sultan's authority. The Jazulite idiom of the saint as political leader died a natural death in the failed messianic revolts of Abu Himara and al-Hiba, and in the co-optation of Sufi brotherhoods by the French protectorate. *Salafiyya* became the only viable language of Moroccan political opposition, and the sultan became a new locus of Moroccan sovereignty. The sultan came to embody the sovereignty of Morocco in international treaties and in the protectorate agreement of 1912, a construct that Moroccan nationalists would appropriate to demand reforms in 1934 and independence in 1944.

The disintegration and reintegration of Morocco as a polity was experienced in and through the human body. As the first resident general of France in Morocco, Lyautey used the corporeality of Muslim holidays, court rituals, and the sultan's person to naturalize his state and reconstruct the sultanate. At Cocard Hospital, doctors used the physical forms of saintly healing to introduce French medicine to Muslim populations. Colonial power attempted to write a new political script for Morocco through the body, but the Muslim body remained a place of memory and of potential resistance, to French rule and to the centralized state.

CHAPTER 4

FRÉDÉRIC LE PLAY IN MOROCCO?
THE PARADOXES OF FRENCH HYGIENE
AND COLONIAL ASSOCIATION IN
THE MOROCCAN CITY, 1912–1937

WALKING THE MARKETS OF MOGADOR, the physician Charles Bouveret remarked that "certain bakers whose ovens are located a distance from the place of sale have natives who are dirty and often infected with sickness transport the breads. I saw a Jew with conjunctivitis carrying breads in his arms such that pus from his eyes was spreading across the bread."[1] Haj Masgini, a Muslim member of the Municipal Hygiene Bureau (Bureau Municipal d'Hygiène; BMH) agreed: "[The vendors] put the bread right on the ground, where dust and even mud are spattered on it."[2] Together, Bouveret and native elites regulated food, founded a tuberculosis clinic and a milk dispensary for European, Jewish, and Muslim infants, and funded medical visits for children in Mogador schools.[3] The Muslim carpentry guild master volunteered to vaccinate his own family in public in order to persuade the Muslim residents of Mogador to accept smallpox vaccination. "We will collaborate with you every time," he told Bouveret. "Just call upon us."[4]

The Moroccan colonial city was the site and laboratory of Lyautey's *solidarisme*, his social vision of the French colonial policy of association. Lyautey drew his hygiene policies from republican Paris, where sewers conquered water to eliminate cholera, the boulevards of Baron von Haussmann cleared slums to unify the urban space into a rational civic body, and city hospitals and clinics implemented the rights of the revolutionary "citizen-patient" in state health care and welfare.[5] Colonial humanism was to be an application of Third Republican welfare to the colonies, adapting theories of the engineer, social reformer, and founder of the Société Internationale des Études Pratiques d'Économie Sociale Pierre-Guillaume-Frédéric Le Play (1806–1882) to Africa and Asia. As Le Play argued that social engineering through health, housing, and family policies would integrate the working classes into a harmonious, elite-directed social body,[6] so Resident General Lyautey envisioned a technologically advanced colonized city to integrate the colonized to France by "recognizing natives' rights and serving their interests," respecting their cultures, involving them in decision-making, and improving their lives with hygiene and environmental sanitation for a mutually-beneficial *mise en valeur* of human and natural resources.[7] When Lyautey created the bureaus of municipal hygiene on November 1, 1912, he included Muslim and Jewish native elites as members in order to create an interracial French civic culture, as Bouveret explained: "All these measures, which, in the beginning, offended old habits, obviously excite some animosity from those who believe—almost always wrongly, without doubt—that their interests are injured; but the private interest must always disappear before the general interest. It is an absolute dogma."[8]

But public hygiene did not function in protectorate Morocco as it did in France. The state-of-the-art medical, parasitic, water, and environmental technologies so beneficial in the metropole often exacerbated disease in the empire rather than curing it. The BMH often created social division, provoked resistance, and privileged colonial economic interests at the expense of native health. These outcomes arose from the paradox of French colonial welfare itself, for a state not a republic provided health care to a patient who was not a citizen. The French imperial nation-state produced self-contradictory imperatives as Gary Wilder has argued, and colonial hygiene revealed the disjunctures between social, medical, legal, urban, and state bodies, contradictions that generated disease, nationalism, and eventually tore Greater France apart as an imperial body.[9]

The paradoxes of colonial hygiene can be traced through four diseases: malaria, typhus, bubonic plague, and typhoid. Epidemics in Morocco reveal the contours of the French colonial city in its urban planning, social life, commerce, and politics. Malaria informed the geography of French colonial settlement and the definition of human and physical environments. Typhus lay bare the violence beneath Lyautey's superficial rhetoric of cultural preservation for Islamic cities (*mudun*) and the actual limits of colonial control over native bodies. Plague challenged the technocratic modernity of the new French colonial cities and illustrated the constructedness of white European settlers as a "civilized" and "modern" population. Typhoid revealed the dysfunction of "shared colonial governance," for municipal sewers became a fault line between European and Muslim civic bodies and ultimately gave rise to Moroccan nationalism.

If French colonial hygiene did not always improve Muslim health, it did provide tools for Moroccans to critique French rule and to imagine a new political society. Historians have located the origins of North African nationalisms with Moroccan university students in Paris, modern civil servants, North African workers in France, or graduates of modern military academies. But colonial urban hygiene was an incubator and catalyst for popular nationalist consciousness in Morocco itself. The hygiene that Lyautey intended to win Moroccans to France often provided instead a graphic demonstration of colonial violence and inequity. Public hygiene generated crises and opportunities; Moroccans appropriated French municipal institutions to fight for resources, demand the benefits promised by France in the Treaty of Fez of 1912, and conceive their political rights through the body's health itself. The Moroccan nationalists Muhammad Hasan al-Wazzani and 'Allal al-Fasi did not merely originate in Fez, they were produced by Fez—the politics of the colonized Moroccan city.

THE MANY CONTRADICTIONS OF LYAUTEY'S PROTECTORATE HEALTH SERVICE

Lyautey's oft-repeated dictum "Give me a doctor and I'll give you a battalion" reflects his conviction that modern medicine rendered the use of violence virtually unnecessary; he made doctors the vanguard of his invading armies and responded to the 1912 Fez uprising with new clinics:

> One of the best means to extend our influence in the country is the development of medical assistance, especially in the region of Fez, where we are in almost immediate contact with rebellious tribes and other tribes who have joined our cause recently and whom we can attract through our doctors. It is the reason why I created mobile native infirmaries accompanying all our troops when I arrived in Fez . . . But one must neglect nothing in Fez itself . . . each quarter of the city must have a dispensary and an independent one for the Jewish quarter.[10]

Lyautey's vision was a technologically advanced medical service gentle to Muslim religion and culture, for "the action of the hygienist, rather than being imposed, must constitute a means of pacification."[11] To obtain the latest science, Lyautey recruited the foremost metropolitan specialists as his *conseilleurs techniques*, but he rejected the centralization of French republican medicine, which he called "parliamentarism"—"meetings of the full orchestra for each minor modification."[12] Instead, Lyautey envisioned a lone, Arabic-speaking "doctor of action" who would adapt positive science to native life through constant surveillance of his territory: "What I want is for the entire surface of Morocco to be divided between a number of doctors who are mobile . . . No corner of the country should escape his gaze: I see him not in an office, but in an automobile, in an inquisitorial search for everything related to hygiene. Thus conceived, this institution would be of limitless effectiveness."[13]

But Lyautey's ideas were grander in theory than fact; his decentralized vision did not translate to a workable public health system. The metropole expected Morocco to be self-supporting, and Lyautey's fragmented medicine-on-the-cheap lacked even the ability to collect global epidemiological data. Decentralization, intended to avoid "too many reports, too much accounting, too many hospitals and not enough hygiene and real assistance,"[14] shifted financial responsibility for medicine to the regions;[15] only the Institut Pasteur, Cocard Hospital, and the Pharmacie Centrale received direct support from the Résidence.[16] The *médecins-chefs* in each region—Fez, Meknes, Rabat, Casablanca, Mazagan, and Marrakesh—were obliged to be statisticians, hospital administrators, fund-raisers, and clinicians.[17] Municipalities bore the cost of native and European clinics, which had ballooned from 1.2 million francs in 1914 to 12 million by 1921.[18] The military chief of municipal services (CMS) exercised near-absolute power over city budgets, commerce, land, police, public works, municipal salaries, and city ordinances.[19] The CMS could refuse the doctor even essential funding for personnel, pharmaceuticals, and equipment. After repeated clashes with his CMS, the BMH doctor René Martial of Fez quit in 1923, writing to the Résidence: "If the hygienist is not friends with the CMS, nothing is possible . . . Hygiene must be unified . . . The BMH must become an institution of the state."[20]

Lyautey also failed to define the protectorate's relationship to its "citizen patients." Whereas France provided medical care as a citizens' right, Lyautey used it as a colonizing strategy: "The natives are quickly conquered by the doctor . . . The day when a notable, a *caid*, or any poor suffering devil decides to see the French doctor and leaves cured, the ice is broken."[21] To maximize political effect, Lyautey created numerous rudimentary native clinics over a vast geographic area, a tactic that drew doctors' anger: "'Native Hospitals' are a pompous designation for these dispensaries . . . which lack laboratory, x-ray, laundry, or isolation ward. [The doctor handles] . . . hundreds of typhics, dysenterics, the malarial, the contagious of all sorts, operates on hernias, fractures, cataracts . . . He must be pharmacist, midwife, surgeon . . . even the sixteenth century did not see such an organization!"[22] Torn between republican medicine and Lyautey's policy of association, French doctors developed a health service of apartheid. Each of the three "races" in Morocco—Europeans, Jews, and Muslims—had a segregated hospital tailored to its level of "civilization." Native hospitals were for "Muslim and Jewish Moroccans, Algerian Muslims, Tunisians, natives of AOF and AEF, Arabia, Syria, China and Indochina," and European hospitals for "all peoples who, by their degree of civilization, can be assimilated to the inhabitants of Europe."[23] Lyautey did not provide republican medicine even for Frenchmen, for Europeans had no right to free care, and the protectorate had not planned for women, children, the elderly, or the handicapped. Catholic charities, the wives of the resident generals, and the Red Cross provided European families with tardy and piecemeal social welfare.[24]

Lyautey claimed to preserve Islamic cities in theory but altered the material bases of Islamic social solidarity in fact. Before the French conquest, *hubus*, or Islamic religious endowments, provided for street hygiene, education, water, and aid to the poor.[25] The French introduced city councils, hygiene bureaus, collective city budgets, and a new Ministry of Religious Endowments for *hubus* property. The jurist Louis Milliot was sent from the École de Droit d'Alger to "rationalize" *hubus* property in the city of Fez, where he discovered a web of social interdependence. Intermediate forms of property allowed the poor, single women, the handicapped, the elderly, and Sufis to be housed without payment. One *hubus* building could include several types of property: money ownership (*manfa'*), the right of *gza* (rent), of *galsa* (presence of one's possessions), of *miftah* (right of the key), and of *istikhraj* (residence after restoration).[26] French legal reform created absolute property and facilitated the alienation and sale of *hubus* buildings, which allowed a mass eviction of the poor and the collection of lucrative money rents.[27] The conversion of *hubus* property to private property helped to create what Janet Abu-Lughod has called "caste cities," a process that secularized and commoditized space in the Islamic city. The Muslim body was thus unmoored from sacred geography, detaching city residents from traditional place and modes of Moroccan historical consciousness.

A PICTURESQUE ROTTING MIASMA, ENVIRONMENTAL PLANNING, AND THE ISLAMIC CITY

French literary figures, explorers, diplomats, and tourists exulted in the Fez *madina* as a medieval Oriental fantasy, a "city which jealously guards its millenarian soul," "a last refuge from the [modern] world," a mysterious labyrinth, "a mass of terraces whose contours vanish in the evening vapor like a shroud enfolding the dead."[28] Hygienists saw not romance but raw sewage, flies, animal corpses, and disease: "The streets, made for camels not for carriages, are rock-paved alleys like torrent-beds, which serve mainly for drains, sewers and cesspools: here every kind of festering offal offends eye and nostril, from poultry-feathers and kitchen-slops to corpse of rat and cat—dead baby not being wholly unknown."[29] Lyautey's young urban planner Henri Prost was charged with creating European cities of modern industry beside carefully-preserved Islamic cities. But dark, congested, garbage-infested places were first thought to cause malaria, and the Second Empire French urbanist Georges-Eugène von Haussmann cleared such "miasmas" from Paris with his large, light-filled boulevards. Prost's urban planning for Morocco strategically adapted Haussmann's hygienic principles to separate Europeans from Moroccans, a spatial design that viewed European settlements as islands of health in a sea of disease.

After the discoveries of Alphonse Laveran (1889) and Ronald Ross (1897), Pasteurian hygienists knew that malaria was caused not by garbage but by a parasitic organism carried inside the anopheles mosquito, transferred from sick persons to healthy ones by the insect bite. In 1913, the Résidence called malaria "the most important disease in Morocco requiring prophylaxis"; doctors reasoned that a distance of two kilometers, the mosquito's flight radius, would protect colonists from the human "disease reservoir."[30] French "new" cities (*villes nouvelles*) were thus founded at a distance of two kilometers from Moroccan cities (*mudun*), a space dubbed the "*cordon sanitaire*," or "quarantine line." Malaria was a matter of maps, wrote the French-Algerian Pasteurian Edmond Sargent, and the physician must be both "epidemiologist and cartographer."[31]

Sargent saw Moroccans as a disease environment rather than a patient population; they were "fresh flesh for new anopheles, the malarial germs which they then transport to the European city." Sargent palpitated the spleens of Moroccan children not to treat them, but to measure the endemic infection in the human disease reservoir: "Infected at a young age, never treated, [the child] tolerates the parasite and the infection becomes chronic, causing the spleen to enlarge, sometimes becoming enormous."[32] Moroccans were indeed carriers—the spleen index of tribes south of Marrakesh was 95 percent positive for endemic infection[33]—and Sargent ordered swamps drained, weeds burned, mosquito-infested water covered in petrol, and quinine given to natives "only in the infected areas where there is a European agglomeration to defend, because we defend the French above all."[34]

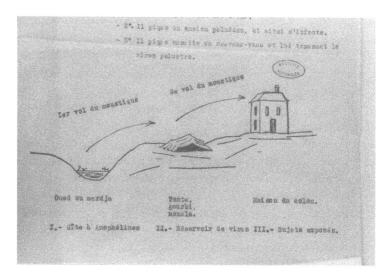

FIGURE 4.1. Spatial mapping of malaria transmission from swamp to native "disease reservoir" to "exposed subject," the colonist. (Archives Nationales de France, Paris.)

Like Sargent's hygiene, Prost's urbanism assumed natives to be an environment, not a public. Prost separated Europeans from natives with the ideal two kilometers in Fez (see Fig. 4.2), but for Rabat, a *cordon sanitaire* could not be created because European entrepreneurs had already built working-class neighborhoods on land adjoining the *madina*. Prost thus "enclosed" the *madina* with boulevards, opening the spatial interval to movement, air, and light.[35] Design was not determined by hygiene alone; the boulevards also displayed the picturesque *madina* walls for touristic consumption. In the city of Fez, the Bu Julud portal was at once visually appealing and useful; it was originally cut into the *madina* wall to open the rebellious Tala'a neighborhood to rapid military intervention but became a symbol of the traditional Fez *madina* (see Fig. 4.3).[36] Hygiene illuminates why a socially-minded modernist and Musée Social member like Prost would plan for the European population to expand in the new *villes nouvelles* but not provide land for the Muslim population to grow in the *mudun*.[37] Prost did not plan for native society because he did not plan for Muslims as a public, even within their own cities. The *madina* was treated as an aesthetic experience for Europeans: "[We] conserve the physiognomy of the *madina* . . . [It] gives such splendid views from our Modern Cities."

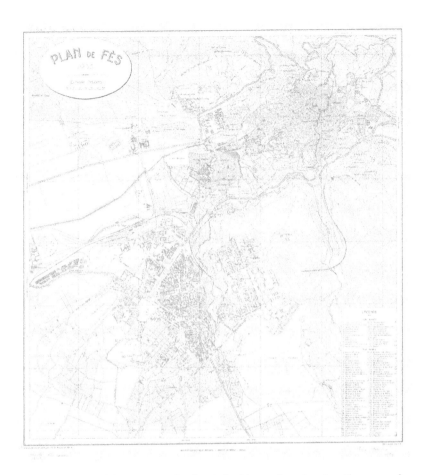

FIGURE 4.2. Map of Fez, an example of malaria-driven urban planning. The areas of native settlement (Fez al-Bali, Fez Jdid, mellah) are separated from the European *ville nouvelle* by the two-kilometer "*cordon sanitaire*." (American Geographical Society Library, University of Wisconsin–Milwaukee Libraries.)

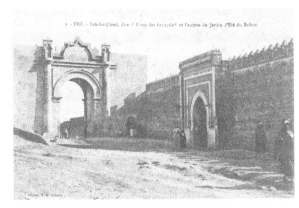

FIGURE 4.3. The Bab Bu Julud portal was at once picturesque and practical, opening the Fez *madina* to rapid French military intervention. (Postcard, author's collection.)

Prost's planning and Sargent's prophylaxis reveal urbanism and hygiene as technocratic systems that must be designed for a public, not universal goods easily transferable to colonial contexts. French doctors protected European cities by circulating through the native countryside with mobile hygiene groups (*groupes sanitaires mobiles*, or GSMs); but with only one doctor for 20,000 people, the GSM's first purpose was to collect morbidity data.[38] The European fortress-city was not a sustainable model, and epidemics would soon oblige hygienists to recognize Moroccans as social beings and negotiate directly with the native body.

THE UNRULY NATIVE BODY: TYPHUS AND
THE LIMITS OF COLONIAL CONTROL

The eradication of typhus in Morocco should have been a triumph of Pasteurian medicine. Charles Nicolle won the Nobel Prize in Medicine (1928) for discovering the transmission of typhus by the louse. The French imported the Clayton apparatus, a boiler/shower system that heated water to 120°C and greatly diminished louse-borne disease in shipping around the world (see Figs. 4.4 and 4.5). But technologies are only as effective as the organization of people, law, and space in which they are applied, and colonial authorities responded to typhus in Morocco with an invasive hygiene police, detention, and the forcible confiscation of dead bodies. Fierce Moroccan resistance to hygiene forced doctors to abandon force in favor of recognition and to grant Moroccans status as political subjects. The diseased, unruly, hidden Moroccan body itself forced authorities to include Moroccans in the "public" of "public hygiene."

In 1912, drought, war, and starvation forced thousands of Moroccan peasants from the southern Sus and Tafilelt regions to the cities of the north. General Deschamps described the Susi Berbers he saw: "The poor things fall to their knees at our passage, begging for alms . . . We have seen several groups dead from starvation, principally children."[39] The Casablanca CMS wrote in 1913: "Dragging their filthy rags in the streets, unable to stand upright, reduced to skeletons, the poor of every age flood Casablanca and propagate morbid germs, which make one fear the explosion of an epidemic."[40] The Résidence worried, "This report does not mention the intervention of the doctor, but one must suppose the local service has not grouped these poor together without submitting them to an indispensable medical examination."[41] To protect themselves, Moroccan municipalities quickly erected "de-lousing stations" outside city limits in 1914–1918, into which police herded "starving natives or those without

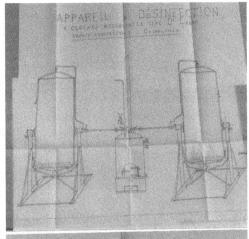

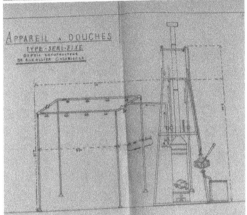

FIGURE 4.4. The Clayton apparatus, boiler and shower system (the latter encased in a tent). (Archives of the Bibliothèque Nationale du Royaume du Maroc.)

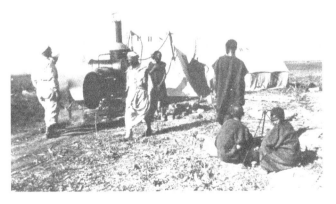

FIGURE 4.5. The Clayton apparatus in the field. ("Rapport annuel du GSM de Fès, 1932," Archives of l'Institut National d'Hygiène, Rabat.)

resources," where they were stripped, showered, rubbed with benzene, and deported to their presumed "country of origin."[42] Procedures in the lazaretto were quite invasive, as one doctor wrote: "It is difficult to maintain even a de-loused population free of parasites . . . investigation by the doctor revealed a perfectly live louse in the vagina of a woman fresh from de-lousing."[43]

With typhus, Lyautey's respect for the Islamic city vanished in a series of *dahirs* from 1915 to 1924 that opened Muslim homes, mosques, shrines, *fanadiq* (caravanserai), and cafés to a search for the louse.[44] Infected natives were forcibly interned in lazarettos, whereas Europeans were informed of "the pressing interest to shower and disinfect one's clothes."[45] The *dahir* of December 8, 1915, authorized the police to condemn and bulldoze native housing; an entire *"village nègre"* was razed in Settat in 1929, and the 1,200–1,500 inhabitants were obliged to construct new housing for themselves without compensation.[46] Dr. Fournial of Marrakesh wrote of the *madina*: "The city-dweller at the bottom of his twisting alleyways is difficult to access and the sick hidden in impenetrable regions are impossible to number."[47] The *funduq* (singular of *fanadiq*), as a lodging-house for Muslim travelers, was regularly raided, "These establishments where numerous natives coming from different points of the territory stay can become dangerous foyers of infection."[48] In Marrakesh, the BMH burned the Moorish cafés of Jma' al-Fna' square and replaced them with tents—"easier to sterilize."[49] Hygienists asked the Résidence to install delousing showers inside the shrines of Mawlay Idris in Fez, Ben 'Isa in Meknes, and Sidi Ben 'Ashir in Salé, to sanitize crowds of visiting pilgrims.[50]

Not surprisingly, Moroccans hid their sick and dead from the municipal hygiene authorities. *Funduq* owners hid infected guests, families hid their relatives, and employers hid their employees.[51] In 1925–1926 in Marrakesh, an infected Muslim prostitute and four children hid from quarantine in a saint shrine of the cemetery, and Jews of the mellah smuggled infected persons from house to house to escape detection by the police: "Everything is done to elude the team that has come to seize the patient. He is passed from room to room, from house to house until coma renders dissimulation impossible. But at that moment it is too late, the dying man has spread contagion all around him, and nine families have been infected."[52] Dr. Braun of Casablanca organized a service of four doctors to examine corpses at 9 a.m. and 4 p.m. each day—a policy "especially indispensable for natives, which will allow us to know the causes of mortality and avoid epidemics"—but Muslims buried their dead clandestinely.[53]

A 1918 Résidence circular required a BMH permit for burials and stationed police at the gates of Muslim cemeteries to catch "illegal" corpses.
A city order of 1923 required *muqaddimin* of city quarters to report epidemic disease, but the Rabat BMH doctor complained: "Of the 65 cases
of typhus in Rabat none were signaled by the *muqaddems* . . . Typhus
gains and develops in the urban centers, because we lack information and
the native chiefs do not follow orders."[54]

Moroccan resistance prevented the collection of accurate morbidity
data: doctors did not know who was sick, where, and with what. A general report for Morocco in 1925 admitted: "Death statistics for natives
. . . have no scientific accuracy." Many cities had no death statistics at
all for Muslims in the period 1912–1925[55] or else statistics derived solely
from Muslim deaths at the hospital: "No hypothesis can be established
for cause of death of natives; of 2600 deaths we only know [those who
died in hospital]."[56] The Marrakesh BMH doctor remarked dryly, "The
1921 report claims that the natives have 12.5% mortality, slightly more
than Norway and less than England . . . The result alone shows that it is
totally inaccurate."[57]

To overcome resistance, French hygiene authorities increased the use
of force. After rural mobile hygiene units detected typhus among Zam-
mur tribes near Rabat, raids were conducted "day and night."[58] Police arrested natives entering at the city gates and escorted them to the lazaretto
for delousing, in Meknes, 10,082 in March 1926 alone.[59] In Marrakesh,
armed troops surrounded Jma' al-Fna' square at midnight and vaccinated
10,000 people at gunpoint.[60] But force was not enough for a medical system to work, and a Salé administrator warned:

> This measure, stopping poor and dirty people as they arrive to the city
> and taking them to the de-lousing station, is bringing the city to the verge
> of revolt. The natives recruited as hygiene agents at the city gates con-
> stantly commit errors, thus oil sellers, charcoal sellers, workers from the
> port, the railroad, employees of the pasha, and Zemmouri tribesmen who
> have come to buy sugar are taken to the station with no explanation . . .
> I cannot be responsible for the consequences . . . the quarantine must be
> stopped immediately.[61]

The Rabat BMH physician agreed, "The medical defense of a city against
typhus is not a *uniquely medical problem*. It is above all a question of *information and authority*."[62]

To obtain information and authority, hygiene authorities were obliged to grant Moroccans a greater voice in municipal decision-making. Dr. Fournial of Marrakesh planned to raid the mellah to catch Jewish beggars seeking alms on Shabbat, but a thousand beggars disappeared: "All the houses opened . . . [and] the entire population . . . gave them asylum."[63] After three months of the epidemic, Fournial met with Jewish community elders to explain typhus transmission and request cooperation. Jews brought their sick to the hospital, created a Jewish Charity Bureau, and requested school showers, a new public market, and new housing.[64] Necessity forced French authorities to bring Muslim and Jewish elites into city government, where they gained a new voice in city politics and used the French colonial state to advocate for their communities.

FRACTURED WELFARE, NATIVE BOURGEOIS, AND THE MUSLIM CHARITY SOCIETY

Traditionally, Muslim Moroccans cared for the poor at mosques and saints' shrines, but massive rural in-migration overwhelmed the shrines and flooded the streets. In 1905, wealthy Fez notables paid for two *funduq* and fed more than 4,000 people per day.[65] In 1914 in Rabat, "native poor sleeping in the street are brought to two *habous* buildings of the El Had portal, visited by the doctor and given hot bread."[66] In Casablanca, ten Muslim notables created three shelters and local housewives brought old blankets, hot food, and tea, but twenty-five to thirty people still died each day.[67] The 'Alawi sultans distributed wheat to urban residents in times of famine, and the French had provided food during the famines of 1914 and 1921.[68] But rather than create state mechanisms for the Muslim poor, the protectorate pressured Muslim bourgeois elites to create private charity societies on a European model to care for the Muslim poor. The Rabat notables of 1914[69] became the Muslim Charity Society of Rabat by 1927,[70] and the Protectorate "pushed a Native Charity Society to constitute itself" in Casablanca[71] and Meknes.[72]

Hubus had been decentralized and fragmented; individual donors endowed *hubus* for specific goals like cleaning the streets, housing widows, teaching the blind, or maintaining public baths, mosques, shrines, flour mills, and *maristans* (hospitals).[73] By contrast, the charity societies centralized and coordinated all *hubus* revenues using the city tax apparatus. A *dahir* of April 12, 1913, constituted the Fez Muslim Charitable Society and funded it with revenues from *hubus*, a voluntary tax on halal meat, and private donations.[74] Charity societies often centered around a saint shrine; the Charity Society of Sidi Ben 'Ashir in Salé received 13,000 francs from *hubus*, 12,000 francs from the municipality, and 5,000 francs from the Direction of Civilian Affairs in 1922.[75] By 1931, Casablanca, Meknes, Oujda, Rabat, Salé, Fez, Marrakesh, Taroudant, and Sefrou had Muslim Charity Societies[76] that supported low-cost housing, medical care, Qur'anic schools, girls' embroidery schools, orphanages, and *hubus* buildings converted to medical dispensaries.[77] Native Jewish charity societies (*hebrot*) were already well-organized and provided food, work, and burial services for poor Jews.[78]

Muslim Charity Societies became instruments of a new Moroccan bourgeois elite and nationalist organizing. Moroccan elites used the charity societies to promote private interests—protection of their workers, promotion of the family's local business, and personal reputation—but the protectorate foresaw political uses. In 1934, the societies were offered funding if the French regional military authority could sit on the board and the CMS could act as treasurer.[79] In December 1937, the resident general tried to outlaw Muslim public charity collections in order "to avoid protests which tend to develop in the Moroccan milieu and which present a political character,"[80] but the nationalist Ahmad al-Manjira openly used the societies to support nationalist schools of the "Carnet Vert" like that of Ahmad ibn Haj Saddiq al-Marrakashi.[81] Thus, the Résidence did not integrate the Muslim elite into a composite Franco-Moroccan social body. Instead, colonial welfare generated the Muslim charity society, an entity outside the protectorate state, which Moroccan elites used to organize and reconceptualize Islamic social solidarity itself.

FLIES AND SHANTYTOWNS, NATIVE LABOR, AND THE COLONIAL HYGIENIST

Flies land on raw meats exposed all day to the sun, wrote Dr. Bouveret, thus native butcher shops needed awnings, washed metal carts, and zinc-covered countertops.[82] He attributed "numerous cases of ambient dysentery and typhoid" to spoiled fish and to soup vendors, who "exercise their commerce without authorization in foul places with disgusting materials."[83] In 1925, Bouveret presented a municipal circular requiring all persons exercising the profession of baker, butcher, *charcutier*, fishmonger, or pastry chef obtain a license from the BMH physician in order to practice their professions.[84] Now the BMH would decide which artisans could practice, what shops could open, how food was to be prepared, and the conditions of sale, contrary to Lyautey's explicit instructions not to interfere in native food and drink.[85] Bouveret's hygiene standards increased costs for native guilds of food production; shops that could not make the expensive improvements were forced to close.[86] In Meknes, the BMH had to approve goat-herders and cheese-makers; the ambulant fish-sellers of Rabat were expelled entirely.

Food in Morocco illustrates an essential difference between metropolitan and colonial *solidarisme*—the integration of labor to the state. In France, Louis-René Villermé's study of the working classes led Le Playist reformers and Third Republican elites to provide low-cost housing and state support for workers; civil authorities mitigated the authoritarian tendencies of hygiene in French cities.[87] But in Morocco, hygiene authorities enjoyed a free hand and ignored the Résidence's social concerns. In a 1924 report, the sociologist Louis Massignon warned that a politically dangerous Muslim laboring class would emerge if Moroccan guilds continued to weaken: "If the corporations diminish . . . it is the entire social life of cities which is threatened . . . Instead of artisans, there will be only day laborers without cohesion or family stability, ready for all kinds of disorders."[88] The protectorate tried to preserve native guilds with a Sous-Commision d'Artisanat, Artisan Councils, an Office of Indigenous Arts, and Prosper Ricard's Department of Fine Arts and Historic Monuments.[89] But municipal laws of 1914–1918 and urban hygiene regulations contributed to the erosion of the economic viability of Moroccan guilds.[90]

Hygiene regulation further penalized Moroccan artisans by privileging their local European competitors in traditional industries: brick making, tanning, soap making, iron forging, carpet weaving, cement making, rag selling, and food processing. Pierre Sorbier de Pougnadoresse, secretary-general of the protectorate, warned that the *dahir* about industry of August 25, 1914, should not be applied to native crafts;[91] but by 1925, most cities had zoned native *fanadiq*, tanneries, and potteries to industrial quarters outside the cities.[92] The BMH doctor in Rabat complained that impenetrable smoke from the pottery ovens impeded pedestrians from walking in the Bab Zaers quarter,[93] and Bouveret declared the native tannery in Mogador "foul, stinking, and nauseating."[94] The spatial separation of the stages of production was a burden for native artisans, who depended on *suqs* (city markets) for both raw materials and the sale of finished goods. Leather dressers, dyers, slipper makers, bag makers, bookbinders, scabbard makers, and saddle makers suffered from the expulsion of Mogador's leather market in 1926.[95] The BMH in several cities expelled the Moroccan trade in rags, bones, and horns, but allowed Europeans to pursue the same trade inside the city.[96] European factories were often given a virtual carte blanche to pollute in native residential quarters, despite the vigorous complaints of native residents.[97]

Indeed, colonial hygienists demonstrated a remarkable failure to recognize Moroccans as labor at all. When rural Muslim migrants flooded the

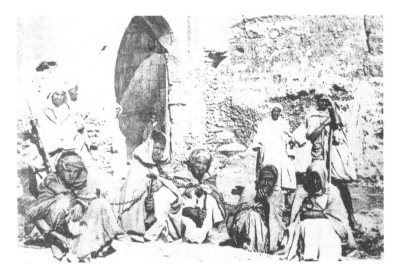

FIGURE 4.6. Moroccan prisoners breaking rocks to pave a road. (Reveillaud and Bel, *Maroc pittoresque* [1919].)

northern cities and erected makeshift shantytowns,[98] doctors declared the new arrivals "a public danger, an incubator for flies, and the place from which all the parasites, fleas and lice originate that infest the city."[99] In Rabat in 1923, the BMH doctor wanted the shantytowns Jabli and Ak-kari destroyed: "These are unemployed men whose wives and mistresses pollute the city with prostitution . . . a population of about 2000 [lives] in a state of disgusting filth . . . each hut has, in addition to numerous sick persons, animals of all kinds."[100] In 1922 Mazagan, the doctor wanted the straw huts burned, "the vehicle of all epidemics." In reality, these rural migrants were the workers of new European industries; Moroccan intermediaries (*"caporaux"*) hired the new arrivals from workers' markets, *muqqaf* (literally, "place of standing").[101] The BMH doctor in Marrakesh noted: "In Djma al-Fna square . . . poor day-laborers sleep and eat in the Moorish cafés of the square. They go every morning to Moqef where employers come to recruit them."[102] Yet the BMH razed shantytowns and deported their rural residents, ironically deporting the colonial labor of new French industry back to the Moroccan countryside.

The protectorate also missed the opportunity to recruit native civil servants to support the French empire. Native prisoners were the first protectorate municipal workers, considered both free and expendable, and they built roads, dredged sewers, burned garbage, caught rats, sprayed DDT, and cleaned markets in a chain gang (see Fig. 4.6).[103] Unemployed Moroccan artisans were also put to work on public works in order to prevent labor unrest.[104] And the new city administrations opened public service to populations previously excluded—Jews and Berbers—and created new jobs such as hygiene inspector and night-soil pit emptier.[105] For the first time in Moroccan history, a Moroccan Jew, David Attar, became a *makhzani* (policeman) in Fez. He later served as a meat inspector in Jewish slaughterhouses for the municipal veterinarian.[106] His family was potentially integrated into the protectorate state, for his widow collected a governmental pension from the municipality after his death, rather than an allowance from the Jewish charitable society (*hebrot*).[107]

CIVILIZING THE MODERN CITY:
BUBONIC PLAGUE AND WHITE WELFARE IN RABAT

In 1912, Lyautey moved the capital of Morocco from Fez to coastal Rabat—the seat of the French Résidence, the jewel of Henri Prost, where graceful Franco-Mauresque civic buildings displayed French dominion in impressive architectural forms.[108] Évariste Lévi-Provençal pronounced Rabat "a masterpiece, famed throughout the world, of successful town planning and architecture."[109] But in 1914, a French colonial wife described her Rabat neighborhood in less impressive terms: "Half-Moorish homes of an idiotic style, yellowing laundry limp on clotheslines, roving dogs, dirty white children, large stupid roads that lead nowhere, piles of garbage, soaking rains, typhus, flies, malaria, dysentery . . . lamentable agglomerations of wood and corrugated metal . . . Garbage collects in all the corners and gives off a pestilential odor."[110] Photographs of Rabat in 1912–1920 reveal the vast gulf between an ideal modern Rabat of architectural plans and the actual Rabat lived by European residents: wooden shacks, vacant lots, garbage, stagnant water, and unfinished construction.

"Imported civilization" creates a special insalubrity in Rabat, wrote the BMH physician Pean: "There is a constant parade of men, animals and vehicles . . . the dust . . . covers our country with a cloud purple or gold by turns, a cloud containing all microbes."[111] Europeans dumped chamber pots into the street, adding to the "dusts of Rabat," the dried fecal matter of "men and animals, whites and Negroes, colonists with dysentery and Frenchmen with typhoid fever, Algerians, Malagaches, Congolese . . . All those who lived in the colonies have a rendezvous in Morocco."[112] Lice, fleas, mosquitoes, and rats nested in the wooden shacks of the *ville nouvelle* and feasted upon garbage piled at homes and on the coast, for Rabat dumped its waste into the Atlantic Ocean, from which it floated back to shore. In 1938, the Rabat BMH physician regretted, "European cities, contrary to what one would think given their recent construction, now have these festering slums (*îlots insalubres*) like our old cities in France."[113]

"Modern" Rabat consequently suffered the most medieval of diseases: bubonic plague. Plague swept the city in 1912, 1915, 1916, 1917, and 1929; Dr. Perrogon marveled, "Rabat, city of gardens, is the only city of the empire unable to rid itself of the plague."[114] Stranger still, plague seemed to afflict only Europeans: "Not a single case was found in the native city, though it has ancient sewers which house a multitude of rats."[115] The victims were primarily Spanish workers[116] who lived in wooden shacks in the new quarters of Rabat: Catalan, Petite Sicile, Océan, and Oukassa:[117] "In the house, there is an old grandfather sleeping on a camp bed, using old trousers as a pillow, and the interior of his shack is full of garbage and chicken debris . . . the old man, who lived in deplorable hygiene, was contaminated 8 days after the [plague vaccination] . . . He died from the malady."[118] Janet Abu-Lughod has argued that the Rabat *ville nouvelle* was a modern city of technology, whereas Muslims were confined to a neglected, crumbling Arab *madina*.[119] But the bubonic plague betrays the dark underbelly of "French modern" and the imperial imperative to invent the European population as a human edifice. To build a modern *ville nouvelle*, the protectorate needed to remake its residents as a civilized white population, one morphologically and culturally distinct from Moroccan natives.

"The population of Rabat, especially the European population, is composed of low-class Spaniards and Italians who are totally ignorant of hygiene," wrote the Rabat CMS in 1917.[120] Rabat expanded rapidly from 700 European residents in 1912 to 7,000 in 1916 and to 16,628 in 1926;[121] in 1919, the European population numbered 4,549 Frenchmen, 1,817 Spaniards, 1,269 Italians, 126 Anglo-Maltese, and 218 others.[122] Contrary to the urban separation planned by Prost, Spaniards often lived in Muslim *fanadiq* in the *madina*, sometimes ten persons to a single room: "These people have no furniture and sleep on straw pallets, thus we are reduced, in a place too infested with fleas, to . . . throwing out the renter, putting his wash on the Clayton, and burning the mattresses."[123] The BMH condemned several such buildings, such as number 25 rue Driba: "Inhabited by Europeans . . . House in very bad condition, rooms of habitation in ruins, W.C. nonexistent. A hole dug in the middle of the courtyard serves this purpose."[124] In the *villes nouvelles*, European companies like the Société des Constructions Mixtes in Rabat rented shacks to Spanish workers at exorbitant prices: "[The plague victim] was found in an agglomeration inhabited by 100 persons with thirteen horses, chickens, pi-

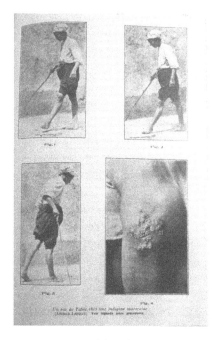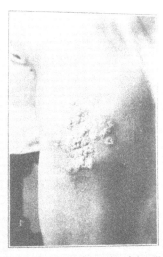

FIGURE 4.7. Spanish and Muslim bodies are blurred in the pages of the French medical journal *Maroc médical*, which reused a single photograph to represent a native Moroccan woman with "civilized" neurological syphilis (*left*), and, in a different article, a Spanish woman with leprosy (*right*). (*Maroc médical*.)

geons, etc. . . . no glass windows, earthen floor, unspeakable W-C with bedpans left to spread materials on the ground and drinking wells."[125] Although Rabat passed a series of laws to demolish wooden shacks and kill rats, the bubonic plague persisted in Rabat.[126] Doctors blamed Spanish habits, especially cohabitation with domestic animals:[127] "These Spanish families . . . live in incredible conditions of filth one cannot imagine. An Arab, no matter how miserable he is, lives more cleanly."[128]

Spaniards brought plague to the white city, doctors reasoned, because they transgressed the civilizational divide between Europeans and natives. Several French observers referred to Spaniards as "half-Moorish," and Remlinger of the Institut Pasteur diagnosed a Spaniard with "Arab syphilis" because he was "brown-skinned, of Andalusian descent . . . Arabic-speaking, and traveled with Arabs."[129] The Service de Santé et d'Hygiène Publique (SHP) considered Muslim and Spanish bodies so similar that the French medical journal in Morocco, *Maroc médical*, reused a single photo of a woman's body to "show" a Spanish woman with leprosy and a Muslim woman with syphilis (see Fig. 4.7). Like Muslims, Spaniards avoided vaccination and their doctors concealed cases of infectious disease from French authorities.[130] Spaniards and Muslims also fraternized in municipal work and housing.[131] Plague had previously been a disease of the Muslim countryside—in 1911–1912, plague killed 14,000 people in the Dukkala—but Spaniards were accused of introducing the disease to the city: "[They are] in close contact with the indigenous population . . . and without family hygiene."[132] To eradicate plague in Rabat, doctors proposed to separate, educate, and "civilize" the Spanish.

The champion of the white family was the wife of Resident General Lyautey, a Red Cross nurse and widow who arrived in Morocco with French troops in the 1907 Casablanca invasion and married Lyautey in 1910.[133] As Mme. Lyautey, she brought a deep commitment to European infant and maternal health; between 1913 and 1914, infant mortality for European babies in Casablanca was 75 percent,[134] affecting more babies of southern European than French origin.[135] Mme. Lyautey opened a *"goutte de lait"* (milk dispensary) for European mothers in Rabat in 1913 and added a maternity hospital in 1914; she also sponsored crèches, maternities, orphanages, tuberculosis dispensaries, and "sun gardens" (*jardins de soleil*) for anemic children across Morocco.[136] To provide nurses and funds, she introduced the Association des Dames Françaises (part of the French Red Cross), the Union des Femmes de France, and the Société de Secours aux Blessés Militaires to Morocco.[137] She coordinated Catholic charity and municipal funds to raise 300,000 francs and open tuberculosis clinics in Fez and Casablanca.[138] The protectorate contributed funds to these charities—1,481,750 francs in 1929—but until World War II, family medicine remained the province of private, mostly Catholic charities.[139]

Mme. Lyautey collaborated with French doctors to reform the European child, a "weak, anemic . . . delicate organism eminently receptive to diverse infections, tuberculosis in particular."[140] In a 1922 textbook, doctors Charles Bouveret and Pierre Vallery-Radot instructed European schoolgirls in the science of cultivating children, *puériculture*.[141] *Puériculture* was a pillar of French metropolitan eugenics after 1871, when French social Catholics, nationalists, and republicans rallied around the need to cultivate healthy babies in order to prevent population decline and provide France with soldiers against a fertile, expanding, militaristic Germany.[142] White women in the colonies were expected to provide a healthy procreation for the metropole: "France has the right to count on the vital energy of her colonies; it is our duty, in the prolific countries like Morocco, to render infant mortality as low as possible."[143]

In Morocco, colonial *puériculture* focused on separating whites from natives with "civilized" motherhood. The Moroccan heat was believed to exhaust the white mother and dry up her milk supply, but Bouveret and Vallery-Radot warned against using Muslims as wet-nurses: "Remember, engrave it profoundly in your memory, that most native women are syphilitic, and thus eminently dangerous."[144] White infants were to drink sterilized milk from the *goutte de laït* to prevent "infectious cholera-like gastro-enteritis." *Puériculture* disciplined mother and infant; the civilized mother nursed on a regimented schedule, unlike the lazy Moroccan. She brought her baby to the doctor, whereas the native mother was negligent and her infant died of infection.[145] As in France,[146] doctors visited white schools; on Avenue Foch in Rabat, the inspector found the students to be dirty, anemic, and myopic, lunching on a thin soup prepared from three kilograms of meat for 104 children. European fathers founded a Ligue Marocaine d'Hygiène Scolaire on October 14, 1921,[147] and Rabat instituted a social worker liaison to visit European homes in 1927.[148] But in the metropole, family welfare programs were generously funded; mothers enjoyed state family allowances, free hospital birth (1892), a health plan for the indigent poor (1893), and four weeks of paid maternity leave before and after birth (1913).[149] French *puériculture* in Morocco was an unfunded mandate administered by private charity rather than public welfare from a centralized state.

Protectorate welfare developed tardily as a response to white labor organization. In 1916, the chief of administrative services declared welfare a local matter rather than the duty of the Résidence, and a circular of October 16, 1923, created Municipal Assistance Boards to hear white appeals for support.[150] But European functionaries—teachers, postal workers, and customs agents—formed labor associations to demand social services. The Association générale des fonctionnaires du Protectorat was created on May 10, 1919, and the Union amicable des travailleurs du livre de Casablanca was created on July 10, 1919.[151] When Lyautey eliminated free health benefits for state functionaries in June of 1922, Europeans complained in the socialist newspaper *La Vigie Marocaine*: "Public assistance is not organized in Morocco, where social problems seem to have little interested the public authority . . . At the same time, poverty is developing in this country with terrifying rapidity, as the Charity Societies of Casablanca demonstrate. . . . In the current state of [metropolitan] French legislation, one has the right to assistance from the state, department or commune . . . [Lyautey's administration] shows a spirit unfamiliar with social questions or a formal will not to create social institutions."[152] Europeans in Morocco imported French trade unionism: Moroccan teachers affiliated themselves with the Confédération Générale du Travail (CGT) and the Ligue des Droits de l'Homme et du Citoyen in 1922; branches of the Section Française de l'Internationale Ouvrière (SFIO) were founded in Casablanca, Marrakesh, Meknes, Fez, Oujda, and Safi; and a Syndical Union of Morocco was created on June 22, 1930.[153]

To counter white labor unions, the protectorate created a Central Assistance Board in 1929. Non-French Europeans had created private ethnic mutual aid societies—the Société Générale d'Union et de Mutualité des Corses au Maroc, the Centre Espagnol, and the Communauté Grecque[154]—but by 1930, the ethnic societies had disappeared.[155] As the following letter from a Spanish boy in Rabat shows, non-French Europeans appealed directly to the protectorate for social assistance: "I am the oldest of a family of eight children—most very young—and the few days of work my father, one of my brothers and myself can do provide us just enough to live. Work is our only resource; and you will understand all my good will to pay this hospitalization cost, [however] need and debts on my family force me to ask you, M. le Chef de Service, to exonerate me from this tax of 144 francs . . . signed, Eulogio Henche."[156]

But colonial welfare even for whites was *bienfaisance* (charity), rather than *assistance* (welfare), a right of the French republican citizen. In the late nineteenth century, western European countries developed national visions for their citizenries through state welfare, but the self-contradictory goals of French colonial welfare in protectorate Morocco fractured the population by race. Native Jews received aid from traditional Jewish *hebrot* societies, the French Alliance Israélite Universelle, and the Oeuvre de Secours aux Enfants (OSE).[157] The Muslim poor were aided by Muslim charity societies. Race welfare produced a divided politics; the Alliance Israélite Universelle and Zionist charities prepared the ideological ground for the massive Moroccan Jewish emigration to Israel, Canada, and France after 1945, and Muslim Charity Societies became instruments of *Istiqlal* nationalist organization and action.[158]

NOT A DROP TO DRINK: COLONIAL SEWERS AND THE RACIALIZATION OF TYPHOID

From the fourteenth century, the imperial cities of Morocco enjoyed sophisticated water systems; accounts of Fez describe water in public baths (*hammamat*), sewers, and the fountains in streets, mosques, schools (*madrasat*), shrines, Sufi lodges (*zawiyat*), and prisons. The River Fez was canalized in a complex network of *rettara*, or water canals,[159] to irrigate private gardens, provide water in homes, and power the waterwheels of more than three hundred flour mills.[160] A corporation of sewer-cleaners (*qwadisiyya*) maintained the subterranean canals that were lined with ceramic tiles to protect clean supplies and carry away waste.[161] City residents could draw water from public fountains or buy from traditional water-sellers, who sold copper cupfuls from goatskin bags. In the early twentieth century, the city of Fez had an abundant 3,000 liters (792 gallons) of water per second per city resident, compared to only 150 liters (40 gallons) per second for contemporary Philadelphia, London, or Paris.[162]

Since the city's fountains, baths, sewers, and toilets were *hubus*, the city administrator of *hubus* was charged with their maintenance. The sultans expanded the water systems; in the late nineteenth century, Sultan Mawlay Hasan had the French renegade 'Abd ar-Rahman design a canalization of River Fez to supply the quarter of Fez Jdid.[163] To settle an 1884 water dispute, the sultan convened the sewer-cleaners guild, *hubus* officials, three millers, and Qarawiyyin scholars of the "jurisprudence of water."[164] The *makhzan* also cleaned the city streets by opening dams at the river's head, a spectacle that impressed European visitors in 1877:

> When the filth, piles of garbage and animal corpses accumulate in the streets to the point that they threaten to block traffic, [the *makhzan*] opens the gates at the top of Fez Jdid which hold back the waters of the river and lets it flow through the city. It descends, crashing, and carries with it all the garbage, often also live animals, furniture, merchandise, etc. because it's usually in the middle of the day, at the moment of greatest commercial activity when they do it, and of course, without telling anyone. Passers-by, merchants, and customers see the water coming and get out of the way as best they can, but it must be said that it doesn't appear to disturb them especially.[165]

Imperial cities had traditional water systems, Tangier and Mogador had European-designed water systems, and even a small town like Settat had a public water supply.[166]

By contrast, the French protectorate did not plan adequate water systems for its new European cities. In the French *villes* of Rabat and Casablanca, most homes had night-soil pits and outhouses in 1916, and the Hotel de la Résidence in Meknes and the Restaurant du Palmarium in Rabat "relied on water brought by Arab water-carriers and pumped into reservoirs."[167] The shallow pits that Europeans dug as toilets in the Rouamezine quarter of Meknes polluted the subterranean water table, contaminating drinking wells with fecal matter in 1923.[168] As a consequence, Spanish, Portuguese, and Italian workers suffered higher levels of typhoid than did natives.[169] In a Mazagan report of 1925, the European workers' quarter reported a high level of typhoid, though city water supplies tested clean for the bacillus.[170] Doctors conjectured that Moroccans must enjoy a congenital immunity to typhoid infection, but a Safi doctor realized that the difference lay in water access: "The old medina has a network of sewers and benefits from the first street fountains . . . By contrast, the Trabsini, a new [European] quarter with rectilinear streets at least 6 meters wide, has provided 26 deaths by gastro-enteritis of a total of 52 deaths for the quarter, or 50%. This is because Trabsini does not yet have sewers or water."[171]

Before the French occupation, most water was *hubus* property, but a *dahir* of July 1, 1914, designated *hubus* as "public property," and French authorities used the law to divert water from Moroccan cities to new European *villes*.[172] In Casablanca, the River Mallah was canalized in 1914 to provide European quarters with 16,000–18,000 cubic meters (4.23 million to 4.75 million gallons) of water a day.[173] New water supplies allowed the Casablanca *ville* to progress from chamber pots to home night-soil pits to a *tout à l'égout* (sewer) system. In Rabat, the 'Ain Reboula was diverted (1913–1923) to give the *ville nouvelle* 2,500 cubic meters (660,000 gallons) of water.[174] In Meknes, the fresh 'Ain Tegma spring produced 2,500–3,000 cubic meters (660,000–792,000 gallons) of water for the *ville* in 1923; the *madina* was left with the polluted River Bu Fakran, which the CMS judged "too expensive" to clean.[175]

In new sewer systems, Moroccans were required (and often unable) to pay for sewer hookup and the repair of ancient systems. The dilapidated open sewers of the Jewish mellah in Rabat exposed fecal matter to the air, and the BMH doctor worried about a potential future epidemic. In 1916, the BMH replaced the mellah sewers with covered cement canalizations, an 80,000-franc project that Jews were required to finance with loans and a tax of 25 francs per meter of sewer. Jewish residents were also required to pay to redirect mellah sewage from the Bu Ragrag River into the new collector sewer.[176] The building of new sewers was focused in European areas; in 1925–1926, thirty kilometers of new sewers were built in European Rabat, compared with thirteen kilometers in the *madina*.[177] Modern sewers were not extended to the Meknes *madina* as of 1934, but the CMS told Muslim residents that they could execute the works themselves at a cost of 152,110 francs.[178]

Clean water became a commodity too expensive for poor Moroccans. The Muslim Ben Slama Street in Rabat refused to pay the sewer tax in

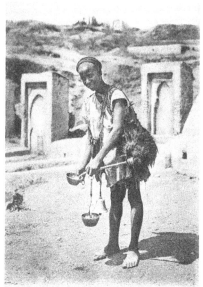

7038   *MAROC. - Scènes et Types. - Marchand d Eau. - LL.*

FIGURE 4.8. Postcard of a Muslim water-seller, posed for tourist consumption in a cemetery. (Postcard, author's collection.)

1924, and its residents lost access to water altogether.[179] The new native industrial quarter in Rabat constructed by Muhammad Rifai al-Kostali in the *ville* had no fountains or sewers because the Muslim homeowners could not afford them.[180] In 1938, the BMH physician in Rabat regretted that French water management had caused clean water to become a "luxury item" for natives: "How can we conceive a better bodily hygiene [for our protégés] when water is so parsimoniously distributed to public fountains or canalized to homes at prices which prohibit usage?"[181]

As the European water systems improved, Europeans became healthier and Moroccans sicker. By 1924, typhoid among Europeans in Casablanca had been reduced by 50 percent and in Mazagan by 66 percent.[182] By contrast, poor Moroccans drank from home cisterns and public toilets and often irrigated their vegetable gardens with sewage water. Native gastrointestinal disease began to rise: Mogador reported 100 typhoid cases among natives in 1926, and the BMH doctor in Kenitra observed that dysentery struck only the native market and town.[183] The Meknes BMH doctor wrote of the *madina* water source, the River Bu Fakran, "very soiled bacteriologically, the waters pass through canals of lamentable decay . . . Typhoid reigns all year long."[184] Typhoid among Europeans in Meknes decreased from thirty-seven cases in 1922 to twenty-one in 1923 because Europeans left the *madina*, "escap[ing] the harmful effects of . . . Bou-Fekrane," but ambient dysentery among Muslims increased from 450 cases in 1929, to 570 in 1932, to 4,173 in 1935.[185] French authorities attributed native typhoid to Muslim habits, especially traditional water carriers (see Fig. 4.8), who "soil the water with their feet . . . BMH agents have observed these native porters filling their bags from the animal watering trough and distributing the water to the inhabitants of the Kabibat neighborhood."[186]

The stabilization of modern water systems in Morocco is a story yet to be written, one of water towers, reservoirs, pumps, and dams. Still, the initial introduction of sewers did not decrease native waterborne illness. In European and American cities of the nineteenth century, bourgeois elites and hygienists were reluctant to undertake expensive reforms to benefit the poor, but as Charles Rosenberg and Richard Evans have shown, waterborne urban epidemics ultimately forced hygiene reform and

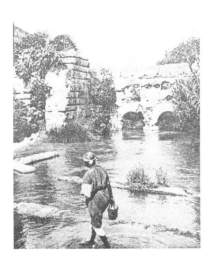

FIGURE 4.9. An example of pre-protectorate Moroccan water engineering of the River Fez, west branch. After passing through the sultan's palace and moving the turbines of the royal armory (*al makina*), the waterwheel (*above left*) raises the river water to an aqueduct that serves the palatine city of Fez Jdid. (Reveillaud and Bel, *Maroc pittoresque* [1919].)

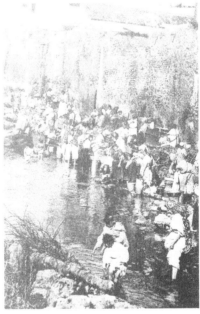

FIGURE 4.10. Public waterways were the source of drinking water for the poor in Moroccan cities. Here Jewish women in Sefrou wash laundry in the River Aggai (Reveillaud and Bel, *Maroc pittoresque* [1919].)

the public provision of clean water.[187] By contrast, in Morocco, the colonial separation of races into two cities—*madina* and *ville nouvelle*—impeded the unification of a municipal sewer system and made waterborne illness a disease category tied to race.

DON'T MESS WITH FEZ: A CITY, ITS WATER, AND THE MOROCCAN NATIONAL MOVEMENT

On August 3, 1929, Lieutenant Huot, an officer of native affairs in Fez, received three students whom he judged "a future problem . . . tending to nationalism or even Communism," but he listened to the request of Muhammad Hasan al-Wazzani, 'Allal al-Fasi, and Muhammad al-Fasi for a *baccalauréat* degree for Moroccan students, because they came with Muhammad Ben Jallul, president of the Indigenous Chamber of Commerce, member of the Fez city council (*majlis*), and, in Huot's words, "a traditionalist of quality who orients himself to progress but understands that evolution of young Moroccans must be prudent and measured."[188] Local politics in Fez brought wealthy elites like Ben Jallul to support young Fez nationalists; they first came together to fight for water access and health care for Muslim families, then expanded their collaboration to a national struggle. We consider hygiene and nationalism, the city of Fez and her famous sons.

To pacify Fez after 1912, Lyautey created the Fez *majlis* of seven appointed and eight elected Muslim members, and a Jewish section of six elected and three appointed members.[189] These wealthy merchant elites were hand-selected by the French to collaborate in a Franco-Moroccan governing elite. As General Gourand wrote in 1912: "The municipal assembly is an element of contact between us and the population, the notables are elements of order and progress. We must count on their influence and popularity to avoid the return of the events in Fez of April." Still, he worried: "We could be very bothered the day one of its members, trying to create difficulties for us, turns to the text [of the *majlis*] and asks us to apply it."[190] Among the 1912 *majlis* members were Haj Tahar ben al-Amin, the owner of a house in London, Haj Hadi Ghallab, who traded in French Algeria, and the British protégé (and translator for the British consulate) Hamza Tahiri; none of these men had ever previously served the state.[191] But hygiene struggles and *majlis* participation transformed merchants into civic leaders. In 1930, *majlis* president Muhammad Lahlou used his protégé status to blast the French: "Let us place naked poor persons on the path of the Spanish High Commissioner, so he can see how the French treat the [Muslim] poor."[192]

Hygiene led Ahmad ibn ʿAbd al-Wahhab Tazi and his brother Muhammad from private life to *majlis* participation. In 1919, the European Maroc-Metropole Company sought to install a *usine d'équarrissage* (knacker's yard) on *hubus* lands of the *madina*, with a second facility for drying animal blood and hides. Ahmad Tazi, who was the *hubus* administrator and a resident of the quarter, protested its foundation "on behalf of the inhabitants of Keddan quarter," but he agreed to entrust the municipality with "the defense of their interests."[193] In operation, the factory's nauseating stench was intolerable, but the chief of municipal services dismissed multiple complaints as the "psychological problems of a few individuals," and "not a political issue."[194] In response, Tazi invited the BMH doctor René Martial to evaluate the factory and report his findings to the *majlis* in its January 1923 meeting, after which nineteen *majlis* members addressed a petition directly to Resident General Lyautey:

> The foul smells from this factory penetrate the mosques and houses in our quarters, which include several thousand inhabitants. These smells prevent people from walking in the streets of the quarters and spoil the meat destined for the consumption of the entire city of Fez, because our slaughterhouse is across from this factory. The Muslim religion declares the odors of cadavers impure. The physician of the BMH has visited the place several times and declares the current location of the factory contrary to public hygiene.[195]

After Lyautey demanded an inquiry, the factory was closed. This experience politicized Ahmad's brother Muhammad Tazi, who became the *majlis* delegate for his neighborhood (the ʿAdwa district), and Muhammad later served as pasha of Fez in 1932. Ahmad was elected to his brother's former *majlis* seat in 1927, which he held until 1944.

The struggle for water led these bourgeois Fez *majlis* members to nationalist politics. The River Fez traditionally supplied the *madina* with water and hydraulic power. In 1914, the Résidence granted a monopoly over electrical energy to the European Compagnie Fasi d'Électricité[196] and reserved use of the waterfalls at the river's tributaries Wad Hamiya, Wad Bukhareb, and Wad Shrasher for its turbines.[197] In 1915, the municipality ceded water from ʿAin Shqaff, a subterranean feeder stream of the River Fez: 2,500 cubic meters (660,000 gallons) to French military camps and

12,500 cubic meters (3.3 million gallons) to the *ville nouvelle*.[198] Consequently, water levels in the *madina* dropped and some sewers dried up in
1915; water levels were dangerously low in 1920, 1923, 1924, and 1925.[199]
Thirty-seven notables on behalf of "Your Subjects of Fez" petitioned the
sultan for redress, claiming the river as the private property of Fez inhabitants —a people's ownership granted by Idris II and validated by fourteenth-century histories, royal *dahir*, and Islamic legal precedent.[200]

But the River Fez had been so weakened by 1929 that it could no longer meet the electricity needs of both European and native Fez, a result
of ever-increasing demand and water diversion to colonial agriculture.[201]
The director of public works proposed redirecting all water from the river
to the CFE (electric company) turbines at night. After their vigorous protests were ignored, the Fez *majlis* collected 50 francs from each Muslim
household to pay a 20,000-franc retainer for a French lawyer; members
organized protests at mosques, and they sent a letter of complaint directly
to the president of France.[202] Ahmad Tazi and the merchant Muhammad
Marnissi organized a petition that garnered 500 signatures, including that
of the future nationalist 'Allal al-Fasi.[203] To diffuse popular unrest, the
French invited Moroccans to participate in a committee charged with defining the authorized uses of the River Fez.[204] But popular Muslim anger
grew in the summer of 1932 as water trickled by at 0.53 meters (1.7 feet)
per second at Tawila bridge[205] and nightly water stoppages directed the
river to CFE hydroelectric turbines.[206] Tahar Diouri, the owner of two
public baths in the Shrabliyyin quarter, wrote an angry newspaper exposé
evoking disease, Islam, and civic rights:

> Beware typhoid, beware dysentery, beware malaria, beware fires! . . .
> On the pretext that it supplies the Compagnie Fassie d'Électricité . . . the
> northern slope of the madina is deprived of drinking water and public
> baths and mosques are forced to close their doors, for the Muslim religion
> cannot be celebrated without water for ablutions . . . The inhabitants of
> the city have only stagnant, dirty water to drink, excellent carriers of ty-
> phoid and dysentery . . . For pity's sake, a drink, a drink.[207]

Water disputes introduced future nationalists to local social problems and to the plight of the Muslim poor. In 1923, Ahmad Tazi's young
brother 'Abd al-Qadir wrote a letter to General Decherf after learning
that a CFE employee refused *madina* residents access to water and beat
the mosque *mu'addin* who intervened on their behalf: "From what quarter, my General, comes this tyranny? Is this evidence of correctness and

humanity?" He added, "Be assured that we alone are the people of this country . . . and that you are only with us as guests charged with a civilizing mission."[208] After ʿAbd al-Qadir was exiled to Rabat as a subversive, his fellow students ʿAllal al-Fasi and Muhammad Hasan al-Wazzani formed a secret nationalist society.

Opposition to the *Dahir Berbère* of May 16, 1930, brought nationalists and *majlis* members together in a 1930 delegation to the sultan and in the Comité d'Action Marocaine (Kutlat al-ʿAmal al-Watani), which presented its *Plan de réformes marocaines* (1934) to the French minister of foreign affairs, Pierre Laval, in Paris, Sultan Muhammad V, and Resident General Henri Ponsot.[209] The *Plan* did not reject the protectorate but demanded its true and faithful implementation. Its authors noted that the "apprenticeship in democracy in its political, social and economic domains" promised by France was in reality a regime of "two weights and two measures," where Frenchmen enjoyed superior schools, hospitals, and political liberties at the financial expense of a legally inferior Moroccan majority.[210] The *Plan* proposed to realize Lyautey's colonial Le Playist vision for Morocco by "prevent[ing] the proletarianization of the [native] working masses and help[ing] those who know misery in all its forms," for "hunger and injustice are the worst enemies of social peace and entente between peoples."[211] The *Plan*'s "true" protectorate was an expanded universal welfare state of new hospitals and medical clinics open to all, in which the assistance reserved for European children would be extended to Muslim families.[212]

Although the *Plan* focuses on the elite concerns of its bourgeois authors, it alludes to a yet-undefined notion of social justice. Morocco suffers a "profound political, social and economic malaise" whose remedy requires the state provision of food, medicine, and welfare for Moroccans, though the *Plan* has no explicit political rationale for a welfare state and no definition of Moroccan social rights. At any event, the *Plan* was rejected in 1934 and the Comité d'Action Marocaine was outlawed by vizierial decree on March 18, 1937.[213]

But water led urban crowds to define Moroccan social rights for themselves and to assert their sovereignty as political subjects. When an *arrêté viziriel* of April 12, 1937, proposed to divert water from the Meknes *madina* to European farms, two thousand Muslim notables representing "the entire population of Meknes" addressed petitions to the sultan and the resident general. To the sultan: "Your subjects of the city of Meknes" ask for water, "the base of our life and our sacred religious acts . . . We take refuge in Your Majesty."[214] To France: "[We] call upon the justice of our protecting government," the "love of equity and the defense of Humanity valued by the free children of France," "an attentive ear to the cry of tens of thousands of men who suffer in their spiritual and material life."[215] The nationalist al-Wazzani framed the water dispute as a national question in his newspaper *L'Action du peuple*: "We and all the Moroccan population stand with Meknes to defend its fundamental rights over the waters of Bou Fakran."[216]

On September 1, 1937, marching crowds in Meknes cried, "Water or death!" "Not a drop for the *colons!*" Five men were arrested: Muhammad Barrada, Driss Manumi, Ahmad ibn Shaqrun, Muhammad Ben Azzou, and Madani Slawi. The next day, a crowd marched under the banner "We want the liberty of our brothers and our water" and soldiers of the Foreign Legion opened fire, killing eleven demonstrators and wounding sixty.[217] After nationalists detailed the events in the press and called for a response to the "night of Bou Fekrane," popular riots erupted in Casablanca, Fez, Rabat, Oujda, Marrakesh, and Meknes from October 25 to October 27. French troops occupied the Fez *madina*, and the Résidence arrested and exiled the nationalist leadership—'Allal al-Fasi, Muhammad al-Wazzani, Muhammad Lyazidi, and Ahmad Makwar. Nationalists framed local hygiene as a national issue, and water shortages mobilized the Moroccan public behind a nationalist platform.

DISEASE AND NATIONALISM, AN URBAN CONCLUSION

The radical socialist *député*, minister of colonies, and former governor-general Albert Sarraut drew his 1921 interwar vision of Greater France as a colonial welfare state from the purported successes of Lyautey's Morocco.[218] But Lyautey's colonial public health service was a structure of contradictions that produced mixed results. Rather than salubrious cities of Franco-Moroccan governance, Moroccans experienced racial apartheid, unequal water access, invasive police, higher morbidity than Europeans, and a divided welfare. Third Republican *solidarisme* proved impossible to re-create in the colonial context, for hygienists viewed Moroccans as an environment, a separate race, and a health hazard, but not as a sovereign people. Welfare fractured the population by race and created three different polities—French, Jewish, and Muslim. The protectorate's medical system also complicated the practice of medicine itself for French doctors, who often battled colonial industrial interests and the military in order to protect native health. The decentralization and fragmentation of the medical service prevented doctors from collecting epidemiological data, compiling population statistics, and formulating effective global medical policies. Despite these difficulties, French sanitation, DDT, and water management did greatly reduce environmental-factor epidemics like typhoid, dysentery, cholera, typhus, plague, and malaria over the *longue-durée*.

The promises and failures of French hygiene produced not Franco-Muslim *solidarisme* but nationalist politics and a new *civisme* in Muslim Moroccan cities. Moroccan bourgeois elites became urban civic leaders and learned to deploy multiple identities. Muhammad Gassus, for example, was a member of the Fez BMH, a *majlis* representative, the uncle of 'Allal al-Fasi, and the namesake of a *salafi* "free school." As Moroccan workers learned trade unionism from the SFIO and joined *Istiqlal* "Muslim unions," so Moroccan city dwellers learned a language of civics, nation, and social rights from water stoppages, disease, and quarantine experienced in the city itself.[219] Finally, the people's needs brought the legitimacy of protectorate itself into question. As Muslim elites searched for redress and variously petitioned the sultan, the resident general, and the president of France, the paradox of protectorate became visible. Who governed Morocco, and in whose name?

The Moroccan nationalist *Plan de réformes marocaines* of 1934 has been viewed as the work of French-educated university students who used French and Islamic modernist ideas, but its authors formulated the *Plan* largely through local experiences with colonial governance in the cities of Morocco.[220] The young nationalists seized upon the municipal council as the democratic form for Morocco[221] and demanded elected councils at every level of government, including a national *majlis* of Moroccan Muslims and Jews[222] with an expanded franchise.[223] The Tetouan newspaper *Al Hayat* viewed municipal councils as "a first step to a parliamentary regime" and a national constitution, a guarantee of "the political and civic rights of citizens and [a] limit [to] the power of authorities."[224] And Moroccan modernity, according to the *Plan*, was a state-directed, centralized system of public health and welfare.

HAREM MEDICINE AND THE SLEEPING CHILD: LAW, TRADITIONAL PHARMACOLOGY, AND THE GENDER OF MEDICAL AUTHORITY

IN 1921, THE EDITORS OF the premier journal of French medicine in Morocco, *Maroc médical*, complained to their readers that the Muslim Moroccan matron undermined the French doctor: "[She is] known to be hostile to us and to put pressure on the patient to turn from our orders to her own remedies—leg of frog or earth from the cemetery."[1] To discover her secrets, the doctors commissioned the wife of a French colonial officer, Aline Reveillaud de Lens, to observe her Muslim female neighbors in the harems of Meknes and report on their medical practices. First appearing as a series of eleven articles in *Maroc médical* from 1922 to 1923, de Lens's work was published collectively as *Pratiques des harems marocains: Sorcellerie, médecine, beauté* (1925):

> In a new pot, boil water, oil, bits of bird, carrot seed, lavender, cumin, Marrakesh poppy and a piece of chameleon. Filter with a wool rag. Have the child drink it until he vomits, then rub his body with the residue in the rag. The matron cauterizes his arm, his fist and his head with a piece of rue wood and covers him until he sweats. The next day, the mother urinates in her hand and spreads the liquid saying, "I reject sickness!" She also urinates into a glass and says, "I have found the remedy!" She adds cumin, leaves the urine overnight, and feeds it to the infant for three days.[2]

The Muslim woman worried French doctors, not only because of such iatrogenic practices, but also because she exercised superior authority to diagnose sickness, administer remedies, and select healers for the family. To gain access to secluded Muslim women and to enter this female medical world, protectorate doctors were obliged to engage French women to act as medical intermediaries. Mme. de Lens's study reveals the gendered nature of medical knowledge in Morocco and the place of women at the intersections of colonialism, medicine, law, and subjectivity.

French doctors also criticized native women's healing because they sought to inscribe the Muslim body into law. Modern governmentality builds its power on the body,[3] and nineteenth-century France licensed one medicine in order to extend state power over individual bodies, homes, marriages, and intimate family life.[4] As Jacques Donzelot has argued, metropolitan France made the "transition from a government of families to a government through the family" by training mothers as its "state-approved nurses."[5] But such mechanisms were useless in protectorate Morocco, where the colonial state was officially forbidden from interfering in the Muslim family, traditional healing, or Islamic law. Worse, native women enjoyed superior medical authority in childbirth, family pharmacology, and *médecine légale* (legal expertise about states of pregnancy, injury, birth, and death), areas in which the French doctor claimed expertise. French doctors resented Muslim women, whom they saw as medical rivals, sorceresses, and the principal obstacles to opening Muslim homes to French civilization.

Gender exposes the messiness of medicine as applied colonial practice; we do not find colonizer versus colonized, but French male doctors resenting their female colleagues, Muslim men fighting their wives in Islamic courts, and French women using Muslim gender seclusion to build colonial careers. Moroccan traditional medicine was itself gendered, for Muslim women mediated between several scientific systems: the Greco-Islamic tradition, "spiritual" saintly healing, and "Prophetic medicine," the popular medical genre codified by Islamic jurists. The introduction of foreign colonial doctors brought French and Muslim gender systems into open conflict as French doctors sought to push Muslim women out of medicine and confine them to private homes ruled by patriarchal authority. Despite its claims to universality, French Pasteurian medicine was a field of gender struggle, with multiple nodes of power and authority.

THE *QABLA*, THE ʿ*ARIFA*, THE ʿ*ADALA*: WOMEN'S MEDICAL AUTHORITY IN MOROCCO

Historically, women "knowers" (ʿ*arifat*) were official medical authorities in the sultans' courts and administrations. The sultans appointed ʿ*arifat* to manage the female insane asylums and the women's prisons (*Dar al ʿArifat*).[6] In the royal harems, the court ʿ*arifa* delivered the sultan's children and provided women of the harem with medical care.[7] A sixteenth-century manuscript describes the duties of Bint Ibn Lajjo, *'arifa* to the ladies of the harem of the Saʿadiyyan dynasty: "[She] showed the domestic personnel how to cook and prepare food, what must be the hours of meals and the services of which it is composed. She taught the women of the harem how to dress, perfume themselves, and have mattresses of silk and cushions and cloaks ornamented with embroidery."[8] Dr. Linarès first entered the Moroccan harem at the request of Sultan Mawlay Hasan's *'arifa*, to treat the ladies and children for heat prostration. Her authority transcended the gender boundaries of the harem, for when the eunuchs unsheathed their swords, she cried, "Are you mad? This isn't a man—it's a doctor!"[9]

Women were the only legitimate Muslim legal voices in gynecology, childbirth, and female health. North African Maliki Islamic law courts accepted testimony regarding the state of women's bodies only from female witnesses, or *'adalat*.[10] In nineteenth-century Morocco, women testified in legal cases of "polygamy, marriage, buying female slaves, 'milk parenthood' [relationships formed by nursing] . . . and the conditions of legal divorce."[11] In Berber customary law courts (*'urf*), women were also considered the only acceptable medical experts in female health.[12] The fourteenth-century sociologist Ibn Khaldun devoted a chapter of his *Muqaddima* to the midwife and her "art of birth," a science "indispensable to society":

> The art of birth . . . is exercised almost exclusively by women, because the law permits them to look at natural parts of the persons of their sex. The woman who does this operation is called the *qabla*, a term which indicates that she receives the child the mother gives her . . . The midwife helps by palpitating the mother's back and the fleshy parts behind, across, and below the womb. In this way she seconds the efforts of the mother to push the child out . . . When the child is out he is still attached to the womb by a cord which ends at his navel . . . The midwife cuts it so that nothing is superfluous and neither the intestines of the newborn nor the mother's womb are harmed, then she closes the wound with cautery or other method she judges appropriate. As the bones of the child are still soft and flexible . . . and as the child can become deformed by passing through the narrow opening, the midwife massages and straightens his limbs so they take their natural form . . . Then she palpitates the mother gently to remove the membranes that enveloped the child and which sometimes are slow to exit. One must prevent the muscles from constricting before the body is free of the membranes, for if they remain, they will putrefy and communicate an infection to [the mother] that results in death . . . [The midwife] rubs the body of the infant with oil and astringent pow-

ders to remove the humidity left by the womb . . . The midwife also cures the abrasions of the vagina caused by the efforts of the child . . . Midwives are best at treating such problems and the illnesses of nursing infants, better than doctors. For a nursing infant's body is only a "potential body"; he becomes an "actual body" only after his weaning.[13]

In the Moroccan family, women were midwives, pharmacists, and medical diagnosticians. "*Qabla*" translates literally as "she who receives," and midwifery was an action women provided for one another rather than a formal profession. Fez residents remember *qabla* as a fluid identity: "In those days one woman neighbor used to come and be *qabla* for the other";[14] "If there is a woman pregnant and giving birth there is a *qabla* she can come, but if she is not there, then one neighbor can be *qabla* for the other . . . and they do it without money."[15] One midwife delivered all the women in a family, sometimes several generations of the same family, but few midwives could earn a living from midwifery and often engaged in other work like *tayyaba* (she who heats water in the public baths), *kiyyasa* (she who scrubs customers in the public bath), and embroiderer of slippers. A male nurse at the modern 'Umar Idrisi Hospital recalled his own mother's midwife:

They didn't let anyone in the house except for the *qabla* . . . midwife of the family. We had for us the *tayyaba* of the *hammam*. A girlfriend of my mother, when we saw that she was in labor, we went to her house and knocked on the door at night . . . she was living in the *quartier*. You're living here, and he's living there, whenever you need her, you go knock on her door.[16]

Another man remembered:

At midnight or at one in the morning . . . we tell her the house of so-and-so, they need you. She goes to their house, she wears her *jallaba*, and the slippers, and she does the ablutions of prayer. And she comes to deliver, maybe a day, maybe two days, maybe three days. She is lodged, fed, drinking, sleeping, until it is solved with them.[17]

Women from conservative families sometimes gave birth alone with no midwife.[18] A Fez resident remembered that his mother held onto a wooden post until she gave birth to a baby girl, and then she cut the umbilical cord herself with a sharpened reed.[19]

Though Moroccan society recognized the *qabla*'s expertise, *qabla* was not a profession. All Moroccan laborers, from butchers to prostitutes, were organized into corporations. By contrast, *qablat* had no guilds, no contracts, no fixed fees and often bought food and supplies for poor families, as one *qabla* in Fez explained: "Look, now . . . for him that gives, God give him good fortune. And for him that doesn't give, I don't ask him for anything. Or he that doesn't have money, I buy things for him, and I bring it to him. And I do it for God, and my Lord helps me."[20] *Qablat* had no formal medical training, unlike *atiba'* (physicians) and barber-surgeons, who received a certificate (*ijaza*) from a master. Who, then, was the *qabla*? She was a true popular healer, a woman who developed a reputation for birth practice and mastered herbal, physical, and magical remedies for mother and baby. Midwifery was an oral corpus of knowledge passed between generations of women.

"Midwife" was also a religious and family identity; children called their midwives *mima* (grandma), and the family invited the midwife to the child's naming ceremony, his graduation from Qur'anic school, and his wedding.[21] Many *qablat* described delivering babies as a religious obligation. After delivering a thousand babies, Fez midwives had a party called *'urs al-hajja*, or "wedding of the lady pilgrim to Mecca." Descendants of the Prophet Muhammad (*sharifat*) such as My Khaddouj of the Fez Jdid neighborhood delivered several children, for her lineage brought blessing to ease childbirth. She described one instance: "I asked her, what is wrong Aziza, she said, I won't give birth. And I am carrying many worries. And I don't have anyone . . . I told her, give me your hand. In the morning the girl came out, and she gave birth . . . Oh my Lord, Oh my Lord. That *stwa* [power, wisdom], God gave to me."[22] A known *qabla* was called upon to wash the dead, a function usually reserved for the caretaker (*muqaddim*) of a Sufi shrine. Acting as *qabla* gave a woman a social identity, created a relationship to the children she delivered, and imparted Islamic religious authority.

Moroccan women's "midwifery" thus encompassed different types of authority: legal authority in women's health (the *'adala*), state functionary (the *'arifa*), midwife (the *qabla*), diagnostician, pharmacist, and family healer. However, women's medicine was not professionalized; midwife was a fluid role of familial and religious authority.

WOMAN AS MEDICAL MEDIATOR: GALENIC MEDICINE, PHARMACOLOGY, AND SPIRITUAL HEALING

In 1920, the inspector general of the Protectorate Health Service (SHP) lamented that Moroccan medicine had degenerated to women's superstition and magic, a far cry from the grand science of the Islamic golden age.[23] However, Moroccan women did not preserve an illogical medicine opposed to a rational male "Greco-Islamic" physicians' tradition. The seeming heterodoxy of women's practices—hot foods for cold sickness, fumigations with incense, saintly visitations—arose from the mediating function of women's healing. Women negotiated the intersection of systems of medical knowledge and were the social vehicles of an "Islamic scientific paradigm" in family health. Women applied remedies from the classical Islamic physicians, popular medical advice books ("Medicine of the Prophet"), tenders of the shrines of the *awliya*', and apothecaries (popularly called '*ashab* or '*attar*).[24] Women's practice in Morocco was thus true popular medicine. To recover the elements of women's practice, we use interviews with elderly residents of the Funduq al-Yuhudy and Lamtiyyin neighborhoods in Fez, in combination with colonial-era ethnographies from Marrakesh (1926), Casablanca (1951), and Meknes (1925).

OBSTETRICS AND EMBRYOLOGY
IN ARABIC MEDICINE: AL-QURTUBI

In the literate scientific tradition, Islamic physicians (*atiba*') used Galenic physiology to describe conception, gestation, embryology, birth, and child development. The Andalusian physician 'Arib ibn Sa'id al-Katib al-Qurtubi (d. 980) authored an early Arabic medical treatise on obstetrics and embryology, the *Kitab khalq al-janin wa-tadbir al-habala wa al-Mawludin* (Book of the Formation of the Fetus and the Treatment of Pregnant Women and Newborns).[25] Ibn Sina (Avicenna, 980–1037) developed gynecology and embryology in his *Al-Qanun fi at-tibb*.[26] Abu al-Qasim Halaf ibn al-Abbas az-Zahrawi (Albucasis, c. 936–c. 1013) created the first speculum and a diamond-tipped probe to perform lithotrities on women.[27] The Spanish/Moroccan Ibn al-Khatib (1313–1374) authored *Risala fi takwin al-janib* (Epistle on the Formation of the Fetus), and the Basra scientist 'Abd al-Malik ibn Qurayb al-Asma'i (d. 828) wrote about embryology in *Kitab khalq al-insan* (Book of the Creation of Man).[28] Al-Qurtubi's text is among the most comprehensive—fifteen chapters variously treating the sperm, the penis, the uterus, conception, pregnancy, prenatal care, birth, midwifery, breastfeeding, newborns, and children's diet.

In al-Qurtubi's text, conception is a matter of Hippocratic and Galenic theory, hot and cold, wet and dry, food and "powers."[29] In al-Qurtubi's physiology, men are hotter than women, and women have more blood; problems arise from corrupted blood and excesses of temperature and humidity. A man is impotent because he is insufficiently hot and needs hot

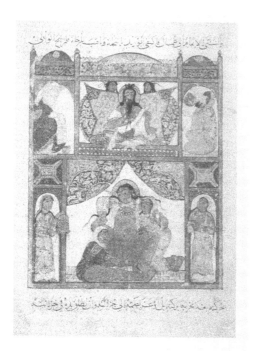

FIGURE 5.1. Illustration of gender segregation in birth. A midwife and women attend the mother on the first floor; the father and physicians are on the second floor, consulting an astrolabe to determine the baby's temperament. (Al-Hariri, *Maqamat*, Baghdad, 1237. Bibliothèque Nationale de France, Paris.)

midity. A man is impotent because he is insufficiently hot and needs hot foods (ginger, nuts, pepper, chicken, saffron) to produce "hot" sperm.[30] A woman fails to conceive either because the womb is too small, she is obese, she has cold in the womb ("the heavy wind"), she retains menstrual blood, or she has ulceration of the uterus. Conception occurs when the uterus is dry enough to close on the sperm. The fetus develops from blood to lump of flesh, then assumes male sex after thirty days or female after forty, augmenting each day from the mother's blood and the air of the mother's breath.[31] Al-Qurtubi, like the Italian Pietro d'Abano, theorized that heat emitted by the stars affects fetal development.[32] But al-Qurtubi's text reveals little knowledge of the clinical practice of childbirth, which he leaves to the midwife: "When the pains increase, the midwife must be compassionate, delicate in her work, supplied with instruments and knowledge, with long practice in birth . . . She must keep her fingernails short to examine women, seize the fetus . . . If the cervix is narrow, descended in the vagina and very wet, this shows the imminence of birth and rupture of membranes."[33] As an illustration from the *Maqamat* of the Baghdad scholar al-Hariri (1237) suggests, male Arab physicians left the mechanics of birth to women (see Fig. 5.1).[34]

Colonial ethnographies, interviews conducted by the author, and contemporary anthropology suggest the enduring influence of Galenic ideas in Moroccan women's medical practice.[35] Birth is still a matter of the humors: heat opens the uterus and cold closes it. A midwife told me: "She is cold, all women, when she is giving birth, you do a scarf for her, you heat her up. You heat it over a brazier of hot coals. That heat, the uterus climbs up with it, the baby stays pushing, and the uterus opens."[36] To close the womb, another *qabla* introduced sugar into the vagina: "When we finish this, and he sleeps with her, he finds her again closed, like a virgin . . . sugar is like a *jabira* [poultice that gathers a wound]."[37] After birth, midwives belted the mother so that the womb would return to its place; if the womb remained "open," the cold could strike or the organs could "fall." Other Galenic notions, such as "dirty blood" (morbid atrabilious humor), also appear in physicians' texts and women's practice.[38] Al-Qurtubi writes, "Blood remaining in the uterus corrupts the sperm" and prevents conception.[39] In Morocco, a new mother was fed "hot foods" to expel [dirty] blood from the uterus—pullets, ginger, garlic, olive oil, *m'hamsa* (a small pasta), cumin, clarified butter, and *sellou* (pounded nuts). A Fez midwife told me: "This heats her up and she sweats, blood and dirt go out."[40]

Moroccan midwifery also reflected the unity of body and mind in Galen's thought. According to Galen, blood bears the mother's "psychological power" from the brain to the body; thus, a pregnant woman's thoughts were believed to influence the development of the fetus. Al-Qurtubi warned that upsetting a pregnant woman could cause her to abort.[41] Moroccan midwives told me that upsetting a birthing mother during delivery could also cause abortion, hemorrhage, or a retained placenta:

If she were *m'asaba* (angry, irritated) or she has her mother-in-law who fights with her, or with her husband, or she gets scared . . . when she gives birth, she stays angry, she has an inundation, it gives her a hemorrhage . . . [If the baby is dead], I lie to her and tell her he is only fainted, I have to do that until she is free of the placenta, so the placenta falls out of her, so she is not afraid, because . . . the placenta will climb up in her.[42]

The mother's thoughts were thought to influence the child's morphology, a notion Western physicians called "maternal impression." Birthmarks are still called *tawhima* (imagining, dreaming, wishing) in Morocco.[43] Pregnant women looked at gazelles in order to give the baby beautiful eyes, and avoided camels to prevent the formation of a harelip.[44]

But how did women access Galenic physiology, if many Moroccan women were not literate before the postcolonial era? There were two vectors of knowledge transmission: Islamic law and popular medical texts. Jurists introduced Galenic physiology to the public through legal opinions, and popular medical texts simplified the high tradition for a general audience. Male healers, especially apothecaries, disseminated the literate tradition to women. Scholars of Islamic popular medicine note similarities between popular practices in Saudi Arabia, Iran, Turkey, and Morocco; these similarities result not from a single "Islamic society," but from a single literate medical tradition and its living relationship to popular practice.[45]

TRANSMITTING HIGH TO LOW: LAYMAN'S GUIDES, THE APOTHECARY SHOP, AND THE LAW

The Moroccan reading public could access the ideas of "high" philosophic medicine through popular medical texts. "Medicine of the Prophet" books provided a simple overview of the four humors, hygiene, illness, remedies, and health recommendations of the Prophet Muhammad. In Morocco, the most popular of these texts was the *Kitab ar-Rahma* (Book of Mercy in the Art of Curing the Sick), by "Sidi Siouti."[46] Local authors wrote about specific ailments in works such as "Explanations of Hadith of the Prophet about the Stomach as the Site of Sickness . . . and the Origin of all Sickness of the Cold," or about particular remedies, as in "Praise Poem on the Benefits of Mint [*Na'na'*]," and "Limits on the Benefits of Medicinal Powders."[47] Another genre was the layman's medical guide, organized from head to toe. "Efficacious Talismans for the Health of the Body of Man," by 'Abd Allah Sidi Muhammad ibn Yusuf ibn Khalsun, promised its readers "a condensed book in medicine which will spare you the doctor."[48] Sexual and erotic advice books such as "Masterworks of the Bridegrooms and Entertainment of the Brides," by 'Abd Allah ibn Muhammad al-Tijani, provided information about pregnancy, conception, and abortion.[49]

Among the popular Moroccan manuscripts about birth is the "Risala 'ilm amrad an-nisa' wa tawiqhunna 'an al-habl" (Epistle in the Science of the Sicknesses of Women and That Which Prevents Them from Pregnancy), an anonymous Arabic text of gynecology and obstetrics conserved at the Bibliothèque Générale de Rabat. Included in a sixteenth-century physician's personal reference book,[50] the "Risala" simplifies Galenic physiology and provides plant names in the Berber language and the

Fez dialect of Arabic. Measurements are given to assist an inexperienced buyer at the apothecary's shop:

> In the name of God, the Beneficent and the Merciful.
>
> Know that the woman is prevented from conception by eight maladies. The first is the reverse wind, the second the wind of the interior, the third is the wind of air, which can be either the wind of air in parturition, or that which resembles it, and the fourth is the heavy wind, and this form is in the side, [a pain] like the cutting edge of an earthenware jar, in the place where the spleen is.[51] And as for the other four, the first of them is when the womb (*um awladha*) is dry, or if it is closed and seizes the sperm and throws it [back], or if it is open, or if it is inclined toward her left hip, and each one of these illnesses has its symptoms and its signs and its suppository (*sufa*) and what is appropriate to it, as it was presented, and it is God who knows.[52]
>
> As for the reverse wind, one takes for it, with the blessing of God the Highest, 'arq aykar and celery seed and the seed of *khalal* and fennel and caraway and white sugar in equal parts, they are finely crushed, and the powder is inhaled for seven days.[53] And symptoms of the reverse wind are that the sufferer has in her belly a wind that makes a strong rumbling noise, and it can be caused by her eating poison, which is not digested. And this is its remedy, which is described and known. And as for its *sufa*, it is peony and lavender and cumin and grilled salt and myrrh, and after being pulverized, these are kneaded into a paste in the grilled yellow of an egg, and she wears it [i.e., as a vaginal suppository] after purification, because it is suited to her, if God the Highest wills, and it is He who knows.[54]
>
> As for the wind of the interior, its symptoms are that the sufferer is terrified by fire and has a great pain in her head [literally: is hung by her head].[55]

Women could access the pharmaceutical literature by patronizing the apothecary shops and receiving instructions from the literate druggist. Herbal shops were sites of translation between texts and women; women in Fez frequented especially the shops of Hamda ibn Shaqrun, descendants of Abu Muhammad 'Abd al-Qadir ibn Shaqrun (d. 1727), author of the *Shaqruniyya*, a verse composition of pharmacopoeia and dietetics. Dawud al-Antaki's pharmacopoeia the *Tadhkira* also specifically addresses infertility and pregnancy. Antaki advises, "To prepare [the womb] for the reception of sperm by resolving the cold and heavy winds . . . crush a piece of garlic and cook it in clarified butter, then take nut of *bua*, saffron, cinnamon, a hundred *sa'ila* of each, half of it is mixed, sifted and [she wears it in a vaginal suppository] in the afternoon."[56] A Lamtiyyin resident recalled, "We did that *dawa' bildy* [native medicine]. You see, it was my mother who did it for us . . . She buys those herbs, she fixes them, she drinks them."[57]

Jurists also contributed to a synthesis of Greek science and Islamic society. When faced with questions of parental relationships, the permissibility of contraception, the biological basis of "milk relations," and the *idda*, jurists found Galenic embryology to be useful.[58] As Basim Musallam has shown, the four embryonic phases in Galen's *De Semine* correspond neatly to passages on human conception in the Qur'an. The passages on embryology are Sura 22:4 and Sura 23:12–14: "We created man of a quintessence of clay. Then we placed him as semen in a firm receptacle. Then we formed the semen into a blood-like clot; then we formed the clot into a lump of flesh; then we formed out of that lump bones and clothed the bones with flesh; then we made him another creation. So blessed be God the best Creator" (23:12–14). Jurists justified fusing Galen and the Qur'an through a hadith of the Prophet Muhammad: "Each of you is constituted in your mother's womb for forty days as a *nutfa*, then it becomes a *'alaqa* for an equal period, then a *mudgha* for another equal period, then the angel is sent, and he breathes the soul into it."[59] Galenic physiology provided a biological science for juridical responses to questions about abortion, inheritance, marriage, divorce, and paternity.[60]

The example of breastfeeding illustrates the dissemination of Galen's economy of blood to the public through legal opinion. The physician al-Qurtubi warns against nursing while pregnant, because the menstrual blood meant to feed the fetus will rise to the breasts and become milk, depriving the fetus and producing a weaker milk for the nursling. Islamic jurists adopted this theory to discourage nursing women from becoming pregnant, warning mothers that a pregnancy would render the nursling *ghayl*, or congenitally weak.[61] The popular "Medicine of the Prophet" texts repeated this warning to the public, cautioning women that a *ghayl* child would become a weakling unable to defend himself even as an adult.[62] The same term ("*ghayl*") appeared in ethnography collected in Marrakesh in 1926; the French physician Françoise Legey observed that women in Marrakesh called the nurslings of pregnant mothers "*ghayl*" and described a jealousy between fetus and nursling: "When a nursing mother becomes pregnant, her milk is pernicious to the nursing child, because they think the amniotic fluid mixes in the milk. It becomes bad because the fetus is jealous and wants his mother to himself. They say, 'jerdaa-el-khial,' nursing milk mixed with amniotic fluid."[63]

Galenic physiology thus filtered down from the high medical tradition to women's practices through jurisprudence, popular pamphlets, and the herbalist's shop; these were the social vectors for the dissemination of medical knowledge.

NEGOTIATING THE SPIRIT WORLD: PROTECTING BABIES FROM *JINN* AND THE EVIL EYE

Muslim women had to negotiate the spirit world of *jinn* and the pernicious energies emitted by the soul of an envious person, the "evil eye," to which Ibn Khaldun attributes "two-thirds of the cemetery."[64] New brides, virgins, and babies were believed to be especially vulnerable to envious humans and *jinn*, as Legey recorded: "Evil genies are always ready to harm [babies] . . . Um Sibian, 'the mother of boys,' hits and pinches [babies], making them cry without stop until the day they die of convulsions. To remove the evil of Um Sibian, one places babies under the protection of the Regragi saints, whose descendants make an image of Iblis [Satan] with a piece of yeast and attach it to the chest."[65] Neonatal tetanus was called "*zagaz*," a *jinn* who could be expelled by bleeding the child from his belly.[66] In interviews, Fassis attributed infant strabismus and withered limbs to the *jinn*: "[If the *jinn* sees a pretty baby] he will change it. Either [the baby] will cry a lot, or he will make his hands crooked, or he will cross his eyes."[67] *Jinn* possession could also render a woman sterile, as an herbalist explained: "When *jinn* occupy a woman, they are mostly in her sex organ. They eat the dirt from her, it enters her if someone writes [an amulet] for her, then when she walks across it, the *jinn* comes up and enters her, or if she masturbates at night, the *jinn* comes."[68]

Women negotiated spiritual healing from *jinn* illness by bringing their families to healers. In Meknes and Fez, the ʿIsawa and Hamadsha Sufi orders performed trance to drive out the *jinn*, and epileptics spent several days sleeping at the *zawiya* of the Nasiriyya brotherhood in Tamgrout for cure.[69] *Shebba* (alum) and *harmel* (*Peganum harmala*, or African rue) were placed in a small sachet attached to the crib to protect newborns from *jinn* and the evil eye, the harmful energy of envious persons. Fez residents explained: "*Shebba* and *harmel* for the Eye. So that whoever sees him, nothing will hurt the baby. Ah yes, the eye of the Son of Adam that sees him and does not say, God bless him . . . And there are those women who don't give birth . . . and her eye stays, it stares with that baby."[70]

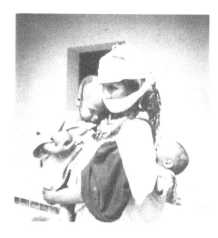

FIGURE 5.2. A mother holding a child with a "saint haircut." The head was usually shaven except for one lock placed in the style of the saint. ("Rapport annuel du GSM de Fez, 1932," Archives of the Institut National d'Hygiène, Rabat.)

Qur'anic amulets were also used to protect babies, for as Ibn Taymiyya advised: "Among the greatest weapons to exorcise the *jinn*" is the verse *Ayat al-Kursy* (2:255).[71] In Morocco, one dried the umbilical stump and sewed it into a pillow with *shebba*, *harmel*, salt, a small knife, and *Ayat al-Kursy*.[72] The baby was called *Embarak* (blessed) or *Mahjub* (the hidden one) until his name day, when his angels were given responsibility for protecting him.[73]

Saints' shrines specialized in particular ailments: "Sidi Frej" for mental illness, Mawlay Ya'qub for skin diseases, Sidi ben 'Ashir for eye disease and dyspepsia. Mothers consecrated their children to a particular *wali* by sacrificing an animal and having the shrine *muqaddim* cut the child's hair in a style identified with the *wali*.[74] In case of sickness, mothers brought the child back to the *muqaddim*, who repeated the haircut to consecrate the child to his saint anew.[75] The *muqaddim* was the "spiritual apothecary" of the shrine and gave women "spiritual pharmacy"; for example, the *muqaddim* of Sidi ben Azuz in Marrakesh cured tubercular adenites by spitting on them.[76] For the "Persian fire" (impetigo), women in Marrakesh prepared a paste of cinders from Sidi Fares's grave and saliva from the shrine's *muqaddim*, which was applied topically.[77]

Many "women's remedies" embodied *baraka* in a substance, which could then be touched or ingested. Midwives had birthing women deliver on the skin of a sheep sacrificed during the Feast of the Sacrifice ('Aid al-Kabir, or 'Aid al-Adha), because it carried God's blessing, or *baraka*: "The day of judgment, a sheep killed at 'Aid al-Kabir will bring on his back him in whose name he has been sacrificed."[78] A Fez family explained: "That slaughtering of the *mouton*, there are two things in it. First there is the name, and then there is what we call a good act of charity. When the woman gave birth, we slaughter a sheep and we say O Lord, praises to God that nothing bad happened to the woman."[79]

Thus, Moroccan midwives drew upon multiple medical languages—Galenic physiology, legal medicine, and spiritual knowing. What appeared to French doctors as a haphazard collection of folk practices was in reality the complex intersection and application of different systems of medical knowledge.

THE ETERNAL *BLESSÉE*, THE MUSLIM SORCERESS OF FRENCH *SOCIOLOGIE*

The French sociologist Edmond Doutté did not see Muslim women as healers at all. Instead, he argued that Muslim women were sorceresses, driven to magic by a primitive society that feared woman as the "eternal *blessée*," the "bleeding one." Woman's menstrual pollution excluded her from official religion and access to the sacred. To compensate for her social inferiority, woman therefore returned to power under the cover of "[heretical] magic, which becomes for her a religion of an inferior order."[80] Doutté argued that Muslim women were sorceresses who inverted Islam to call on Satan and pre-Islamic Berber gods, urinated on the Qur'an, and parodied prayer and pilgrimage. In his Marrakesh ethnography, Émile Mauchamp collected one magical recipe for "moon paste":

[The sorceress] buys a new kneading-dish during the day . . . and visits all of the homes of the genies with it: slaughterhouses, toilets, cemeteries, and saint tombs, as well as synagogues and mosques, of which the genies are the guardians. She takes water of the seven springs or covered wells . . . The night of the full moon, between midnight and one a.m., she darkens her right eye with kohl, puts blush on the right cheek, a bracelet on the right arm, an anklet on the right foot, and braids a lock on the right. Then she goes alone to the cemetery, puts the dish on the ground, strips naked, and runs holding a reed with a little green flag attached, asking the spirits of darkness to make the moon descend for her. In the dish she has put the water of the seven fountains. Then one sees the moon mount to its zenith and descend into the dish. Immediately a storm is unleashed, the water foams and spills over. . . The sorceress collects this foam. At the same time, benzoin and coriander cook in a neighboring pot, and the sorceress commands, "I want you to serve me for good and for evil." When the tube is full of foam, the sorceress puts out the incense fire and spills the water on the ground: the liberated moon rises slowly in the sky.[81]

Moroccan men feared their wives' magic and showed French doctors the bezoar antidote they kept to counter the poisoned food one might be served by angry wives after one's extramarital dalliances.[82]

Women's oral traditions collected by Aline de Lens in 1925 seemed to validate a view of Moroccan women as practitioners of sorcery:

> In antiquity, old women wanted to seize the Devil.
>
> What can we do to attract him? They asked themselves. The Devil always arrives during a dispute, so the old women started insulting each other. The Devil arrived. Then the shouting turned to sobbing.
>
> "What's wrong?" asked the Devil.
>
> The old women responded, "The Devil is dead!"
>
> "That is a lie! I am the Devil."
>
> "He is dead, we tell you. You, we don't know you."
>
> "I speak the truth!"
>
> "Enter into this glass vial and we'll believe you."
>
> He entered and the women quickly stoppered the vial.
>
> "Let me out!" He shouted.
>
> "By Fire! We won't let you free!"
>
> "Bitches! Female camels! Prostitutes!"
>
> "You! One-eyed person! Possessor of a single hair!"
>
> "O my daughters! Deliver me and I will help you!"
>
> "How can you help anyone, you, the Father of Evil?"
>
> "I will teach you how to prevail over men."
>
> The old women agreed, and he taught them sorcery, as well as the art of curing illness.[83]

French doctors sought to eliminate women's traditional practices and to restrict Muslim women to the private sphere of the home, and to a more "appropriate" role as the subjects of their husbands.

But the protectorate agreement forbade direct interference in the Muslim family. France was able to avoid giving Muslims citizens' rights because questions of Islamic personal status (marriage, divorce, inheritance) were governed by *shari'a* law. A Sénatus-Consulte of July 14, 1865, found "Muslim status incompatible with French law."[84] Dean of the Algiers Law Faculty Marcel Morand argued that the decision to leave the Muslim family to *shari'a* jurisdiction would show North Africans "[the legislator's] respect for their religious beliefs . . . or at least . . . make them more easily accept our domination."[85] Though French jurists considered the Islamic family oppressive to women, Octave Depont warned that French family law was "diametrically opposed to the natives' social state" and would "breed revolution" in North Africa.[86] Resident General Lyautey agreed. Having seen the destructive effects of direct colonial rule in French Algeria, Indochina, and Madagascar, he vowed to protect Islamic civilization in Morocco.

Lyautey proposed "women for women," French women to introduce obedience, virtue, and science to the Muslim family. This notion began in 1885 with the military ethnographer–turned–Catholic missionary Charles de Foucauld, who requested "semi-nomadic White Sisters" for Tuareg women: "Their devotion, their gentleness, their spirit of sacrifice would have the happiest effect."[87] At the Congrès Coloniale Française in 1904, the physician Georges Samné enthused, "Don't you see the great value of a French woman in such a milieu, in families and schools? What an admirable moral role to play! What educative power!"[88] Nuns in France had been used to introduce Third Republican hygiene to suspicious peasants in the French countryside.[89] For Morocco, French women would provide access to secluded Muslim women outside the legal limits of the French protectorate.

"WOMEN FOR WOMEN"?
THE LADY DOCTOR IN FRENCH MOROCCO

The first maternal and infant health programs in Morocco were Catholic charity programs directed by the resident general's wife, Mme. Lyautey. In the procolonial journal *France-Maroc*, Mme. Lyautey announced that France had introduced social welfare to Morocco, an idea hitherto "unknown in Islam."[90] But Mme. Lyautey's maternity served primarily Europeans; between 1922 and 1933, 4,437 Europeans and 553 natives gave birth at the clinic, and most of the native mothers were Jews.[91]

Yet French doctors needed access to Muslim women in order to implement public health measures. Pierre Lapin, director of the Institut Pasteur, complained that tuberculosis spread in the secluded Muslim home: "We can clean the streets . . . but we can do nothing about hygiene in the household where man spends half his life and woman her entire life."[92] As smallpox raged in Mogador in 1926, Charles Bouveret begged Muslim families to accept female vaccinators inside the home.[93] In Casablanca, Dr. Frédéric Bienvenue claimed that Muslim children had a high mortal-

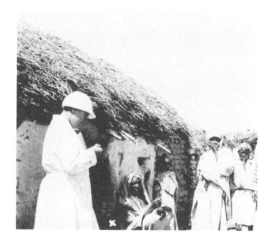

FIGURE 5.3. "Mlle. le Dr." Langlais investigates a typhus outbreak among the Awlad Yarra, 1932. The white *x* indicates the first typhus victim in the village. ("Rapport annuel du GSM de Fez, 1932," Archives of the Institut National d'Hygiène, Rabat.)

ity rate caused by native mothers' irrational practices: "Here is a remedy for 'green diarrhea:' vinegar, calcified alum, 'méah' (a kind of gum with tar and cardamom) and a little of the mother's urine. What constitution is robust enough to resist such medications?"[94] Doctors argued that Muslim women themselves needed rescue from native midwives; Dr. Somnier of Mogador demanded French intervention in 1922: "Midwives leave the placenta in the uterus, producing a dangerous infection. We have a woman in the hospital now who is on the brink of death from a mishandled birth."[95] The director of Native Health for the SHP, Mauran, grudgingly agreed in 1912 that female doctors would be necessary in order to access Muslim women.[96]

Lyautey opened a call for female doctors at the Paris École de Médecine in 1913. Maneesha Lal has argued that European women doctors used the secluded native woman to claim a unique imperial role for themselves, and indeed, female physicians like Mlle. Dr. Marianne Langlais did enjoy greater professional opportunities in Morocco than did women in the metropole.[97] Langlais led a rural vaccination team across Morocco, became the first head of epidemiology at the Institute d'Hygiène, and served as chief physician for the native hospital of Rabat.[98] Of the seven women physicians who served in the Protectorate Health Service (SHP) in 1922, all but one were of foreign origin and became French citizens only through colonial service in Morocco.[99] But these women saw themselves as rational scientists who alleviated women's suffering, rather than as female colonizers whose gender gave them a unique "woman's colonial mission."

Women doctors in North Africa were often obliged to battle the colonial state in order to provide medical care for native women. In Algeria, Françoise Legey, the pioneer of Muslim women's health in North Africa, pressured Algerian Resident General Jonnart to let her open the first all-woman clinic for natives in 1902: "They gave me . . . in rue de la Bombe in Algiers, two rooms next to the jail for the prostitutes. I had them whitewashed, disinfected, and installed myself there, after telling the population that I would come for two hours in the afternoon three times a week and receive patients for free. The first day, five came, and after a little while, six hundred!"[100] The Ministry of Foreign Affairs recruited Legey in 1910 to Morocco, where she served as the first female doctor; she was stationed in Salé, Mazagan, Marrakesh, and Casablanca. The women who joined Legey also advocated for native women's health; Dr. Eugénie Delanoë demanded a school for native midwives and milk dispensaries for Muslim infants, "a duty for every country, every nation, for whom children are the power, the honor and the future."[101] Dr. Sarah Broido attacked the closed state brothel system of the protectorate; any native woman suspected of prostitution could be arrested as a "clandestine prostitute," subjected to a mandatory vaginal examination, and incarcerated in a brothel. Broido and the Union Française pour le Suffrage des Femmes de Casablanca demanded an end to the closed brothel system as a violation of human rights.[102]

Women doctors also identified iatrogenic native practices and rallied Moroccan elites to support public education and hygiene reform. Delanoë encouraged new mothers to stop lining their infants' eyes with kohl, a reform that reduced the level of trachoma infection in the city of Mogador by half by 1936.[103] Moroccan notables were impressed with French women doctors and requested them expressly. The grand vizier asked Delanoë to deliver his wife's child and train his own servant as a birth attendant.[104] The Jewish population of Mogador raised 30,000 francs to create a milk dispensary for Jewish infants, and the Jewish community in Meknes outlawed Jewish traditional midwives in favor of French-educated midwives with diplomas.[105] The sultan asked municipalities to regulate Muslim barbers after learning that unclean razors exposed children to tetanus, syphilis, and ringworm.[106] Pasha Thami Glawi invited Legey to create a dispensary for native children in Marrakesh in 1921; her dispensary had attracted 41,879 consultations by 1923.[107] She added a maternity clinic in 1927 with a labor room, an operating room, and three recovery rooms: twelve beds for Muslims, six for Europeans, and twelve for Jews.

Legey presented French obstetrics in an all-female environment; 266

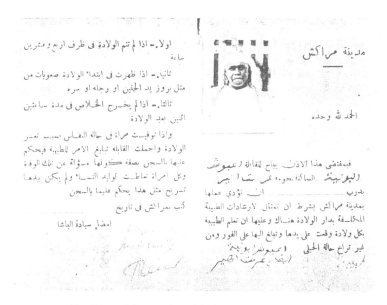

FIGURE 5.4. Identity card for a native midwife in Marrakesh, signed by Pasha Thami Glawi. (Françoise Legey and A. Décor, "L'assistance aux femmes en couches à la maternité indigène de Marrakech," *Bulletin de l'Institut d'Hygiène du Maroc* [1932].)

Muslim women gave birth at the clinic between 1927 and 1931.[108] But Legey recognized that her Muslim patients were mostly poor and marginal women; most of the Muslim population still birthed at home with a midwife. To improve conditions of home births, Legey requested and was granted the authority to license all native midwives in Marrakesh. She described the candidates: "It was a parade impossible to imagine—deaf, blind, even paralytic women. Half were eliminated and forbidden to practice under pain of imprisonment. 125 were kept."[109] *Qablat* were required obtain an identity card from the maternity and to inform Legey in cases of stopped labor, proincidence of the umbilical cord, breech presentation, or retained placenta. If a woman died in childbirth, the midwife would be held legally responsible for her death. Legey appointed one midwife as leader (*muqaddima*) of each city quarter and invited all the *muqaddimat* for a six-month clinical training at the maternity. Although it is difficult to gauge the impact of Legey's efforts, forty-five Muslim babies orphaned by their mothers in childbirth were registered for bottles at the Marrakesh milk dispensary in 1929. In 1931, there were only seven such babies.

Legey viewed Moroccan native midwifery through the prejudices of the French medical profession, perhaps a consequence of her experiences. She was called to native births only in desperate cases of severe infection, hemorrhage, and urethral, rectal, or vaginal tearing: "After six or eight days of labor, if God has not delivered the woman . . . sometimes the European doctor is called to intervene. Is it necessary to say in what conditions? The child is dead and the woman is exhausted, infected . . . It is impossible to describe the state of the miserable ones who arrive [at the maternity] with uterine rupture or hemorrhage."[110] Legey never attended normal Muslim home births because the French doctor was usually consulted as a last resort.[111] She thus joined her male colleagues in condemning the Moroccan *qabla*'s traditional practices as "purely magical" and iatrogenic.

GENIES, POISONS, AND HAREMS: THE FRENCH WOMAN AS MEDICAL ETHNOGRAPHER

French women were deployed to reveal the Muslim harem to the medical gaze. This was possible because Lyautey's rule created a culture of Franco-Moroccan sociability, unlike the racially segregated colonies of Algeria and Indochina.[112] As French officers dined with Moroccan notables, their wives entertained the ladies of the harems. The protectorate exploited this female intimacy; the Service of Public Education (Instruction Publique) recruited Amélie Marie Goichon to report on the Muslim bourgeoises of Fez; Georges Hardy hired Mlle. Burtley, Mme. Driss-Amor, and Mme. de Pressigny to study Muslim children; Émile Lepinay, the editor of *Maroc médical*, commissioned Aline de Lens to report on the medical practices of her Muslim neighbors.[113] In the introduction to de Lens's *Pratiques des harems marocains* (1925), Lepinay enthused: "Mme. A. R. de Lens knows how to make old women speak, and it is their secrets, collected with a thousand difficulties, that she brings to our readers."[114]

French women's ethnographies revealed a Muslim female world of exorcisms, supernatural disease, poisons, and phlebotomy. De Lens described often-familiar ailments, but with etiologies in which *jinn* caused sickness, either by "striking" the victim or by possessing him. Sorcerers could invite possession by feeding their victim a poison called *ta'am* ("food"), composed of bones and excrement: "The couscous rolled by the hand of the dead, Ftel-el-Miet, mixed with the bones of the dead (crushed), *assa foetida*, fallen hair reduced to cinders, powder of dried Taranto, wood of fig finely pulverized, this is at the base of all magic drugs administered unknown to the victim, to give him a lingering illness

. . . This is Taam. All tubercular patients, all maladies of fever, all cancer patients are Mthaoum, which is to say they have eaten Taam."[115] A hadith of the Prophet describes such foul substances as the "food of the *jinn*."[116] A contemporary *fqih* explains that *ta'am* brings *jinn* to feed in the victim and cause illness through the victim's own *jinn* familiar:

> The *jinn* knows the *qarin* [spirit familiar] of the victim through his name and the mother's name—the *jinn* and the *fqih* write the amulet together, and the type of the *qarin* (earthy, watery). The *jinn* is the one who says how to make it. The result is that the *jinn* influences the *qarin*. When the *tu'kal* [*ta'am*] enters the stomach, it sticks to it. The *jinn* eats it, lives with it. The *jinn* knows what he needs to live with the victim and influence his *qarin*. Then he tells the *qarin* that if he wants to rest, he must look at a particular person, the person with the amulet, for example. The *fqih* writes an amulet for the woman to wear to the man who has ingested the *tu'kal*, and he will love her.[117]

Muslim women appear in harem ethnographies as the practitioners of *jinn* magic. Legey wrote that women avoided places of *jinn* residence: "The most dangerous time of night is between 11:30 p.m. and 2:30 a.m. One must not go to the street, toilet, kitchen, bath, fountain or wells. This is the moment the Maezt Dar l'Oudou, the goat of cabinets, occupies these places."[118] To clear *jinn* from a room, women threw *shebba* and *harmel* in the corners and chanted, "Harmel is sacred, O Prophet of God."[119] Legey described Muslim women as the family intermediaries who brought children to saints' shrines and Sufi orders. She relates a scene of Gnawa *jinn* exorcism akin to the *zar* healing cults of Sudan:

> The [Gnawa] master calls to the genies in the body of the possessed person and says, "Come little friends, we only want your good and all assistance is favorable to you." The players of the rattles laugh ecstatically, rolling eyes full of promise to the genies. They offer a meal to all the devils and the assistants. This meal is composed of milk, dates, and sugar thrown on the ground and in all places familiar to devils. At this moment, the scene turns into delirium. By this ceremony of offering, one has attracted in each spectator, in each rattle player, a genie familiar who will work on exorcising the sick person and attracting the evil devil, who kills her little by little.[120]

Harem ethnography also revealed a battle of the sexes. De Lens recorded recipes "to give a deflowered bride the appearance of virginity," "assure a husband's fidelity," "bring misfortune upon a co-wife," "augment the size of the breasts," and for the frustrated mother-in-law, "detach a newly married son from a too-beloved new wife." For dominance in marriage, a new bride should urinate postcoition into her hand seven times and pour the contents into her husband's tea. As she pours, she should repeat:

I made you drink my water
So you do not see but by my eyes
You do not hear but by my ears
You do not speak but by my words![121]

To make a husband stop beating her, his wife added hyena brain to his soup. To augment his desire, she conserved a date in her vagina for seven days and served it to him in his food. To render her spouse as pliable as "the dead body in the hands of the washer of the dead," she disinterred a fresh cadaver and prepared her husband's food with its hands. Doctors reported from the field: "We learn from M. Allal Abdi . . . [that] two women were surprised at night in the cemetery digging up a cadaver to prepare a couscous with his hands destined for one of their husbands. The dish would supposedly produce the effect of a love potion and give him a boundless love for her. The results were quite different—he divorced her."[122]

FROM WOMEN'S MAGIC TO FRENCH PHARMACEUTICAL

But a close examination of de Lens's ethnography reveals a women's pharmacology not dissimilar to that of France. For "eye malady," de Lens records the instruction "rinse the eye with copper sulfate." French physicians cauterized the swollen eyelid of trachoma infection with copper sulfate, in order to prevent the eyelashes from curling inward and scraping the cornea. To prevent a child from inheriting her syphilis, a Moroccan mother dipped wool in mercury and tied it to her wrists and ankles, a treatment quite like the mercury-based "grey oil" that French physicians prescribed for syphilis. French colonial administrators and pharmaceutical companies eagerly "bioprospected" among native remedies in Morocco, for botany was "big science and big business, an essential part of the projection of [Western] military might" in the colonies.[123]

The Irish naturalist John Ball created the first modern European compendium of Moroccan plants in 1878, but it was Professor Émile Perrot of the École Supérieure de Pharmacie de Paris who organized a study of Moroccan plants for the 1900 Exposition Universelle in Paris.[124] Perrot noted that natives in India, Sierra Leone, Siam, Cambodia, and Brazil had independently discovered "chaulmoogra oil," a leprosy cure derived from trees classified in the (now-defunct) Flacourtiaceae family. French colonial administrators discovered that Cambodian natives had used chaulmoogra to create a "veritable leprosarium" in the forest of Khel-Chey.[125] Since British and American pharmaceutical companies made fortunes from chaulmoogra oil, Perrot hoped to make a similar find in Morocco. An Interministerial Committee of Medicinal Plants and a National Office of Primary Materials for Drugs, Pharmacy and Perfumes were constituted in Paris in 1918, and Perrot created its Comité Marocain in 1920.[126] Perrot reported that Morocco could be a major producer of perfumes (orange flowers, thyme oil, geranium rose, sweet marjoram) and medicinal plants (black mustard, thymol, saffron, opium, linen, psyllium, henna, castor oil, cedar, cade and thuya tars, henbane, datura, rue, safflower, ash, galingale).[127]

Military pharmacists helped to form a botanical society, the Société des Sciences Naturelles au Maroc, and collaborated with field officers of the Direction des Affaires Indigènes (Department of Native Affairs) to collect and test the medicinal substances used in Moroccan women's "magic." Aline de Lens recorded the following for "the sickness that comes to children at the time of flowers": "The matron makes two incisions behind the right ear of the child and rubs them with tar, then coats the inside of the nose and mouth with tar. She then kills a serpent, cuts off its head, encloses it in a hollow reed . . . and suspends it from the caftan of the little patient." Moroccans spread such cedar tar on the mucous membranes to fight smallpox, psoriasis, and inflammation. The pharmacist-major René Massy tested native tar preparations and found that tar made from *Cedrus atlantica manetta* (Atlas cedar) was a powerful antigonorrheal agent, which he suggested could replace cade oil (made from *Juniperus oxycedrus*) and Santal, an expensive medication imported from India.[128] The pharmacists Pierre Fourment and Henri Roques tested the bark (*souak*) that women used to scrub and whiten the teeth, and discovered that it had analgesic, exfoliant, and antiseptic properties.[129]

Colonial scientific societies attracted French pharmaceutical companies to Morocco, which founded commercial laboratories and factories to exploit Morocco's botanical and mineral wealth. The Établissements Lafont founded a pharmaceutical factory in Morocco in 1927. In 1933, the Coopération Pharmaceutique Française de Melun founded a branch in Casablanca, and the Établissements Byle et Comar created Laboratoires Laabi in 1941. By 1949, there were eight private French pharmaceutical laboratories in Morocco.[130]

PATRIARCHY STRIKES BACK: THE LAW, THE LABORATORY, AND THE CONQUEST OF WOMAN

After the era of Lyautey (1912–1925), law and science converged in an attack on Muslim women's medical knowledge. French physicians wanted medical authority, Muslim men wanted to circumvent women's legal expertise, and the protectorate wanted to enter the Muslim family. These interests came together through the laboratories of the Institut Pasteur and the new Institut d'Hygiène du Maroc (1930), inaugurated under Resident General Lucien Saint by the president of the Conseil Supérieur d'Hygiène in Paris, Léon Bernard; the directors of the Instituts Pasteur in Algiers and Tangiers; and the director of military medicine for the Troupes de Maroc. The IHM was created to centralize epidemiological information, educate the public in hygiene, coordinate large-scale environmental projects, design "social hygiene" programs, and provide laboratories of forensic anatomy, microbiology, and toxicology for the legal needs of the state.[131]

The French laboratory offered visible "scientific" evidence to replace the knowledge of native midwives and the need for French women as intermediaries. At first, Muslim men invited French female doctors to examine their wives, but they soon requested French laboratory tests directly for legal cases of inheritance, paternity, marriage, and divorce. Moroccan rural authorities voluntarily sent viscera to the new IHM toxicology laboratory of Dr. Albert Charnot (Le laboratoire de toxicologie et de recherche médico-légale) to investigate suspicious deaths. Colonial power expanded through science, but it was Moroccans themselves who were the agents of its expansion. As Moroccan men and women visited the laboratory for medical testing, they introduced positive knowledge of the Muslim body to Islamic courts, jurisprudence, and the family.

The first battle between French and Islamic law took place literally in the body of the Muslim woman. Historically, Berber courts combined codes of local custom ('urf), with Islamic law (shari'a), a disorganized legal system that privileged powerful families and senior patriarchs.[132] French Native Affairs officers warned that young Berbers would soon revolt against the despotism of the rural Berber courts.[133] But in an address to the French Senate on May 28, 1912, Raymond Poincaré underlined that French governance must not centralize law in Morocco and create a nation; the particularities of Berber society should be preserved in order to keep Morocco politically fragmented.[134] French authorities first tried to separate and govern Berbers and Arabs under two separate legal codes with the *dahir* of September 11, 1914, a policy culminating in the notorious *Dahir Berbère* of May 16, 1930.[135] This direct approach provoked nationalist protest, and the Résidence was forced to withdraw the 1930 *Dahir*. Nevertheless, Georges Surdon of the Institut des Hautes Études Marocaines explained in his lectures of 1928–1929 that France must seize this opportunity to replace Islamic law with secular law by "reforming" Berber customary law courts: "The Berber has maintained himself thus until the present and has not been Arabized . . . This is why we must collect Berber custom; not to codify it, but to conserve it so it is not absorbed by the *shari'a* . . . Custom, in the presence of a code, is fated to disappear. In Morocco, there are two written laws: Islamic law of revealed origin and French law. It seems preferable to see custom absorbed by French law rather than by *shari'a*."[136] To govern rural Berber areas without extending Islamic law or strengthening the sultan's state, Lyautey "codified" Berber law and reorganized the Berber court system.[137]

French Native Affairs officers considered Berber law to be more permissive for women than Islamic law, and contrasted the unveiled Berber peasant woman in the fields with the cloistered urban Arab lady. In the Ichkern region, French officers found that local notables referred to women older than seventeen as *tadjalt* (nonvirgin) rather than a *taârimt* (virgin). When Lieutenant Denat asked for explanation, he was told, "Every type of wheat finds a buyer."[138] The Aït Harakat of Guelmous accepted children born to their wives in their absence: "A proverb says, '*Aïn tioui targa i bab iîger!*' 'Everything brought by the channel [of irrigation] becomes property of the owner of the field.'"[139] Divorce could be consensual, and the Ichkern allowed the wife of a missing husband to take a lover if she did so discreetly.[140]

In reality, Islamic law (*shari'a*) and Islamic courts gave women and children more property rights than did Berber *'urf*. Islamic law gave women the right to inherit property, which most Berber courts did not.[141] Children inherited even if their parents' marriage were "considered absolutely null by the unanimous opinion of the doctors of the four schools of Islamic law."[142] By contrast, Berber courts favored male litigants in family matters. Among the Ichkern, a husband could divorce his pregnant wife in her seventh month, deny paternity, and be absolved of child support.[143] He could also claim the children of his ex-wife almost indefinitely.[144] In one case among the Aït Harakat tribe, the man Haddou Ou Assou divorced his wife, Itto Qasso, in 1927. Six years later, after Itto had remarried and given birth to a boy in 1934, Haddou claimed the child and won custody: "I thus addressed my complaint to Pasha Hassan. He . . . invited my ex-wife to prove by twenty witnesses that the claimed child belonged to Mohh [her current husband]. The twenty witnesses refused, and at their insistence, I consented to reduce their number to five from among the closest relatives of the woman. These are: Qasso, Itto's father, her step-mother Taffon-Bihi and her nephews Allou-n-Hamid and Asso-n-Basso, who refused to swear for her."[145] Robert Aspinion reported that the Ber-ber court would reject an ex-husband's claim only if the woman's relatives supported her or if Muslim midwives could offer expert testimony about her pregnancy.[146]

The French found a point of entry with "the sleeping child" (al-raqid), an Islamic legal concept.[147] The sleeping child was a fetus "frozen" in the breast of his mother, where he could remain sleeping for up to five years, according to Maliki jurisprudence.[148] For women, the raqid was very use-ful; a child born late, during a husband's absence, or after his death was considered legitimate and entitled to inherit. The raqid prevented unilat-eral divorce (talaq), because according to the Qur'an, a man cannot di-vorce a pregnant wife before she gives birth, after which he owes her two years of maintenance for breast-feeding.[149] A divorced woman could thus receive up to five years of maintenance by claiming a raqid pregnancy, and a widow could delay the division of her husband's succession by de-claring herself pregnant at his funeral; any child born within the five-year delay period would consequently inherit. Shari'a and Berber customary courts left the diagnosis of the raqid to the woman herself, her mother, or a midwife.

The legal concept of the raqid dates from the early Islamic period. To delimit the duration of pregnancy, jurists turned to the Qur'an, the Prophet Muhammad, and the first four (rightly-guided) caliphs. The Qur'an sets the minimum gestation period at six months in Sura 46, but the maximum gestation period was open to debate.[150] The Caliphs 'Umar, 'Uthman, and 'Ali recognized four- or five-year gestation periods.[151] Ca-liph 'Umar settled matters of female biology by considering the expert counsel of old (wise) women:

A woman who had lost her husband and who did not think she was preg-nant when he died observed the ritual idda of four months and ten days and remarried after the legal delay. She remained with her new husband four months and a half, then she gave birth to a viable child. Her husband came to find 'Umar al-Khattab and told him. 'Umar convoked the old women to have their opinion on this delicate case. One of them told him, "I will inform you about this woman. She lost her husband while she was pregnant and her menstruation continued during her pregnancy. Her son froze in her belly, because her period continued during her pregnancy; the

sperm of the new husband awakened the child and he reassumed growth."
ʿUmar believed her and gave the newborn the name of the first husband.[152]

Subsequent Maliki jurists such as Khalil ibn Ishaq al-Jundi, Ibn Abu
Zayd al-Qarawani (d. 996), and Ahmad b. Yahya al-Wansharisi (d. 1508)
used Galenic embryology to support the five-year gestation period.[153] Al-
Wansharisi argued that the raqid went dormant because of excessive cold
and could be awakened by the "hot" sperm of copulation:

> What to decide about a woman who claims to be pregnant for four years?
> A woman can remain pregnant for five to seven years, if she is not submit-
> ted to copulation. And Allah knows better than anyone. The child con-
> tracts in the lining of the womb like a chewed mouthful contracts [in the
> mouth], because when the mother undergoes copulation again, the fe-
> tus swells up again anew. Glory to Allah the Creator, the Omniscient! . . .
> When the pregnant woman finds she has her menses, these have for effect
> the shriveling of the child in the womb. On the contrary, if the woman
> does not have her menstrual flow, the child is growing normally.[154]

In the Morocco of the twentieth century, French physicians were in-
credulous that shariʿa judges could believe such a "physiological absur-
dity."[155] Doctors saw the raqid as a woman's ruse to avoid divorce, and
Dr. Delanoë commented wryly, "Every sterile woman claims to have a
[sleeping child]."[156] But Denat, the Native Affairs officer among the Ichkern, noticed a sincere belief in the raqid: "The women themselves—we
have already indicated the conditions in which they believe themselves to
have a sleeping child—firmly believe that they are on the verge of being
mothers for several years . . . some keep absolute faith. I cite the case of
a notable, member of the Customary Berber tribunal of Ichkern, who already has three young children from his wife. For ten years she declares
she has a sleeping child. He believes it absolutely and it would be delicate
to make him recognize his error."[157] Qablat described the sleeping-child
fetus as a soft, mobile mass in the belly, unlike the rigid uterus of gestation.[158] To awaken it, the woman heated her body by eating a chicken
baked with honey, ginger, garlic, thyme, myrtle, lavender, mint, and nut-
meg, by visiting the steam baths, and by having sex with her husband.[159]

The laboratory gave Berber male litigants a new opportunity to challenge Muslim women's authority in birth. When the Institut Pasteur offered the Friedman urine pregnancy test in June 1933, the director, Pierre
Remlinger, was delighted to expose women as liars: "In no other milieu

will pregnancy tests provide a greater service than in a Muslim one . . . pregnancy can be an excuse for theft, a way to escape imprisonment."[160] Fathma, thirty years old, claimed pregnancy at the moment of her divorce. Her husband had her examined by a European midwife, who said she wasn't pregnant, and a Muslim *qabla*, who said she was. The *qadi* (judge) sent Fathma to the Institut Pasteur, and Remlinger crowed, "She dropped her act and admitted she had menstruated that very morning."[161] Under the influence of French science, Berber courts in the Marrakesh region rejected the *raqid* in 1931, and the Zemmouri tribe rejected it by 1935. French officers applauded the end of the *raqid* as evidence of Berber "evolution" toward rational thought: "One remarkable factor of evolution is the Customary Court of Appeals . . . Thus, in 1934, in one of its opinions, [the court] decided that, contrary to principles heretofore accepted in the matter, a man absent from the tribe can deny paternity of a child his wife gave birth to when the physical impossibility of cohabitation is established in an irrefutable way."[162]

By contrast, the *shari'a* law courts defended women's medical authority and the *raqid* against the French laboratory. In a 1935 *fatwa*, a Maliki *qadi* affirmed a possible gestation period of four years, and in 1949 a second *qadi* ruled that French laboratory tests were merely "information," not evidence, which would be discarded if in conflict with the testimony of Muslim witnesses: "In the documents where the state of health plays a primordial role, the *shari'a* prefers the testimony of the *'adul*. In these conditions, a doctor will see the *shari'a* reject his declarations, which are nevertheless received . . . but refuted by the testimony of an *'adul* because the latter is 'honorable and irreproachable.'"[163] The court affirmed female *'adalat* as the only acceptable witnesses in pregnancy and interpreted the *raqid* broadly to favor women and children. In a succession case of 1945, a widow declared herself to be pregnant seventeen months after the death of her husband, and the court collected the husband's estate from the first beneficiaries and reapportioned it to include her newborn child.[164]

But Moroccan women themselves soon visited the Institut Pasteur for their own medical needs. In 1935, four women requested Friedman pregnancy tests, one to escape repudiation, two seeking inheritance, and one seeking alimentary allowance.[165] Many Muslim women came to the Institut Pasteur to make health decisions: six nursing mothers feared creating a *ghayl* infant, nine new wives came impatient to conceive, and one woman requested a Friedman before submitting to gynecological surgery.[166] Muslim and Jewish women also asked French physicians to write them certificates of virginity.[167] Visits to the Institut Pasteur uncovered various gynecological ailments; as Dr. Pierre Champagne wrote, "Every woman who believes she has a sleeping child is a patient for us to discover."[168] Women who believed they had a sleeping child often suffered extrauterine pregnancy, retained fluid, amenorrhea, cancer, tumors, ovarian cysts, or prolapsed uterus.[169]

The French laboratory thus provided women with a new framework through which to negotiate legal rights and pursue the healing of their own bodies. Urine pregnancy tests could be used as court evidence or to detect problems correctable by gynecological surgery. Improved health could potentially strengthen a Muslim woman's legal position in her marriage, for *shari'a* allowed a man to annul his marriage if his wife had an obstructed vagina, a torn perineum leading to confusion between the urethra and vagina (fistula), tumors obstructing the vagina, a prolapsed cervix, or a fetid vaginal odor.[170] However, as women appropriated new French medical technologies and gynecological surgeries, they did so at the expense of their traditional medical authority.

TAMING THE SORCERESS IN THE
TOXICOLOGY LABORATORY OF DR. CHARNOT

In 1931, Dr. Charnot created the first Moroccan laboratory of toxicology at the Institut d'Hygiène du Maroc, which he described as a modern-day "Chambre Ardente," the royal court originated by Henry II in 1547 to condemn heretics and later used by Louis XIV in 1679 to catch abortionists and poisoners.[171] Charnot analogized the Moroccan midwife to the notorious Catherine Deshayes, the widow Monvoisin, a midwife accused of performing 2,500 abortions and using the dead fetuses for satanic rituals.[172] In his *La Toxicologie au Maroc*, Charnot described poison in Morocco as a female art, cultivated by elderly Muslim women over years of harem imprisonment.[173] Charnot argued that the vengeful Muslim woman dispatched her male oppressors at the dinner table: "In the stomach of one victim, we found a piece of yellow-orange orpiment [arsenic] the size of a chick pea. This crass subterfuge did not attract attention, thanks to the couscous."[174] Charnot also claimed that the Moroccan sorceress despised the French doctor, for though Muslim men confessed to him easily, Muslim women hid their secrets: "A native was poisoned by the root of *Atractylis gummifera* [a Mediterranean thistle]. This root was presented to the accused, a wife of the victim, who swore on the Qur'an that she knew neither the name nor the properties, but a few days later, from the bottom of her prison, she threatened an Arab of her village with her vengeance. She accused [him] of telling the *roumis* (French) about '*Addad*' [*Atractylis gummifera*] and the poisonous properties of this root."

Sorcery was quite simple according to Charnot; at base, black magic was a toxin discoverable by chemical analysis.[175] Terrifying items were added to impress the buyer's imagination, "What lady poisoner would be content with a glue thistle when the 'sharifa' can get her the dried blood of an evil man or the urine of a blind woman?"[176] Poisons were widely available in native markets: "One finds orpiment [arsenic] in the boutiques of native druggists, either in crystals, formed of stacks divisible into parallel sheets of a lovely golden or lemon yellow, or a powder."[177] Moroccan beauty aids like kohl eyeliner and *addad* skin exfoliant were poisonous; kohl (an antimony compound) is harmless when applied to the pH-neutral eye but becomes a heavy-metal poison in the acidic stomach, where it dissolves and enters the bloodstream.[178] Charnot developed an encyclopedic knowledge of Moroccan toxins: animal products (cantharides, geckos, toads, vipers), plants (spring squill, opium, rue, belladonna, datura, henbane, glue thistle, mandrake), and minerals (arsenic, sodium arsenate, mercury, copper sulfate, lead, cinnabar), and created his own protocols for unfamiliar toxins like *addad*.[179] Morocco had natural deposits of asbestos, antimony, silver, copper, tin, iron, gold, lead, magnesium, alum, potassium nitrate, phosphates, arsenic, and zinc oxide—a mineral wealth far superior to that of France.

Charnot merely offered toxicology testing; it was the Berber courts who voluntarily sent samples of human viscera, hair, clothing, fingernails, and earth from the victims' graves for analysis. Charnot performed two analyses for Berber criminal cases in 1946, eighteen in 1947, and twenty-one in 1952.[180] Yet a statistical analysis of Charnot's toxicological reports at the Institut d'Hygiène du Maroc reveals that half of the accused poisoners were male and most of the victims were women, contrary to Charnot's own stereotypes.

The larger implications of toxicology can be seen in a case that came before the district court of Had Kourt, which sent the blood, urine, stomach, and lung of one Rkia bint Sellam to Charnot with the following report:

The defendant Said ben Ahmed Souhi . . . brought complaint to Us, declaring that the named Fatna bent Abdelkader quarreled with his wife Rkia bent Sellam and insulted her, "You are worthless, you are humiliated and despised . . ." The women went to the *qaid* to settle their quarrel. Arriving in the *douar* Kebzienne, one of them encountered the husband. He intervened and reconciled them. They walked home.

Under the influence of anger, Rkia Bent Sellam found a plant known as "Dadd" and after cooking it, ate it. This according to the deposition of witnesses . . . The *muqaddam* declared that he was called to attend the death of this woman. After asking her about her condition, she declared she had eaten the plant called "Dadd" and that she was the author of this act. After pronouncing these words, she died.[181]

It is worthy of note that the *muqaddam*, Rkia's husband, and the witnesses *all have the same family name*. Rather than a suicide, the suspicious narrative suggests that the Suhi family of Had Kourt may have poisoned Rkia bint Sellam and used local family connections to cover up her murder. Although fragmentary, Rkia's case suggests that Charnot's toxicology lab extended the reach of the centralized legal state into local Berber society, a biopolitical development that ultimately could be used to prosecute crimes against women.

THE GENDER OF MEDICINE in Morocco touched the legal paradox of French association policy itself in Morocco. The French Résidence was charged with a contradictory task in 1912: safeguard the Muslim religion while instituting "a new regime of administrative, judiciary, educational, economic and financial reforms."[182] Resident General Lyautey was to protect Islamic law, which French authorities thought incompatible with modernity. He was to preserve the Muslim family, which French jurists believed kept women in a state of slavery. To rule without ruling directly, Lyautey created a shadow technocracy charged with "assisting" the Sultan's *chérifien* state. To circumvent the official limits of state power and enter Muslim homes, Lyautey used French women to act as his unofficial intermediaries. Though men dominated the practice of medicine in the metropole, women were often the practitioners of French medicine in Morocco.

The re-gendering of French medicine illustrates a larger principle: colonial medicine was an encounter between different conceptual systems of healing, a complex reality forged by patients and doctors negotiating French and Moroccan medicines as social and cultural systems. This shifting framework provided women with new opportunities and limitations. French female physicians with limited professional prospects in France enjoyed a privileged position in protectorate Morocco. Muslim women could appropriate French science to manage their own health, fertility, childbearing, and legal rights in marriage and divorce. As healers, Muslim women were scientifically syncretic, moving among multiple medical languages and finding in French biomedicine a new array of institutions, healers, and remedies from which to draw. The French codification of Berber law displaced Muslim women as legal-medical experts but generated a "new framework for conflict" that women could navigate.[183]

The urine pregnancy test illustrates the social mechanics of biomedical regimes—how French ideas of the body's truth enter "indigenous" codes of Muslim law. Male doctors at first reluctantly relied upon French women as medical intermediaries, but the laboratory, by rendering visible (or claiming to render visible) the hidden realities of the female body, enabled male colonial physicians to assert their authority directly over native women's bodies. Legal systems are obliged to define human bodies as social entities. The battle between *shari'a* jurists and French doctors over the "sleeping child" revealed a deeper confrontation between French law and Islamic law, both of which aim to develop the potential human person into a full social being.

In adopting French laboratory tests, Moroccans advanced a new idea of truth itself. Replacing the testimony of Islamic witnesses with a laboratory urine test substituted the truth of the human soul derived from *niya*, the purity of faith, with a nonhuman, demonstrable, mechanical, scientific truth extracted involuntarily from physical bodies. This change suggests a moment in a social process of colonial embodiment, one of the multitudinous ways in which Sufi epistemology was displaced and positive science internalized in law and society.

A MIDWIFE TO MODERNITY: THE BIOPOLITICS OF COLONIAL WELFARE AND BIRTHING A SCIENTIFIC MOROCCAN NATION, 1936–1956

IN 1952, THE FRENCH PHYSICIAN Jean Mathieu and the sociologist Roger Maneville interviewed 167 traditional Muslim midwives (*qablat*) to determine their suitability for the "veritable corps of Moroccan midwives" planned for native women by the protectorate health service, with "modern ideas of hygiene and pediatrics."[1] It is unsurprising that the report rejected the Muslim *qabla* as dangerous—obstetricians in Europe also attacked midwives to redefine birth as the physician's province. But for Morocco, the study placed entire responsibility for the social ills of colonial industrialization on the Muslim midwife.[2] And it was the *qabla's* way of thinking that precluded Moroccans from self-governance: "This study will show the wisdom of the Government in making the acquisition of modern culture a prerequisite for Moroccan independence . . . Midwife by definition, intermediary, abortionist, sorceress, adviser, weaver of spells . . . The *qabla* allows us to see, despite the seeming evolution of customs, the immutability, one may say, of the Moroccan *mentalité*."[3] Only when Moroccans discarded the *qabla's* Muslim *mentalité* could they be granted political independence from France: "[When they differentiate] between the domain of religion and the domain of positive knowledge. In a word, when they will have acquired the secular mind."[4]

To achieve the secular mind, the French taught Muslim women to knit, nurse babies, and keep house. The protectorate's *"médico-social"* welfare state, created after the Second World War, was in part an application of metropolitan science to empire; in the nineteenth century, the French state responded to tuberculosis in the French working classes with *puériculture*, the science of raising children. French colonial humanism adapted the *solidarisme* of Frédéric Le Play for use in the empire, as a way to create a French imperial family. But in Morocco, colonial policy makers intended maternal and infant health programs (PMI; Protection maternelle et infantile) specifically to destroy the Muslim *mentalité* and to refashion Moroccans into rational, well-differentiated individuals ready for industrial work. These policies gave rise to a battle between Moroccan nationalists and the French protectorate to define and govern the modern Muslim family. The nationalist leaders 'Allal al-Fasi and Muhammad al-Wazzani defined independent Morocco through an Islamic modernist idea of the welfare state.

Of interest to us here is the field of battle—the Muslim woman's reproductive body. Why did Moroccan independence depend upon birth practice? When and why did the Muslim woman's veiled body become the symbol of an antirational "Muslim mentality," and its uncovering the triumph of the secular republic? In obstetrics, French colonial authorities and Muslim nationalists fought over population control and reproduction, but they also struggled to define both the body in public life and the political subject created by public health institutions.

But can the body talk back? Can the body tell its own truth despite colonial and nationalist biopolitical strategies? Obstetrics and birth in Morocco illustrate the nature of medicine as a disjointed set of epistemologies, practitioners, and clinical practices rather than a discursive monolith—a medicine that can allow the human body to speak its own truth.

THE GREAT AWAKENING: TUBERCULOSIS, URBANISM, AND A NEW SOCIOLOGY OF ISLAM

Nineteenth-century French doctors praised Morocco for its apparent immunity to "*phtisie*," or pulmonary tuberculosis, but in 1922 a Fez native dispensary recorded 1,505 Muslim tuberculosis cases in one month.[5] In a report of 1934, a Rabat doctor called tuberculosis "the primary cause of death for Muslim adults."[6] Yet as late as 1932, the director of the Service de la Santé et de l'Hygiène Publiques (SHP), Jules Colombani, denied that tuberculosis was an epidemic among Muslims in Morocco.[7] How is it that the protectorate "did not see," or made itself not to see, an epidemic of Muslim tuberculosis until the 1940s? This blindness was due in part to the decentralized nature of the colonial health service, which impeded data collection, but the key lay in an early French sociological vision of Morocco as rural, tribal, and static. "Primitive" Moroccans could not have tuberculosis, the great industrial disease of nineteenth-century Europe. Only when the colonial frame of vision shifted with the modernist sociology of Robert Montagne did French authorities "discover" Muslim tuberculosis, recognize Morocco as an industrializing country, and take action in a new colonial welfare state targeting Muslim women and children.

Robert Montagne, a young naval lieutenant–turned-sociologist, trusted his own observations rather than received sociological dogma. In the new industrial port of Mehdiya, he observed that Moroccan traditional life was vanishing rapidly: "Soon," he wrote, "[there] will be only its archeological ruins."[8] Lyautey appointed Montagne to the Institut des Hautes Études Marocaines (created 1920), and made him secretary-general of the protectorate's ethnology and sociology section.[9] Setting out on missions to document millenarian Berber institutions among the Sus, Anti-Atlas, and High Atlas tribes in 1921–1930, Montagne discovered instead a revolution in rural life.[10] Berber tribes were pulling apart; their young men were migrating to the northern cities, and subsistence-farming families were resorting to cash cropping, land sales, and sending sons to the French army to obtain the currency needed to pay new taxes and purchase manufactured goods.[11] Colonel Justinard recorded Berber oral poetry that expressed ambivalence about participation in a cash economy:

> As for tea, you see
> The Christian knows well that you are his enemies
> He hits you with cannonballs of tea
> He ambushes you on the balance of the scale.
> The enemy strikes you in the stomach. He knows well that there
> Death is easy, in the belly where the heart and liver are.
> The Christian strikes, he aims well. He brings bread and sugar . . .
> People of the scale, be deprived of God in the next life.[12]

Protectorate land-registration programs also had the effect of alienating many Moroccan peasants from their lands. Many farmers became agricultural wage labor on their former lands, or migrated to the cities in search of work.[13] The protectorate's "Sociétés Indigènes de Prévoyance," created in 1928, were intended to stem the growth of a rural proletariat, but the SIP failed to study or prevent the mass exodus of rural populations from the Sus, Dra, and Tafilelt regions.[14]

As the director of the Institut Français in Damascus (1930–1938), Robert Montagne developed his own modernist sociology of Islam. In his "L'évolution moderne des pays arabes," (1935), Montagne drew upon the work of René Maunier and Marcel Mauss to argue that European colonial rule forced extremely rapid change on native cultures: "The native is pushed from the level of tribe to city to State, sometimes in a generation or two."[15] Fragile societies crumbled under modern pressures, but Muslim "Orientals" absorbed Western ideas to create "modern hybrids." By understanding Muslims sociologically and directing their social evolution,

France could preserve her North African empire from the threats of pan-Islam, pan-Arabism, and nationalism:

> If we proceed thus, we quickly notice that the Arab countries, Egypt,
> Syria and Palestine, are the epicenter of a vast movement which has waves
> east and west in the Muslim world . . . [but] whatever the politics . . . it is
> only an instant in . . . social life, the social body itself, which is infinitely
> more complex . . . We need sometimes to abandon the complexity of the
> movement, the newspapers and the books . . . to study domestic economy
> and technical evolution.[16]

In 1936, the *recteur* of the Université de Paris appointed Montagne to lead a massive study of Algeria, Tunisia, and Morocco—demography, family, rural life, urban life, language, economics, women, clothing, housing, intellectual and social movements, Islamic institutions, schools, and the press—a project that the Front Populaire government made into the Centre des Hautes Études d'Administration Musulman (CHEAM) in Paris.[17] Montagne's perspective was echoed in new journals such as *Questions Nord-Africains: Revue des problèmes sociaux de l'Algérie, de la Tunisie et du Maroc* (1934–1939) and the *Bulletin Économique et Social du Maroc* (1933–1939, 1945–1987).

In Morocco, industrial expansion during the Second World War took the protectorate by storm, and French authorities focused on its material rather than social consequences. Between 1938 and 1949, the use of motor power in the Moroccan economy more than doubled. In 1933 more than one-quarter of the total value of Moroccan exports was from mining, which passed from an index of 100 in 1938 to 220 in 1949. In 1938, Morocco produced 30,000 tons of fish and in 1949, 93,000 tons. In the same time period, European agribusiness increased exports of fresh vegetables from 25,000 to 50,000 tons and citrus fruits from 10,000 to 95,000 tons.[18] The French saw possibilities for further development in food processing, construction, metallurgy, textiles, and chemicals. In 1947, the French found themselves with a rapid industrial fait accompli, and the first accurate population information would reveal an urban and health catastrophe.

The sociologist Jean Célérier warned that labor migration "creates *serious problems of urbanism, hygiene and police*,"[19] but it was the team of the Native Affairs officer J. Huot and the *lycée* teacher R. Baron who revealed the shocking conditions of the northern cities. In a 1936 study of the Rabat shantytown Douar Doum, 13,352 Muslim Moroccans (26 percent of the Muslim Rabat population) lived in "degrading misery," subsisting on a daily average income of seven francs for a family, "Prostitution allows some women an income . . . The children are dirty, covered in vermin, nearly naked; men and women wear rags."[20] Daily salary was spent almost entirely on a diet of bread, oil, and tea. Residents who could not afford the nine francs per month to rent shacks made of flattened metal tubs (*bidons*) lived in illegal tents and straw huts (*noala*).[21] In the Arab cities (*mudun*), bourgeois homes became overcrowded proletarian tenements. The sociologist André Adam found an average of nine families inhabiting a single-family home in Casablanca, ten persons to a room, with one latrine for all, "Small courtyards become veritable cesspools . . . Many of these alleys are covered with a permanent carpet of garbage on which children, dogs and cats roll among a cloud of flies."[22] He concluded, "[This] is only a fragmentary aspect of an immense event: the birth of a Moroccan proletariat."[23]

Sociologists were also the first to discover an explosion of the Moroccan Muslim population. The protectorate's censuses of 1921, 1926, 1931, and 1936 were inaccurate; areas of the country resistant to French rule until 1931 could not be measured, and Muslim births were not reported to the French authorities. The Muslim population was estimated in 1936 at 5,170,000, for an estimated increase from 1931 of 15.85 percent.[24] The first accurate Muslim demographic information came in 1945, when famine and drought forced Moroccans to register for protectorate-provided food rations, a monthly seven-to-nine-kilogram bag of grain.[25] The 1947 census reported a staggering Muslim population figure of 8,088,600.[26] This data revealed that the population of Casablanca alone had quintupled in twenty years. If that rate of growth were sustained, the demographer Jacques Breil projected that the Muslim and Jewish populations would double in thirty-five years and triple in fifty-five years.[27] Breil judged Muslim workers to be poorly trained, but he observed that Muslims constituted the primary labor force for colonial agriculture, mining, and industry in Morocco.

Shantytowns were not populated by "vagrants," as BMH doctors had believed, but by the new native labor force of French colonial industry. The urbanist Michel Ecochard found that 1,890,000 Muslims resided in the cities in 1950; thus, Muslims had become nearly one-quarter urban by 1950, compared with only one-tenth in 1920. The urbanization process, which had unfolded over 150 years in France, had taken place in Morocco in just thirty years.[28] The SHP would be the last to recognize its brutal health consequences: tuberculosis, malnutrition, and high infant mortality.

The French did not introduce tuberculosis to Morocco, but rapid in-

Table 6.1. Muslim and Jewish Moroccan workers by industry, 1936 and
1947, (000s)

Sector	Muslims		Jews	
	1936	1947	1936	1947
Fishing, forestry, agriculture	1,267	1,521	0.4	2.4
Extractive industries	11	22	—	—
Other industries	155	223	12.6	20.9
Transportation	63	30	2.5	1.2
Commerce—food	58	64	5.1	5.7
Commerce—other	14	78	3.7	20.8
Public service	28	45	1.1	2.3
Domestics	22	124	3.2	5.9

Source: J. Breil, "Quelques aspects de la situation démographique au Maroc," *Bulletin
économique et social du Maroc* 9, no. 35 (October 1947): 133–147.

dustrialization under French colonial rule transformed the disease into
an epidemic. Tuberculosis followed two human vectors: labor migration
to the northern cities and colonial migrant labor to Europe during the
First and Second World Wars. In 1915, the Interministerial Commission
of Muslim Affairs contracted with the Résidence to send Moroccan workers to France and on January 1, 1916, the Ministry of War created the
Service des Travaux Coloniaux.[29] Sixteen thousand Moroccans worked
in France in the period 1916–1919; 15,000 in 1925; 20,000 in 1929; and
10,000–15,000 until 1950.[30] One-quarter of these Moroccans worked in
the Paris region; the rest were in Lyon, Marseille, and Saint-Étienne.[31] In
French mines, munitions factories, and farms, Moroccans contracted tuberculosis from European carriers and advanced rapidly to the end stages
of the disease. The French Ministry of War sent Moroccans home to die
in order to spare the metropole the expense of their care.[32] In his Mogador
hospital, Dr. Bouveret observed the returning workers:

> Our hospital is filled with the tubercular, who arrive at the end stages of
> infection and die here. An investigation allows me to pose the following
> conclusions:
> 1. The exodus of Moroccan workers to the metropole is the most impor-
> tant factor of contamination.
> 2. The workers arrive in France to lamentable hygiene conditions . . . They
> live in the notorious slums of Gennevilliers and such places, where they
> become infected.

3. They are sent back to Morocco without a medical exam and contaminate their families upon return to the household.[33]

In 1917, the Ministry of War claimed that Moroccan workers lived in good conditions, but a study of North Africans in Gennevilliers in 1929 described exhausted, undernourished men in crowded dormitories: "A single window lights this room of 8 by 5 meters, fourteen iron beds . . . separated by a space of a few centimeters."[34] Dr. Mohammed Ben Salem of the Marseilles Franco-Musulman Hospital called tuberculosis "the Muslim plague," for it progressed rapidly to massive, bilateral lung infection in North Africans.[35]

After 1940, doctors began to study tuberculosis in Morocco itself and its deadly impact on children.[36] In a 1942–1947 Casablanca study, Dr. Jean Chenebault found Muslim child tuberculosis "massive, precocious and fatal."[37] Precocious, because 33 percent of Muslim children had positive cutaneous reactions by age one; massive, because 87 percent of Muslim children had been exposed by age eleven; and fatal, because 63 percent of exposed Muslim children died, compared with only 5 percent of exposed European children in Morocco. In 1946, Charles Sanguy found an astounding 28.3 percent Muslim infant mortality rate in Casablanca—one in three babies dead in the first year of life.[38] Tuberculosis is a class disease related to socioeconomic status, because healthy, well-nourished bodies form a calcification around the bacillus to arrest its progress. Muslim children, because of severe malnutrition and difficult living conditions, progressed immediately to the disease state.[39] The pediatrician Jeanne Delon compared malnutrition among the Moroccan urban poor to the starvation experienced by Jewish prisoners in German Second World War concentration camps and identified a new, deadly protein deficiency in Muslim infants that she named "Moroccan Kwashiorkor": "In one or two weeks after weaning, edemas appear in the face, extremities, and feet, serous discharge from the nose . . . dry skin and breakable, discolored hair . . . The evolution is always very serious and rapid towards death."[40]

Finally, a World Health Organization BCG (Bacillus Calmette-Guérin) vaccine campaign conducted from 1949 to 1951 revealed that *the entire country* of Morocco had been exposed to tuberculosis, from Warzazat (54 percent) to Casablanca (97 percent). The WHO vaccinated European children after the Second World War and expanded the campaign to North Africa on October 7, 1948. The FISE (Fonds international de secours à l'enfance) provided vaccines, equipment, and personnel for test-

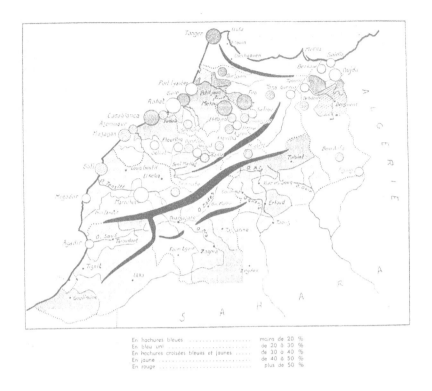

FIGURE 6.1. Degree of tuberculosis exposure in infants in Morocco, 1951. (Gaud, Houel, and Fayveley, "Indices tuberculiniques au Maroc," *Bulletin de l'Institut d'Hygiène du Maroc.*)

ing 1,402,000 Moroccans in the rural south (Tafilelt, Warzazat, Agadir), 1,020,000 in urban areas, and 1,233,443 in mines, dams, and shanty-towns.[41] In urban Casablanca, Fez, and Meknes, infantile exposure exceeded 50 percent, and adult exposure was more than 97 percent; even mining communities such as Khouribga had lower exposure rates than did the industrial northern cities (see Fig. 6.1).[42] Exposure rates in the countryside averaged 20–30 percent, but tribes of intense labor migration showed higher rates, like the Aït Baha of Agadir. Thanks to the new sociology, by 1946 the Résidence realized that the booming industrial growth in protectorate Morocco relied on a native workforce that was starving, exposed to tuberculosis, and living in squalid shantytowns.

But politics were of greater concern to the Résidence than native health, especially after the nationalist *Plan de réformes* of 1934, widespread urban strikes and rioting in 1936–1937, and the presentation of an

Istiqlal (Independence) Manifesto in 1944. Sociologists warned that Muslim tribes and guilds were disaggregating into a rootless urban proletariat "ready for all disorders" and awaiting only nationalist or communist leadership.[43] In France, Moroccan workers joined metropolitan trade unions (CGT, Confédération Générale du Travail), an experience that was the starting point for the Étoile Nord-Africaine and Algerian and Tunisian nationalisms. In Morocco, Muslims joined French trade unions, but in secret. The Résidence outlawed Moroccan unionization with the *dahirs* of 1936 and 1938, and the Section Française de l'Internationale Ouvrière (SFIO) officially rejected the Moroccan bid for independence, but strikes on June 18–19, 1936, in Casablanca included 1,400 Moroccan participants, twice the number of European workers.[44] Authorities in the metropole monitored the contacts of Moroccan university students with the Tunisian *dustur* ("constitutionalists," or nationalists), the pan-Islamic activist Shakib Arslan, Egyptian nationalists, and the Étoile Nord-Africaine of Massali Haj. Roger Maneville, an officer of Native Affairs who was sent on mission to study Moroccans living in France in 1939–1940 and 1944–1946, warned that Moroccan students were "purely engaged in nationalist politics": "Their political evolution, although still incoherent, is nevertheless noticeable. Without doubt, it will not remain long in the theoretical stage. Soon enough, there will be a concerted offensive with the other countries of Arab civilization against our prestige in North Africa."[45]

The French Résidence had believed that Moroccan students could not mobilize rural tribes and bourgeois elites with *salafi* modernist nationalism, but Maneville demonstrated the naïveté of this view; Moroccan nationalist students were already uniting classes in a community welfare center in Gennevilliers, a suburb of Paris. The Association Marocaine de Bienfaisance, which was funded by Muhammad Diouri, a wealthy businessman and signatory to the *Plan de réformes marocaines*, had a board composed of Moroccan students, workers, and businessmen. Medical students and social workers volunteered free care, and the center offered free classes, clothing, day care, summer camp, and meals to poor Muslim children. Sultan Muhammad V intended to travel to Paris in order to inaugurate the center in June 1945, but he was refused entry to France by the Quai d'Orsay. Maneville warned that the center constituted "points of contact between the *évolués* and the laboring masses, a chance to sow nationalist propaganda among workers" that "polluted" migrant workers from the Sus tribes "and will soon bear fruit."[46] The Quai d'Orsay accused Diouri of Nazi war profiteering and arrested him—this provided a pretext to close the center. Nevertheless, France had learned a valuable lesson: nationalists could use the welfare state to unite Moroccan classes behind an independence struggle. This had to be prevented at all costs.

FRANCE AS MUSLIM FATHER? ROBERT MONTAGNE AND THE MOROCCAN PROLETARIAT

For a new policy in North Africa, the Résidence turned again to Robert Montagne, who proposed that France become father to the evolving Muslim family. Montagne had directed French propaganda in the Islamic world during the Second World War for the Service of Muslim Affairs of the CFLN (Comité Français de la Libération Nationale, the provisional government of the French Republic) and for Charles Hippolyte Noguès, resident general of Morocco and commander of the North African Theater of Operations.[47] In 1948–1950, Montagne coordinated a massive project in Morocco of eighty sociological studies conducted by French colonial officers in Marrakesh, Agadir, Casablanca, Rabat, Safi, and Port Lyautey (Kenitra). The researchers included André Adam, René Bazin, Jacques Berques, Roger Maneville, and the physicians Henri de Leyris de Campredon and Jean Mathieu. Montagne himself collected data from sixteen thousand Moroccan workers in Casablanca. This project, published as *Naissance du proletariat marocain* (1952), documented the industrial transformation of Morocco. Casablanca, with 10 percent of the Moroccan population and 80 percent of Moroccan commerce, was Montagne's laboratory of Islamic modernity.

Montagne saw tribal organization disintegrating: "In the proletarian cities, rural civilization is dying . . . In less than one generation, the fundamental institution which supported it is disintegrating: the patriarchal family."[48] He argued that the tribal family rooted Islam, land tenure, customary law, and gender relations; its death would thus free individuals to create a new society.[49] France must lead this Muslim proletariat before it developed class consciousness: "Its soul is being born and will belong to whomever knows how to guide it and love it for itself."[50] The key, Montagne argued, was the Muslim family. Because 30 percent of Muslim women in Casablanca were wage earners, he concluded that a "proletarian matriarchy" was replacing tribal patriarchy, leaving fatherless, hungry, ill-clad boys to become street children and "the criminals of tomorrow."[51] The Muslim father was therefore incapable of leading a modern family and would inevitably entrust his sons to the French schoolteacher: "Be the father of this child. Guide him, correct him . . . I am ignorant and cannot do it."[52] The secret to defeating the nationalist movement, Mon-

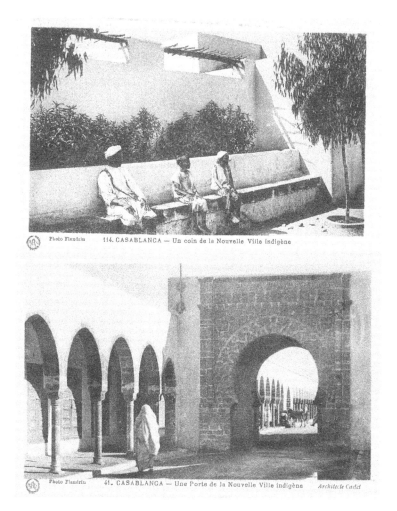

Photo Flandrin   114. CASABLANCA — Un coin de la Nouvelle Ville indigène

Photo Flandrin   41. CASABLANCA — Une Porte de la Nouvelle Ville indigène   *Architecte Cadet*

FIGURE 6.2. Views of the "*nouvelle madina*" in Casablanca, designed to incorporate aspects of traditional Islamic life (*bottom*), yet introduce order, hygiene, discipline, and modern family life (*above*). (Postcards, author's collection.)

tagne argued, was an "immense, concerted effort" of French teachers, physicians, and social workers to become the collective parent to the Moroccan child and his mother: "Each quarter could have its own school, day care, home for boys, workshops to teach women a trade, dispensaries for newborns (for whom maternal ignorance often promises death), a bureau of social welfare . . . Such would be the essential institutions to realize in order to lead to a total transformation of the conditions of life for the Muslim proletariat."[53]

The resident generals who succeeded Lyautey, from Théodore Steeg (1925–1929) to Eirik Labonne (1946–1947) to Alphonse Juin (1947–1951), gradually developed a paternalist colonial welfare state for the Muslim family. Dr. Georges Sicault, director of the SHP (1947–1955), laid out programs to prevent prenatal mortality, stillbirth, and gastrointestinal disorders in newborns, improve health for school children, and provide vocational training and homes for abandoned (street) children, addressing "all causes of morbidity and death that menace populations in their attempts to adapt to the modern world."[54] Le Corbusier student Michel Ecochard designed new, low-quality, mass proletarian housing for Muslims in Casablanca and in Rabat of "scientifically-determined 8x8 minimum housing cells" laid out in rectilinear grids.[55] Colonial modernists created the Casablanca *nouvelle medina*, the "traditionalist high-rises" of the Cité Verticale, and hygienic housing in the shantytowns of 'Ain Chock, 'Ain Sabaa, and Carrières Centrales. Architectural modernism embodied an objective, scientific embrace of technology and hygiene, intended to reform Muslim society and the Muslim family through its disciplining forms.[56]

TEACHING THE MUSLIM MOTHER: ADVOCACY, COLONIALISM, AND OPPORTUNISM 1900–1946

French medical, sociological, and legal authorities had long converged on a view of the Muslim family as an obstacle to modernity. The dean of the Faculty of Law in Algiers, Marcel Morand, wrote of the Muslim family as a primitive social fossil, "It is among all Muslim peoples exactly what it was in the first century *hijra*."[57] This too-strong family crushed intellectual autonomy, Morand argued, and prevented the development of well-differentiated, sovereign individuals. Mauran, the first director of the native health for the SHP (1913), argued that Moroccans were politically immature from the defects of Muslim parenting: "One can say that the nullity of the role of mother of the family, the indifference of the father in education, are the causes of the sociological worthlessness of the young generations; one makes egotists, impulsive persons, effeminates, and slaves of heredity. One does not make citizens."[58] Georges Hardy and Louis Brunot of the Service of Public Education (Instruction Publique) blamed Muslim mothers for the "deficits" of their sons: "Woman's influence dominates in the life of children, and as woman is reduced to intellectual misery in Morocco by seclusion, ignorance, and social inferiority," she perpetuated Lucien Lévy-Bruhl's prelogical mentality, which "limits thought in its least manifestations."[59] Suzanne Bey-Rozet, the director of social work for Morocco, agreed: "The problem of social evolution in Morocco is above all *maternal . . .* the *deficit of the mother.*"[60]

French female doctors sought to teach Muslim mothers a "scientific" approach to childcare, disease, and the body. In her ethnography *Essai de folklore marocain* (1926), Dr. Françoise Legey found that Moroccan mothers inhabited an irrational world of spirits and magic, which, she argued, produced dangerous, unhygienic medical practices:

> If a woman takes her child on her knees and sits outside, she exposes him to a magic illness caused by the owl as it flies over him. This bird can let fall his droppings on the child, who becomes immediately very sick. He loses strength and has diarrhea and chronic ophthalmia.
>
> To protect the child from the night owl, the mother takes a living owl, opens his beak and puts her milk in its mouth, then caresses and kisses it, and lets it go. This makes the owl his "milk brother."
>
> To cure the droppings of the owl, one takes the child to the shrine of Sidi Moussa Zahhaf. Mother and child stay at the *zawiya* and each day the *muqaddam* [curator of the shrine] puts an egg white in the child's mouth. Then he puts wool in egg white and puts it around the child's neck. He puts a stain of tar on hands, elbows and temples. The white is the color of the owl's droppings, the tar evokes the night.[61]

Legey found that Moroccan women used urine, feces, animal tissues, and dirt to cure newborns of sickness, but she argued that Muslim mothers were "gentle, intelligent and obedient" and could be educated, and they "bring babies to see us with a regularity unknown in the Jewish population."[62] The French doctor had a responsibility to rescue the Muslim mother from the barbarous native midwife, according to the obstetrician F. Cismigiu: "Very brutal in general . . . the kablas pull on everything that presents at the vulva: hand, cord, foot . . . They are incapable of recognizing a bad presentation or a narrowed pelvis."[63]

The PMI (Protection Maternelle et Infantile) envisioned the educated Muslim mother as an extension of the doctor in the home and an ally against the "social diseases" of tuberculosis and syphilis. The Muslim home was thought promiscuous, disorderly, dirty, and unhygienic, where bodies, fluids, and genders commingled.[64] If Muslim infant mortality were due "⅓ to digestive problems, ⅓ to the 'congenital peril,' and ⅓ to infection," then an educated mother could separate tubercular adults from newborn babies, treat the fragile skin of *héredo-syphilitic* infants, and prepare clean food free of bacteria and contaminants.[65] Doctors in anti-syphilis campaigns had already convinced thousands of pregnant Muslim women to undergo a series of eight novarsénobenzol (arsenic) injections of 0.15 grams each in order to prevent the miscarriage and birth defects caused by hereditary syphilis.[66] Legey wrote, "A young mother will come to us and proudly present her baby, a rosy little doll, 'Here is the child of the injections.'"[67]

The Service of Public Education focused on instilling the future Muslim mother with rational thought without disturbing her subservience as a Muslim wife; the goal was a woman "modern in her way of living, but respectful of traditions."[68] Hardy and Brunot explained the importance of such education, for they deemed Muslim mothers incapable of teaching their sons civic values: "The essence of the Arabo-Muslim character is selfishness . . . [because] reason is limited to the rigorous application of a code . . . [Morality] develops in a very different environment from that in which French children live . . . Without true liberty, a sense of responsibility cannot take root."[69] French Catholic and lay educators agreed that the education of Muslim girls would evolve the Muslim family, but the French provided little schooling for Moroccan boys and less for girls.[70] In 1913, French schooling consisted of one embroidery workshop for 82 Muslim Moroccan girls, followed by 17 Muslim girls' schools with 3,108 students in 1932, 27 schools with 5,707 students in 1940, and 47 schools with 9,782 students in 1945; the last figure still represented just 0.2 percent of the female population.[71] French teachers argued that girls' schools "bridged the [French and Muslim] worlds," yet Muslim "proletarian" girls were principally taught manual trades like embroidery, homemaking, and carpet weaving in vocational schools. In 1943, only seven girls in Morocco received a diploma equivalent to the one awarded to boys at the elite *école des notables*. In any case, the *dahir* of October 10, 1943, required that Muslim girls' education terminate at the age of thirteen.

French female doctors, teachers, and social workers, together with the wives of Resident Generals Lyautey, Steeg, and Lucien Saint (1929–1933), advocated the application of French *puériculture* to Muslim families. Suzanne Desgeorges, the first French social worker in Morocco, discovered that Muslims allowed her into their homes to vaccinate children during a 1927 Rabat smallpox epidemic. This experience inspired her to propose "a [woman] political agent" to infiltrate Muslim homes "under cover of hygiene and public health."[72] In 1930, the Ministry of Justice cautiously approved: "This delicate mission must be placed under the direct control of Mme. Saint using only first-class French women."[73] The Service of Native Affairs added, "[The social worker] must at no time have the character of a *political agent* . . . Above all, she must not upset the milieu where she works but 'tame' them and attract them to our modern ideas of family."[74] Desgeorges attempted unsuccessfully to spy on the household of the Rabat nationalist Muhammad Lyazidi. After her visits, Lyazidi addressed the following indignant letter to the *contrôleur civil*:

> Since I have been absent from Rabat, a certain demoiselle named Desgeorges visits my household from time to time for reasons I do not know. Last Tuesday she came especially in order to advise me to see a person in the Direction of Native Affairs. I coldly declined her offer, not knowing the relationship that might exist between this lady, who claims to be from the Health Service, and M. Surdon, Director of Native Affairs. I would ask that you indicate to this inopportune visitor that I will no longer admit her to my home without a formal invitation, signed Lyazidi.[75]

Nevertheless, Desgeorges's idea—to use pediatrics to enter the Muslim family—became the basis of the post-1940 French protectorate's *médico-social* welfare state.

Change was on the horizon as early as 1931, when the director of the SHP, Jules Colombani, declared that medicine must "evolve in a social direction" to protect "the indigenous race, the true wealth of the country." After Lyautey left Morocco in 1925, the SHP began to centralize, first with the creation of the Institut d'Hygiène du Maroc (1930). Moroccans were now regarded as a public to educate rather than a disease environment to manage, and the institute's Musée Social developed French- and Arabic-language medical posters, films, and books designed for native health education (see Fig. 6.3). A Service of School Hygiene was created in 1938 under the direction of Dr. Jean Mathieu to inspect schools, create a medical record for each child, and visit private homes in order to investigate the "social origins of disease." In 1946, the SHP created a Service of Social Medicine with five bureaus: Preventive Medicine (eye maladies, syphilis, PMI [maternal and infant health], hygiene education), School Hygiene, Social Services, Administration (orphanages), and Public Welfare, all under the direction of Dr. François Cauvin.[76]

Social Catholics and the Vichy Regime (1940–1944) also laid groundwork for Muslim family health programs.[77] Resident General Noguès accepted the Vichy Service of Youth and Sports (SYS) and its director for

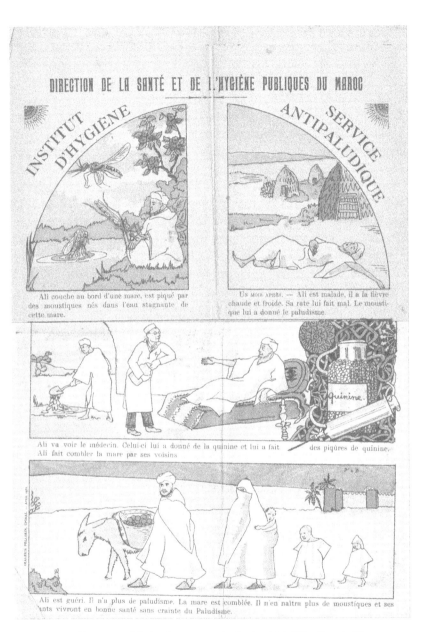

FIGURE 6.3. This 1934 public hygiene poster by the Institut d'Hygiène du Maroc shows the new protectorate strategy: to educate the Muslim Moroccan public about disease, its etiology, prophylaxis, and treatment. (Author's collection.)

Morocco, Jacques Faure (see Fig. 6.4). The SYS-Morocco newspaper *Jeunesse* proposed importing "L'Aide aux Mères" to Morocco, a Paris organization that sent young female *"collaboratrices"* to postpartum mothers in the home. With advice on cooking, cleanliness, and *puériculture*, the *collaboratrice* "penetrates the working milieu."[78] On May 8, 1941, an "École Sociale de Jeunesse" was created in Rabat to train French women in social work, Arabic, Islam, home economics, and hygiene, with a practicum at the Institut d'Hygiène. Vichy's "Travail, Famille et Patrie" ideology produced the Écoles Ménagères (Housewife Schools) for French women in Rabat and Casablanca, and the *dahir* of July 8, 1941, placed all French welfare charities in Morocco (milk dispensaries, orphanages, tuberculosis clinics) under protectorate state authority.[79] Dr. Maurice Gaud (1934–1944), whose position in 1942 was "Directeur de la Santé Publique et de la Jeunesse, Directeur de l'Office de la Famille Française," viewed birth as Vichyite nationalism: "It is not for herself that [the woman] gives birth, but for the national community, a community that transcends her. It is not for the modest personal satisfactions of the present that she suffers, but for the future of the country."[80]

In 1945, SHP Director Maurice Bonjean (1944–1946) proposed applying the Vichy *médico-social* programs originally created for Europeans to Muslim families.[81] Drought, famine, and a resurgence of epidemics in 1940–1945 compelled the protectorate to offer the first large-scale aid to the Muslim poor, and these soup kitchens and tent cities provided a beginning point for protectorate welfare to Muslims.[82] Lyautey's lone *médecin du bled* was finally and definitively replaced by large specialized hospitals, an educative public health, and a bureaucratic documentation of the Muslim child and his family.[83]

The first Protection Maternelle et Infantile (PMI) centers were opened in Meknes in 1948, a "center of *puériculture* and family education" for bourgeois native girls, and a "center of popular sanitary education" for proletarian women in the Borj Mawlay 'Umar shantytown. PMI centers offered Muslim women prenatal and infant care, home visits, and "mother schools," which taught lessons in nursing, weaning, food preparation, housework, and hygiene.[84] By 1952, there were twenty-seven PMI centers in Morocco: four in Rabat, four in Casablanca, one in Fedala, five in Fez, one in Sefrou, five in Meknes, one in Erfoud, two in Marrakesh, three in Agadir, and one in Oujda, with a mobile PMI unit for rural areas.[85] The French intended for PMI clinics to counter nationalist activity, monitor child health, and convince Muslim women to give birth in French clinics.[86] Birth was the moment at which a child entered Islamic society,

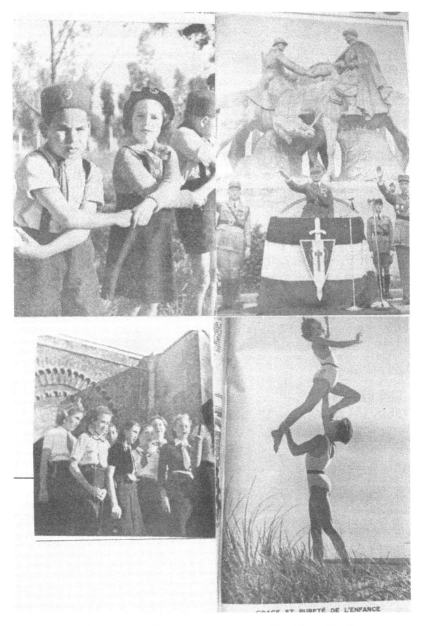

GRACE ET PURETÉ DE L'ENFANCE

FIGURE 6.4. Vichy in Morocco focused on youth, natural health, and family reproduction. Moroccan participation in scouting was limited, but the young Prince Hasan (*above left*; the future King Hasan II) was recruited here as a scout for propaganda purposes. (*Jeunesse*, 1942.)

wrote the sociologist Charles Le Coeur, and the point at which he engaged in the "conflict between ritual and technical thought."[87] Birth was
thus the logical point for French intervention. Born scientifically, the new
Muslim child would be protected from native midwives and the irrational
"Muslim *mentalité*." At stake in French colonial *puériculture*, then, was
the education and constitution of the human subject himself.

MIDWIVES, *MUWALLIDAT*, AND THE
MEDICALIZATION OF MOROCCAN BIRTH

Two images reflect the different approaches to Muslim birth used by traditional midwives and French obstetricians. In the traditional birth photo
(see Fig. 6.5), the birthing mother is seated, supported by a *shaddada* ("she
who holds tight") and a midwife (*qabla*). The mother is actively engaged
in her own labor in an all-female environment, her sex organs draped by
a sheet. In the second image, the mother lies exposed and blindfolded on
a hospital examination table, a passive, blind object in her birth process;
her sex organs are visibly presented to the obstetrical surgeon for his intervention (see Fig. 6.6). The colonizing of birth was not only a transfer
of authority from women to doctors, it was also a positivist unveiling of
the Muslim female body, a rendering visible, readable, and quantifiable.
On the delivery table, the SHP saw the final triumph of French positivism
over "the Islamic mind" and its protector, the Muslim woman. If Orientalism seeks Islam's truth beneath the woman's veil, as Meyda Yegenoglu
has argued, then SHP obstetrics claimed to interrogate, dissect, and conquer Muslim woman in her very flesh, reducing her to the visible, universal, biological meat of "woman's parts."[88]

To destroy Muslim women's healing authority, *Maroc médical* recommended replacing the traditional Muslim *qabla* with a French-trained native birth attendant, the *muwallida*. As Roger Maneville and Jean Mathieu wrote in their 1952 ethnography of Casablanca midwives, native
qablat worked in antiscientific darkness, "The spirit of observation is
rare among these women. As we have seen, birth takes place under a veil,
without the midwife knowing what happens in the vulva."[89] In replacing the *qabla* (she who receives) with the *muwallida* (she who births), the
SHP attempted to redefine birth from mother's sacred act to doctor's medical procedure: "The obstetrical act, which is a physiological act, is surrounded by a very dense halo of superstitions in the Moroccan masses,
maintained by ancestral customs belonging to sorcery, which will only

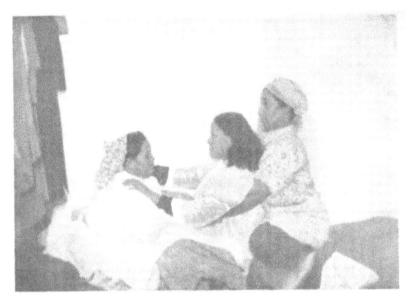

Positions respectives, au moment de l'accouchement, de la qabla, de
l'aide-accoucheuse et de la parturiente qui a dénoué ses cheveux pour
faciliter, dit-elle, sa délivrance.

FIGURE 6.5. Traditional Moroccan Muslim birth. The mother is seated, her back supported by a *shaddada*, and the midwife sits before her. (Jean Mathieu and Roger Maneville, *Les Accoucheuses musulmanes traditionelles en Casablanca* [1952].)

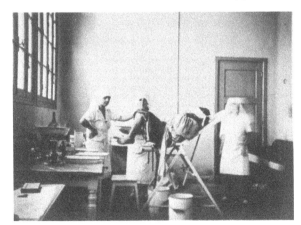

FIGURE 6.6. Biomedical birth of a Moroccan Muslim woman, who is blindfolded on a delivery table. (Archives of the Bibliothèque Nationale du Royaume du Maroc.)

disappear when the battle against obscurantism will have allowed the prejudices to fade away."[90]

However, French efforts to medicalize birth dispelled instead the French "sociology of Islam" mythologies about the Moroccan female body. Nancy Scheper-Hughes and Margaret Lock define medicalization as a reduction of social bodies to purely biological ones, and Cecilia Van Hollen sees medicalization as "biological disorders treated with biomedical interventions on individual bodies rather than with attempts to transform the *social* structure."[91] In Morocco, medicalization detached obstetrics from sociology and allowed French doctors to use purely clinical data to study Muslim birth. Consequently, French obstetricians in the years 1948–1956 began to identify actual problems in Muslim women's health and lay the human and infrastructural groundwork for a postcolonial Moroccan obstetrics. The social history of PMI in Morocco illustrates the distance between the ideologies of colonial policy and the applied reality of medical practice, a space that has produced the maternal and infant health programs of UNICEF, the World Health Organization, and the Moroccan Ministry of Health.

In the early years of the protectorate, French doctors assumed a "pathological Muslim body," a notion derived from the French sociology of Islam. Muslims were thought to be highly sexual, perverse, and therefore syphilitic. The Moroccan woman was believed to give birth rapidly and easily like an animal; the rural woman was described walking into the fields, squatting to give birth, cutting the umbilical cord herself, and resuming work with the baby tied to her back.[92] "Frequent sexual intercourse" and "Arab habits" like sitting cross-legged on the floor were said to "widen" the Arab pelvis, which Dr. Renée Lacascade "documented" in her 1922 Paris medical thesis (see Fig. 6.7). The idea of "easy birth" contradicted the few incidences of Muslim childbirth that doctors actually encountered: "You will find the most unexpected cases of dystocia: [infant] shoulder impacted *for several days* with uterine rupture and fetus passed partly into the abdomen."[93] Native midwives were blamed for all birth complications: "It is not the maternal organism that constitutes a danger at birth; it's the ignorance of the *gabla*."[94]

Once doctors had attended thousands of Muslim births in PMI maternities, however, clinical statistics dispelled both the "syphilitic Arab" and "the Muslim pelvis." Dr. G. Decrop of Tangier reported that only 5 percent of 254 Muslim births showed even a *probability* of syphilis; the Rabat maternity found only 1.8 percent of Muslim patients possibly

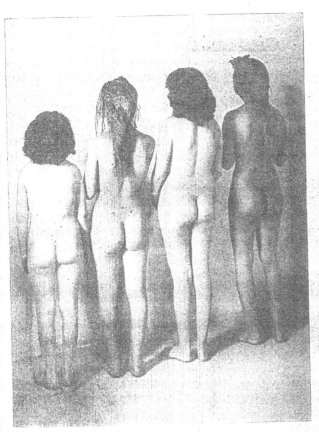

Losange lombo-sacré très aplati.

FIGURE 6.7. The "widened" Muslim woman's pelvis, which the author claims was produced by "Arab habits" such as sitting on the floor and being carried on the mother's back in infancy. (Lacascade, *Puériculture et colonisation* [1922].)

syphilitic, with no infected babies.[95] In Casablanca, only 10 of 1,530 Muslim mothers tested serologically positive for syphilis (0.55 percent).[96] The "wide Muslim pelvis" was also a myth, and rather than easy birth, statistics showed that Muslim women suffered a higher incidence of bad presentations, more maternal mortality, more "narrowed pelvis," and more stillbirth than Europeans or Jews at the Marrakesh maternity over the period 1927–1946.[97] Muslim women accounted for 91 percent of craniotomies, 91.6 percent of embryotomies, all cases of impacted shoulder, and all uterine rupture. Muslim birth was dystocic because, as a Rabat obstetrician observed, "One knows the most difficult cases are reserved for the maternities . . . Of the 13 deaths in 1951, 8 took place on the examining table . . . This makes the maternity more emergency room than normal maternity."[98]

The new visibility of Muslim bodies revealed the devastating effects of malnutrition on childbearing women in Rabat and Casablanca. Obstetricians found a "flattened, corrupted pelvis" in 33 percent of Muslim women, a condition that paradoxically afflicted only multiparous mothers. After birthing several normal children, the woman's pelvis suddenly narrowed during the third, fourth, or fifth pregnancy.[99] X-rays revealed a general decalcification of the mother's skeleton; as each successive fetus drew nutrition from her bones, the mother's bones softened, the pelvis collapsed, and her long bones exhibited the "pseudo-fracture" of Milkmann-Debray-Looser syndrome, a condition normally found in the elderly.[100] Mothers lost further nutrients during the customary year or two of nursing, and many lost the ability to walk. When patients were provided with adequate food—calcium and vitamin D—recovery was "spectacular":

Barka Bent Allal, aged 23. Entered Rabat maternity September 28, 1952 for fourth birth. 1947, first pregnancy normal. 1949, second pregnancy, after fourth month, pains in sacral region that worsened until total inability to walk, which ended after birth . . . 1950, third pregnancy, pain begins in sixth month and immobilizes her. After normal birth she remains bedridden two months. 1952, fourth pregnancy, pain starts in third month, inability to walk. Exam reveals: bad general condition, wasting of large muscle groups, painful manipulation of leg articulations. Pelvic exam shows: narrow pelvis, 8 cm useful diameter, presentation cannot engage, needs cesarean. X-ray reveals: pseudo-fracture in fibulas, pelvic girdle, both femurs, right ribs (2,3,4,5) . . . Treatment: Vitamin D and Calcium. Evolution: Spectacular improvement of general state, disappearance of pain, left hospital walking.[101]

In Morocco, French obstetricians exercised a surgical fearlessness shocking to their metropolitan colleagues. Antibiotics enabled heroic procedures, wrote the Rabat obstetrician Jean Marmey, who advocated "corporeal cesarean section," a bisection of the woman's entire abdomen to lift her uterus from the body. "Thanks to perfect visibility," he enthused, the exteriorized uterus "presents the advantage of easy execution," despite "inconvenient" shock and massive blood loss.[102] Moroccan obstetricians also practiced symphysiotomy, a controversial procedure in which the cartilage linking the halves of the birthing woman's pelvic girdle is bisected to allow an impacted fetus to pass. Obstetricians in France had rejected symphysiotomy in the eighteenth century because it could cause urinary fistula, hemorrhage, and permanent difficulty walking.[103] Alphonse Laffont, professor of obstetrics at the Faculté d'Alger, scoffed at Muslim patients who called French maternities "the places where one operates, and one dies."[104]

Nevertheless, obstetrical surgery solved otherwise deadly birth complications for Muslim mothers and families. Nonsurgical birth should not be romanticized; in Legey's Marrakesh maternity, of the twenty-four Muslim forceps births, fourteen ended in craniotomies for the infant, 1927–1946.[105] Cesareans saved such children; when doctors performed 153 cesareans on Muslim women in Rabat in 1941–1952, maternal mortality was 4 percent and infant mortality 6 percent.[106] As for symphysiotomy, the procedure was (and is) practiced in Africa and Latin America. The Brazilian physician Enrique Zarate revived symphysiotomy in the 1920s because he encountered conditions in Brazil similar to those in Morocco: women arrived at the hospital, after days of labor, exhausted, infected, and near death.[107] Moroccan obstetricians adopted Zarate's symphysiotomy to deliver a mother with an infected uterine cavity, for a cesarean incision would generalize the infection to the abdomen and could produce blood sepsis. Symphysiotomy was also performed to save a live infant whose head was trapped in utero and in desperate cases when speed was essential, but doctors agreed that it was a medical procedure of last resort.[108]

PMI doctors used female French social workers to teach Muslims motherhood, yet expected "rational" French women to transcend childbearing themselves. Male doctors praised Germaine de Staël (1766–1817), who "had a baby and a conversation with equal ease." The Muslim woman, by contrast, was described as a fertile womb with "no life aspirations beyond maternity and marriage" obliged to bear numerous children for the "populationist" Muslim patriarchal family.[109] Charles Bouveret and Pierre Vallery-Radot quoted Pierre Nobécourt of the Paris Medical School, who insisted that motherhood was a physician's science: "[Mothers] are in serious error if, having acquired simple notions of the art of raising children, they forget the insufficiency of their knowledge . . . thus costing the lives of so many tiny beings."[110] None of the young female social workers recruited from France by the PMI were mothers themselves; the SHP *médico-social* director François Cauvin explained that they were to "tame" Muslim mothers for the French doctor:

> [The Muslim woman] will be welcomed into a house that is hers, from which all masculine presence is excluded . . . One will first interest her in the little being she carries in herself; teach her hygiene practices . . . Of course, the evil eye and traditional rites will come up in conversation, the teacher will be asked questions, the responses will dissipate fears. They will allow themselves to be examined as many times as necessary by the French midwife. The delivery will take place in the maternity, and she will return with the newborn to the second section of the school, reserved for young mamas, where she will learn to nurse rationally.[111]

He considered Muslim women too primitive for actual instruction, but he believed they could "repeat gestures" of cooking, sewing, and hygiene modeled for them by a female social worker.[112]

In France, *puériculture* sought to fashion children into citizens; in Morocco, PMI was to inculcate the future native workforce with modern ideas of time and work.[113] The SHP director Bonjean explained, "Moroccans, like all Orientals, place civilization on another level than reason and scientific research; it is to the lower world that the Occidental clings as supreme reality, whereas the Oriental seeks reality in the transcendent."[114] PMI "gestures" would replace religion and women's superstitions with bodily discipline and a time schedule. Muslim mothers swaddled their infants against the body, which, doctors complained, smothered them physically and psychologically (see Fig. 6.8). Instead, the baby was to sleep alone in a sunny, well-ventilated room with arms and legs free to develop his independence. The Muslim woman offered her breast without discipline, "at the least fear, the least cry," and must instead be taught to nurse on a strict schedule.[115] Hygiene would rescue babies from contaminated food and dirty clothing: "Most of these newborns have skin infections, and some succumb to generalized blood infection through the skin."[116]

PMI doctors aimed to eliminate Muslim traditional midwives and thus "esoterism and the occult" from domestic life.[117] The Moroccan man in

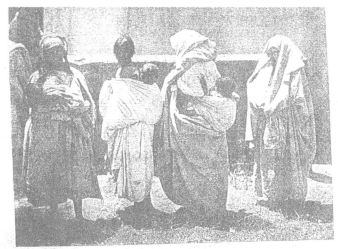

FIGURE 6.8. Muslim swaddling. 1. The baby nurses, he will take his place on the back of the mother. 2. The baby is awake, his mother lifts her *haik* to show him. 3. The baby sleeps covered by the *haik* despite the extreme heat. 4. The baby is forty days old, he is carried in front, draped by the *haik*. (Lacascade, *Puériculture et colonisation* [1922].)

his blue jeans resembled a "civilized worker," wrote Mathieu and Maneville, "but he isn't. Our man still belongs to the Middle Ages, and he is as far from us as the *qabla*."[118] The Moroccan used electricity, telephones, worked in the factory, visited the cinema, and drank Coca-Cola, but returned to a medieval home of Islamic genies, magic, and the evil eye. The French-trained *muwallida* was intended to revolutionize this female Muslim world and unseat her elders with a positivist approach to birth and family life. Unlike the elderly *qabla*, "whose notions of obstetrics never come from observation, facts, or experience,"[119] the *muwallida* observed births, wore sterile gloves, and charted the baby's descent to the cervix.[120] Maneville wrote proudly of a seventeen-year-old *muwallida* who delivered a child for her own mother "without any sentiment of modesty or embarrassment for mother or daughter."[121]

Despite Mathieu and Maneville's intent, their study *Les Accoucheuses musulmanes traditionelles* reveals the *qabla* as a competent midwife with sophisticated techniques. *Qablat* supported the perineum to prevent tearing, used external maneuvers to turn a bad presentation, applied crushed beef ticks to torn tissues as a coagulant, and restarted dilation either by inserting an oiled finger into the vagina, performing Kristeller massage, or putting a wool tampon into the woman's anus. Midwives identified bad presentations: *occiput posterior* (*mqabbel*, or turned), frank breech (*bu faris*), and complete breech (*mqa'ad*, or seated). When Mathieu and Maneville asked about magic rituals such as throwing salt to remove the *jinn*, *qablat* laughed at "charming myths that never existed." Saintly practices were limited to invocations, "O Mawlay 'Abd al Qader [al-Jilani], flap your wings, O Angel of God, deliver the *nfisa* (bride), O Messenger of God."[122] If saints were disappearing from birth, Galenic physiology remained; the mother was tightly belted to "encourage the womb to return to its place" and she was fed hot, blood-generating foods to create breast milk: okra, garlic, cumin, sardines, pullets, ginger, olive oil, *m'hamsa* (a small pasta), clarified butter (*smeeda*), and pounded nuts (*sellou*).

The study also revealed that the *qabla* remained the principal Moroccan authority in birth, even as she accepted French medicine. Mathieu and Maneville complained that even the most "evolved" *muwallidat* accepted the existence of the "sleeping child" and abandoned some French techniques upon graduation in favor of learning *qabla* remedies.[123] In 1949, only 1.49 percent of Muslim women in Casablanca gave birth in a hospital.[124] Though doctors rejected *qablat*, traditional midwives accepted French doctors; *qablat* sent their clients with birth complications to deliver at the French maternities, and if a *qabla* believed a new mother to be syphilitic, she washed the newborn in sterilized water, forbade breastfeeding, and recommended iodized potassium pills from the SHP.[125] Economic conditions were transforming birth itself and the poorest women suffered the classic indicator of industrialization: child abandonment. Mathieu and Maneville recorded the case of a young girl who gave birth alone near a Casablanca shantytown, cut the cord between two rocks, and walked the streets of the New Medina crying, "*Chkun elli ibri l-wuld? Chkun elli ibrghi l-wuld?*" ("Who wants a child? Who wants a child?").[126]

In implementation, the PMI programs were quite different from the ideological designs of the SHP. Noëlle Courtecuisse, a PMI social worker who provided pre- and postnatal care in the Douar Doum shantytown in Rabat (1948–1950), became the PMI regional director (1950–1952). She created five PMI centers in Fez and ten PMI centers in Casablanca after independence (1952–1962). Arriving in Morocco at age twenty-five, Courtecuisse described herself as "senior" to the other social workers: "We were all single, and we stayed single, almost all of us. [The Moroccans] called us 'masoeurwat,' (*ma soeur*, or 'sister'), because we lived in a collectivity, like a convent."[127] The SHP launched public health initiatives like BCG vaccinations, the census, and the addition of powdered fish bones to fortify children's food, but Courtecuisse explained: "We were the agents on the ground." Female social workers created PMI centers as lived reality. "There was no model," Courtecuisse said. "We were the model, each created it according to her manner, her personality, each one did with what she has."

In practice, PMI social workers focused on developing Moroccan female leadership in cooperation with local medical authorities: "What is important for us in Morocco, it is to find the leaders, the women leaders. Because it's not through us that it will happen, it is through the women leaders that the trust of women will be gained." A law of 1950 required Moroccans to declare births to the municipality and present a certificate of vaccination from the PMI clinic, but Courtecuisse relied on personal relationships with Muslim women rather than law to ensure that Muslim babies were vaccinated:

> We noticed that if a woman comes to see us regularly, if it's a woman who accepts our advice, who has a desire to progress, to act. If we have a woman of this sort who invites us to her home—it happened to me often, that one is invited to her home to drink a glass of tea, and she invites her neighbors. And from that moment, if the neighbors come, it shows that she has an influence. Because the neighbors know I will be there, and if they come, then it means they accept [me], and we have tea and cookies, and discuss the problems of children.

The dangerous "matrons" of male physicians' writings are "grandmothers" in Courtecuisse's account, older female relatives who "disagreed about little things, the food for the baby, or when to start eating couscous . . . And for them we [PMI social workers] were little girls, too young to give advice." Courtecuisse gave native midwives silver nitrate eye drops to administer to newborns and a kit of sterilized instruments. She walked the shantytown streets in a white lab coat and called herself *toubiba* (doctor), but SHP doctors disagreed with her methods and accused her of treating Moroccans too much like Europeans: "When I discussed with certain doctors, they found this absurd . . . They said in a country like this, they [Muslim populations] won't understand it. We were not of this idea, because it's through women that we could change the country."

Despite its ideological origins, protectorate PMI constituted the bridge to postcolonial maternal and infant care. Courtecuisse's Moroccan career coincided with the Independence Manifesto of 1944, the coup against King Muhammad V in 1953, and acts of political terrorism, yet nationalists did not attack PMI clinics. *Istiqlal* members attended the 1949 funeral of a social worker in Fez, and the first Moroccan minister of health, Abdalmalik Faraj, invited Courtecuisse to create PMI centers in Casablanca shantytowns and to help open a national school of social work in 1956.[128] When the national school provisionally closed in 1962, the Moroccan prime minister, Muhammad Benhima, wrote, "We had hoped that the social medicine problems of Morocco would be found in the creation of a corps of national social workers . . . It's too bad, for the Moroccan woman and for the country."[129] Many former colonial doctors transitioned to become the global physicians of international health; Georges Sicault, a former director of the Protectorate Health Service, left Morocco in 1956 to join UNICEF, an organization founded by his father-in-law, and to represent the United Nations Children's Fund (UNICEF) to the World Health Organization's Committee on Maternal and Child Health.[130]

The career of Aicha Ech-Channa, the director of the Moroccan nongovernmental organization Solidarité Féminine and the recipient of the 2009 Opus Prize, illustrates the link between PMI and postcolonial Moroccan women's health. In a 2012 interview, Ech-Channa recounted that her first exposure to maternal and infant health was in 1958, working as a seventeen-year-old PMI volunteer in Casablanca. Noëlle Courtecuisse called Ech-Channa to her office and advised her to take the entrance exam for nursing school, though she had no baccalauréat degree. Courtecuisse then interceded with the Moroccan Ministry of Health to obtain a salary and fellowship for Ech-Channa, to finance her studies and to support her dependent family members. Ech-Channa became a social worker and created Association de Solidarité Feminine in 1981, an NGO that prevents child abandonment by providing unwed mothers with job training, housing stipends, medical assistance, and child care. For the Moroccan feminist Fatima Mernissi, Ech-Channa is "like the saints of our traditional madina." She "give[s] us the energy to imagine a luminous Morocco where a reformed state cooperates closely with an energized civil society to assure children's security, regardless of social class."[131]

FOUNDING A SCIENTIFIC NATION:
AL-FASI, AL-WAZZANI, AND THE *PLAN DE RÉFORMES*

On December 4, 1937, a Tunisian nationalist addressed an open letter to the Moroccan nationalist 'Allal al-Fasi, "the great victim of French imperialism," who had been exiled to French Gabon by protectorate authorities: "From your 'place of residence' in this Equatorial Africa ravaged by the tse-tse fly of deadly bites, you [can] meditate upon a great lie that is simultaneously a great hypocrisy, '*La Civilisation*,' which one could more accurately call 'Barbarism multiplied by Science.'"[132] But even as nationalists across North Africa attacked France for her hypocritical "civilizing mission," they adopted French definitions of sovereignty, citizenship, and scientific modernity. The 1935 Congress of North African Muslim Students resolved that "true scientific culture" must be inculcated "into the brains of North-African children" to combat "women's ignorance, heretical [that is, Sufi] practices, and the ignorance of religion."[133] In their efforts to define a scientific Muslim nation, North African nationalists thus continued the French modernist project in Islamic guise. As Abdellah Hammoudi has observed, "When one realizes that an identical project of modernization occupies the center of colonial and nationalist approaches, the opposition between them seems less radical."[134]

The nationalists Hasan al-Wazzani and 'Allal al-Fasi adopted positive science in order to define the independent Moroccan nation-state. In *Al-Harakat al-istiqlaliyya fi al-maghrib al-'arabi* (1947), 'Allal al-Fasi redefined the Moroccan *umma* as a self-determining nation existing from prehistory and known by its "love of freedom."[135] That nation "enlightened and guided Europe in its progression to modern civilization," according to al-Wazzani, by bringing to Europeans the "sciences of Greece and Rome."[136] Yet the nationalists located sovereignty also in the sultan. "By sovereignty," wrote al-Wazzani, "one must logically understand the real right of the sultan to act freely internally and externally . . . the liberty of action of the sovereign as an incarnation of the absolute right of the State: liberty."[137] The *Plan de réformes marocaines* reproached France for failing to respect the sultan's authority *and thus* Moroccan sovereignty.[138]

The ambivalence of a sovereignty located simultaneously in the sultan and the nation was reconciled through a focus on the centralized state itself. Nationalists rewrote Moroccan history to become the history of the Moroccan state. The royal dynastic chronicle *Kitab al-Istiqsa' li akhbar duwwal al-maghrib al-aqsa* of Ahmad Khalid an-Nasiri was adopted as the official narrative of Moroccan history, and the saint-centered, miraculous *Salwat al-Anfas* of al-Kattani was rejected.[139] Moroccan saints like Muhammad al-Jazuli were recrafted as "protonationalists" who had paved the way for nationalism by creating a "religion of the people."[140] In this way, saints, sainthood, and saintly knowing were erased from the narrative of Morocco's history and replaced by a national and dynastic model of sovereignty.

Nationalists needed also to define the relationship of this Moroccan state to the citizenry-as-body. The public health crises of 1937–1956 engaged Moroccan nationalists in a public debate over health, medicine, and a welfare state. Nationalists agreed that Moroccan hunger, epidemics, and poverty were the result of "twenty-five years of exploitation of the native to the benefit the colonizer,"[141] and they first called upon protectorate authorities to guarantee Muslims the same medical benefits given to Europeans.[142] The nationalist Comité Executif argued that human need itself created a right: "It is not fair that the unemployment bureaus aid one element of the population and exclude the other, for hunger and poverty affect all persons without distinction."[143] As early as 1934, Abdalqadir Tazi argued that public welfare should be the basis of a new national Moroccan community: "I address myself to my compatriots moved by religious and nationalist pride: our brothers in humanity, in country, in religion, live like animals in a state of complete abandonment. The government has been powerless . . . to raise them from ignorance and misery. It is up to you, compatriots, to come to their aid, to help raise them materially and morally, for them to follow you and support you in your cause."[144] Nationalists oscillated between Islamic and republican languages for the new body politic; *Al Atlas* (April 2, 1937) looked to the Islamic institution of *zakat* (charity) for social justice, "uniting the rich and poor in moral and material solidarity." But most authors advocated a centralized, state-run welfare (*bienfaisance*) of *hubus* revenues. The *Majallat al-Maghrib* argued that *hubus* should serve the needs of the nation, not the wishes of individual donors, and should be distributed according to a mandatory civil status determined by census data.[145]

The modern Moroccan nation appropriated biomedicine as a right of citizens and a cornerstone of Moroccan sovereignty. *Al Hayat* argued that training Moroccan doctors was essential "to ensure the free and independent life of the nation,"[146] and nationalists called for medicine, pharmacy, law, and literature to be taught in a new, European-style university, the "Institut supérieur marocain."[147] In the *Plan de réformes*, the Comité d'Action Marocaine wanted public health to be reconstituted as a ministry under the sultan's direct authority, the "Viziriat de santé publique," which would multiply hospitals and tuberculosis clinics, install sewer systems, fight venereal disease, educate the public in hygiene, and ensure that a Moroccan majority was represented on Municipal Hygiene Bureaus and the Central Council of Hygiene and Public Health.[148] In 1936, al-Wazzani called for maternities to be created for Moroccan women in all urban centers, and the *Plan* envisioned paid state maternity leave, free pre- and postpartum care, and state allowances for breastfeeding mothers and for

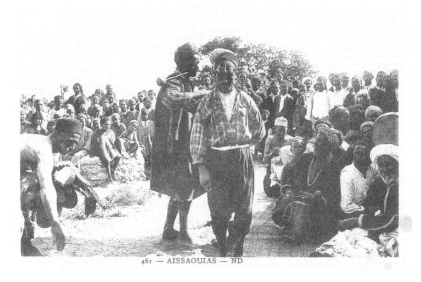

461 — AISSAOUIAS — ND

FIGURE 6.9. 'Isawa healing and the possessed Sufi body were embarrassments to Moroccan nationalists. Here Sufi healing is produced for tourist consumption as a postcard. (Author's collection.)

day care.[149] The first Moroccan minister of health after independence, Abdalmalik Faraj, argued that medicine must be state-directed and centralized in order to guarantee Moroccan unity and independence.[150]

The nationalists attacked Sufi healing as heretical, savage, and unscientific. Al-Fasi and the Qarawiyyin 'ulama' petitioned the sultan to outlaw saint mussems (celebrations for the saints), where "heterodox practices" perpetuated popular ignorance of "pure and noble Islam."[151] The newspaper L'Action du peuple applauded the prohibition of "the contemptible 'Isawa and other similar brotherhoods" and their "barbaric, savage practices" as a "great social reform."[152] Al-Wazzani condemned saintly healing as women's superstition and "public stupidity."[153] Al Alam complained, "[The people] do not understand the necessity of medical care and prevention . . . [Most] believe in superstition, magic and the intervention of angels and Satan in illness and cure."[154] The nationalists recognized a political dimension to Sufi trance, but they were equally embarrassed by the magical, emotional, possessed, unruly, "unmodern" Sufi body itself.[155] To the horror of al-Wazzani, European filmmakers recorded jinn-possessed 'Isawa "as if it were the present style in our country and defined the evolutionary social stage of our people." He protested, "Rather, one should show the other Morocco, the modern Morocco, of a new generation."[156]

Nationalist writers were fiercely protective of the Muslim family yet ambivalent about the forms of its modernity. 'Allal al-Fasi praised the family as the "mother of all social institutions"[157] and described marriage to a Muslim woman as a Muslim man's national duty:

> Muslims, my brothers, do not marry foreigners, for you will be guilty six times; You will be responsible for the forced celibacy of your Muslim sisters and commit a crime against your country. You will introduce a different mentality into your Oriental society and commit a crime against morality. You will introduce impure blood into your race and commit a social crime. You will introduce a foreigner into your home and commit a political crime. In preferring a non-Muslim, you consider passion before religion and commit a crime against religion. By accepting all these crimes, you will swallow your soul and commit a crime against humanity.[158]

The *Plan de réformes* made Muslim orphans the responsibility of the nation under a new Muslim "Conseil Supérieur de Tutelle" of the Ministry of Justice, which would assume control of Catholic schools and orphanages. *Al Akhbar* called for "national" mothers' schools: "If we wish a school for [Muslim] girls, we want instruction based on the Arabic language and the study of household arts, not a museum for tourists or an object of propaganda for a foreign country."[159] 'Allal al-Fasi demanded universal modern primary education for Muslim girls in the Arabic language, and the *Majallat al-Maghrib* proposed training Muslim women to be midwives, nurses, and doctors for women.[160] But the Muslim *délégué* to the Instruction Publique cautioned against unveiling, "contrary to Qur'an and morality," and limited girls' education to the Qur'an, religion, arithmetic, morality, homemaking, and hygiene, a program echoed in the *Plan de réformes*.[161]

Muslim birth highlighted the dilemma of appropriating French science for independent Morocco; as al-Wazzani wrote, "We wish to modernize, while remaining ourselves."[162] A certain A. Sfrioui wrote a passionate 1952 defense of traditional Muslim birth practices in *Maroc médical*, refuting both the sociology of Charles Le Coeur and the claims of French doctors. In birth, the child enters the "social and moral groups of Islam, his family, his locality," and his father "comes to murmur in the ear of the newborn the profession of Muslim faith, 'There is no God but God and Muhammad is the messenger of God,' the formula which will accompany his last sigh."[163] Sfrioui celebrates the henna festival for the mother and the clothing of the baby in a tiny chemise, *mansouria* (robe), *sematta* (belt), and turban. The baby enters society on his naming day, when a sheep is sacrificed and he is presented to the saints: "The little Fassi or Fassiya is thus offered to God and put under the protection of protectors of the city."[164] The Moroccan minister of education (1955–1958), Muhammad al-Fasi, collected Fez women's oral traditions as *Contes Fassis* (1926) in an effort to preserve and celebrate traditional Moroccan family rituals. Yet nationalists could not deny the superiority of biomedical birth, and Sfrioui concludes his article:

> To finish, I confide to you, in secret, that one of my friends, a very evolved Fassi, declared to me recently when his daughter was born, "I just broke with tradition. I had my daughter taken to a clinic where she was cared for without the *qabla*. The '*sabaa*' [first seven days] was reduced to the ritual sacrifice of a sheep."
>
> And I applauded for 3 reasons: the first that he thought at least to keep the sacrifice of a sheep, the second that he spared his neighbors several sleepless nights [of celebrating], and the third, and principal, that the birth was practiced by a doctor.[165]

WITH RAPID COLONIAL INDUSTRIALIZATION IN Morocco, the protectorate began to consider the entire Muslim population as a valuable resource, part of *Maroc utile*. Native tuberculosis led France to deploy a new welfare state intended to preserve the health of the Moroccan population and prevent anticolonial revolution. This colonial developmental strategy was later reprised as the Plan de Constantine (1959–1963) in French Algeria, which was also an effort to prevent national revolution.

The implementation of Protection Maternelle et Infantile (PMI) in Morocco reveals the peculiarities of biopolitics in a colonial setting. As Foucault argues, the "juridico-deductive" strategy of governing must first establish an individual's natural rights and then construct a state to rule him.[166] French physicians imagined a clash between the modern world and their own ethnographic construct—the Islamic *mentalité*. By replacing the Muslim *qabla* with a French-trained birth attendant and teaching Muslim mothers to prepare food, nurse babies, and keep house, French doctors attempted to rescue Muslims from their own *mentalité*. Colonial biopolitics attempted to reconstitute Moroccans as rational political subjects, to protect them as economic resources, and to build from them a body politic to govern.

In Moroccan nationalism, we find an Islamic appropriation of biopolitics; nationalists framed the struggle for independence as a defense of the

Muslim family, the Islamic religion, and the health of Moroccan bodies. In newspapers and the *Plan de réformes*, nationalists used famine and disease as irrefutable evidence of the failure of French rule. Yet nationalists adopted the French positive language of science even as they indicted French colonialism. Nationalists demanded biomedicine as a citizen's right and rejected saintly healing as superstition and *shirk*. The postcolonial Moroccan state has institutionalized its own version of patriarchal power with the *Mudawanna* (1957), a personal status code that renders the patriarchal family the only means by which newborns can acquire full civil status in Morocco.[167] The inscription of bodies into law and bureaucracy is essential to biopolitical power, a project begun by France and continued by the postcolonial Moroccan state after independence.

Yet in postcolonial Moroccan health, we find medical, institutional, and human networks operating according to semi-independent logics; medicine does not necessarily multiply the power of the state.[168] The period 1936–1952 laid the foundations for the internationalization of Moroccan health care and created a human bridge to postcolonial medicine. The patterns of morbidity continue: Morocco reported 104 new cases of tuberculosis per 100,000 persons annually in 2004, with one-fifth of all cases found in Casablanca.[169] The country has adopted the WHO Global Plan to Stop TB for 2006–2015. Malnutrition continues to affect Moroccan reproduction, since the Moroccan food supply still relates to the global economy and international money systems.[170] Health care remains international; the WHO, Red Cross, the United States Agency for International Development (USAID), and UNICEF still cooperate with the Moroccan Ministry of Health.

But in the history of PMI we also glimpse an articulate body, a body telling its truth despite colonial or nationalist biopolitical schemes. In the Moroccan woman's collapsed pelvis and the Moroccan infant's kwashiorkor, the body itself testified. The body itself showed that the destruction of human reproduction in Morocco was due, not to a Muslim *mentalité*, but to a political regime that deprived human beings of the basic right to physical survival.

EPISTEMOLOGIES EMBODIED:
ISLAM, FRANCE, AND THE POSTCOLONIAL

IN 1999, I INTERVIEWED elderly Moroccan patients at a public health clinic in the Lamtiyyin neighborhood, a working-class area in the traditional city (*madina*) of Fez. "Do you want to meet a real hero?" asks Mawlay 'Ali, in his seventies. "My mother is ninety-five years old, and she gave birth by herself." I became a frequent guest at the home of his mother, My Khaddouj, a tiny woman who explained to me that the powers of *baraka* (blessing) given to her by God protect her from illness, keep her hennaed hair free of grey, and allow her to deliver babies safely. At the same time, she describes "falling down" with typhus fever in the 1940s and shows me the milky cataracts spreading in her eyes. The paradox of a body at once healthy and sick, impervious and diseased, spiritual and biological, suggests the multiple frameworks through which Moroccans understand the human body. This fragmented body expresses different and layered ways of knowing—Sufi and positive epistemologies—and the competing models of sovereignty they evoke. It is a historical artifact of the Moroccan experience with French colonialism and an emblem of the Islamic postcolonial condition.

The legacy of French colonial science is most visible in Moroccan nationalism and state public health. To defend Morocco from colonialism, early twentieth-century Moroccan reformers, scholars, and court officials imported the *salafi* thought of Oriental scholars and introduced state reforms guided by European scientific, technological, military, and financial advisors. *Salafiyya*, often misnamed "Islamic orthodoxy" or "juridical Islam," was an intellectual attempt in the nineteenth and twentieth centuries to reconcile positive science, modernity, and secular law with Islam. A *salafi* definition of Moroccan modernity was normative by 1919–1926; thus, the Rif Moroccan nationalist 'Abd al-Karim al-Khattabi led a revolution against Spanish rule to create an independent "Islamic republic" rather than a traditional Moroccan (*makhzan*) state. When Morocco became an independent country in 1956, the King Muhammad V asked many of the protectorate's French doctors and social workers to stay on as employees of the new Moroccan Ministry of Health.

A precolonial Sufi polity is difficult to imagine in modern Morocco, because the diffuse, invisible, miraculous Sufi knowing from which it arises is difficult to reconcile with the extension of a modern, liberal, centralized state. Moroccan nationalists attempted to purge the political arena of Sufi knowing and to substitute positive ideas of law, civilization, nation, social solidarity, and self. Yet Moroccan politics cannot escape Sufism. The Moroccan nationalist movement called itself a *zawiya*, the Islamist Shaykh Yassin of the 'Adl wa Ihsan Party (Justice and Righteous Conduct) claims the Sufi Muhammad ibn 'Abd al-Kabir al-Kattani as a spiritual forefather, and King Muhammad VI uses Sufi language in his public speeches and maintains official connections with Sufi orders. How then is Sufi knowing embodied and reproduced in the postcolonial era?

There is no longer a connection between the built environment and a public memory of the saints. In 2005, I retraced al-Kattani's footsteps through the city of Fez with the help of 'Ali Filali, a teacher at the Qarawiyyin secondary school, photographing the saints' graves in the mosques, houses, gardens, and shrines of Fez. Saint shrines of important families like the Sqalli and al-Kattani are maintained, but most graves have become workrooms, storage areas, or garbage dumps. In Saba' Luyyat (Seven Curves) neighborhood, we ask for al-Miyara, a nineteenth-century legal scholar of the Qarawiyyin Islamic University. A shopkeeper opens a small door in the wall and we enter a shady courtyard; sacks of cement and drifting plastic bags obscure the broken graves of Qarawiyyin scholars. Across the alley, al-Kattani writes that we should find the scholar Sidi al-'Aziz Tajibi, but all we see is a leatherworking shop. When I ask for Sidi al-'Aziz, the proprietor opens a sliding metal cabinet to reveal a stone surface—a saint in the closet. Most of the Sufi *zawiyat* (brotherhoods) are closed or sealed over with cement; a poor family squats in the crumbling *zawiya* of Ibn Suwwal and washes laundry in the marble basin of prayer ablutions. A twenty-eight-year-old Moroccan friend from a *sharifian* Fez family lives in the Fez *madina* but has little knowledge of Fez saints: "Yeah, we have a *sayyid* [*wali*, saint] buried in the floor of our house, but nobody knows who it is. My mom used to send us to Mawlay Idris with raisins and a pin for the school exams. You were supposed to eat each raisin with a pin and ask Mawlay Idris for help. So we ate the raisins and threw the pins away and hit on girls instead. A lot of girls go to Mawlay Idris."

But the Muslim body remains a site of Islamic Sufi knowing, of self-determination, and a potential base of resistance to the modern Moroccan state. Like many Islamic countries, Morocco has a thriving Sufi tradition at odds with its *salafi* nationalism, a reality made visible by the movement of the sick and afflicted between hospitals and traditional healers in a quest for therapy. Traditional healing has not disappeared; rather, there are integrations of traditional apothecaries, midwives, and *awliya'* with biomedicine. The Ben Shaqrun family maintains its traditional herbalist shops in the Fez *madina*, and one of its sons, 'Abd al-Latif ibn Shaqrun, has become chief of emergency services at Avicenna Hospital in Rabat. The saint shrines with natural springs like Mawlay Ya'qub near Fez boast modern medical facilities; the Mawlay Ya'qub shrine now also has a hydrotherapy spa and a five-star hotel. Visitors to the Sidi Harazem shrine have informally named a corner of the park "*laboratoire*," because those suffering from abdominal pain urinate into glass bottles after drinking the shrine's waters to see if kidney stones have emerged.[1] These instances of medical pluralism suggest a persistence of Sufi epistemology in social life through the health and healing of the Moroccan body.

TRADITIONAL HEALERS AND BIOMEDICINE: A CONVERSATION WITH BAHIA IN FEZ

An energetic woman in her sixties, Bahia calls herself a *qabla taqlidiyya* (traditional midwife), which she distinguishes from the midwife of herbal pharmacology, the *qabla al-'ashub* (midwife of herbs). Over a plate of cookies in her Fez living room, she opens a black medical bag to display her sterile gloves ("*ligat*," from *les gants*), disposable razors to cut the cord ("*zazoir*," from *rasoir*), "Sfasfo," (Spasfon, a pharmaceutical drug), "*borbo*" (talcum powder), a metal clamp, "red medicine" to wipe the vulva (Betadine), sanitary pads, scissors, hypodermic needles, bandages, and "Officine" (Roficine, silver nitrate drops) for the baby's eyes, all of which she buys at the local pharmacy. It is not surprising that Bahia delivered nearly as many babies in a single month of 1999 as did the public maternity clinic in the Sidi Boujida neighborhood. Dr. Fouad Bouchareb of 'Umar Idrisi Hospital estimated that 68 percent of women in Fez birthed at home with a midwife in 1999.[2] What is remarkable is that Bahia has appropriated and integrated elements of Western medicine to traditional midwifery practice. She attended a three-day state-run medical training, after which she assimilates biomedical remedies to a *qabla*'s mode of knowledge, a Galenic physiology, and the Moroccan *qabla*'s traditional relationships with women and children.

Bahia's medical knowledge is syncretic; she assimilates modern pharmacology and "microbes" to a Galenic physiology. She holds up a box of antispasmodic suppositories ("Sfasfo") and explains that they open the uterus through "heat," "That heat, the uterus climbs up with it, the baby stays pushing, and the uterus opens." Sterility is caused by "cold, microbes, or sitting in the dirt on the floor of the *hammam*," which she treats by stroking the woman's belly upward with warm olive oil to "open" the fallopian tubes that are "curled shut, curled down, or facing the wrong way." For "cold in the womb," Bahia has the woman insert a wool tampon filled with cumin *bildy* and olive oil, "It heats her up and foul-smelling water starts to come out of her . . . That water swelled up the mouth of the uterus. The swelling went down, the dirt starts to go out, and the water of the man was seized, and she conceived." Bahia clamps the umbilical cord after birth to prevent it from being sucked into the woman: "If she is [scared or shocked], it gives her a hemorrhage, or the placenta will climb up in her. If it climbs, she will need a *cortage* (curettage)." But Bahia also uses the black "seeds of Mercy" that hajj pilgrims bring to her from Mecca: "The womb breathes, and the body, and God gives." Bahia attributes cure itself to God; medicine is only a means (*sabab*).

Bahia retains the *qabla*'s extensive hands-on expertise in birth practice. She palpitates the woman's belly to ascertain the baby's presentation and adjusts it using gloved fingers lubricated with olive oil. For a partial breech presentation, she holds the baby's exteriorized leg, tells the woman not to push, waits for the contraction, then grasps the baby's second leg: "I don't pull or anything. I put a towel on the baby like this. I hold onto him, and I take his two legs like this, and I tell her, breathe. The contraction comes to her and I do the towel. He comes out with his hands like that. All of him comes out except for his head. I should not pull on him until his head comes out." Complete breech is *ty al-kitab* (the closed book), shoulder presentation is *farsi*, and she uses heat to turn a bad presentation: "I do heat and oil and I do a scarf, which I heat up, and I put the scarf on her belly, which heats the baby, and he turns." If he doesn't turn, or if the woman has "narrow hips," Bahia takes the woman to the hospital. Bahia uses Western medical instruments; for babies born "fainted, he doesn't talk," she puts a tiny aspirator in his mouth, "*l'oxygène*, so I take out the dirt (*al-waskh*), and we return to him breath (*an-nafas*)." She uses traditional remedies but explains their mechanisms in biomedical and Galenic terms. The postpartum mother should eat fish, chickpeas, acorns, sardines, walnuts, *bildy* chicken, pullets, onions, parsley, and cinnamon, because "there are *vitaminat* [vitamins] in it, it helps the woman, it cleans out blood, and she rests."

Bahia's career demonstrates that Moroccan midwives (*qablat*) continue their precolonial role as mediators of medical systems and integrate across epistemological, institutional, and cultural lines to provide care for mothers and newborns. As during the colonial period and PMI, women's personal relationships span the divide between European and Moroccan practitioners. Bahia credits a German nurse with encouraging her to become a *qabla*. After Bahia delivered her own sister-in-law in an emergency home birth on the living-room floor, the municipality sent the nurse to her house to follow up: "I told her, I don't deliver for people. But [the German nurse] said no, keep going in your work. Everything you do is good, *très bien*. I told you, she encouraged me a lot." Traditional midwives often provide a first exposure to birth for future Moroccan doctors; a local girl who assisted Bahia in the neighborhood is now an emergency-room obstetrician in Rabat. Bahia chose to give birth to her own children variously attended by a Muslim midwife, a female Christian doctor, a Jewish doctor, and "Monsieur Bat who does *cortage* at Ghissani hospital" for "a baby that died in my belly." She takes her clients to a private maternity clinic if she feels a cesarean section is necessary, but avoids doctors who "cut too quickly" or pressure her to provide clients for lucrative private surgical practice:

> Doctor Z. said, Even if you found that nothing is wrong with her, tell her it is *grave* [serious]. And send her to me, and I will do cesarean. I told him, no, my brother. Me, I don't sin. You take 5,000 dirhams and I take a sin. Why should I do that? . . . They like me, I was with the doctor, I go and open the drawer, I take out the medicine, and I take out shots and I take whatever I want. But when he told me those things, why would I do that? The woman is fine, she can deliver, why would I tell her that? Shame on me. So he can take money?

Bahia's mediation between families, the state, and doctors suggests an integral role that *qablat* could play in the public health service. As we walk the streets, Bahia indicates the children playing, "I delivered that one," "I did those too." The children call her *Mima* (Grandma), and her house is "boiling with small children" at the holidays. Families consult

Bahia for infant ailments, sterility, and sexual problems. In 1999, the Moroccan Ministry of Health incorporated midwives in a semiofficial capacity; after Bahia completed her three-day training with the Association Marocaine de Planification Familiale, she received official birth registration forms, "attestation of birth," and a rubber stamp with her name, telephone number, and the designation "*qabla taqlidiyya*." But as part of a larger effort to professionalize and medicalize childbirth, the Moroccan Ministry of Health ended the state training of traditional birth attendants after 2009, a development that is not necessarily positive for women's health outcomes.[3]

Bahia's syncretic midwifery bridges different medical epistemologies and technologies, suggesting the need for a critical rethinking of scientific categories. Seyyed Hossein Nasr has argued that Islamic and Western sciences are epistemologically incompatible, but we find "Islamic" and "Western" therapies are indistinguishable inside Bahia's black medical bag.[4] As Karla Makhlouf Obermeyer argues, biomedical and traditional birth in Morocco are not dichotomous terms but a flexible and syncretic uncertainty.[5] In the colonial period, traditional *qablat* and French-trained Moroccan women acted as cultural intermediaries—"middles"—translators of colonial medical categories and objects to a Moroccan world of bodies and social practice. It remains for us to undertake Nancy Rose Hunt's archeology of "remains and debris"[6] and to study Moroccan birth as a historically created lexicon of birth rituals, symbolically entangled objects, religious experience, and spiritual phenomena.

MEDICAL PLURALISM AS POLITICAL CRITIQUE

Four gentlemen, all septuagenarians in traditional crafts (tailoring, silk spinning, teapot manufacture, textiles) and lifetime residents of Lamtiyyin quarter, met me in March 1999 at the local clinic to explain health care in Morocco. The men complain bitterly of the failures of the independent Moroccan government to provide social assistance to the poor. The people "don't have money to buy medicines, they rip up that paper [the doctor's prescription], they wait until they die":

> We need to have good care in the hospital. Not a hospital that opens, they turn the light on, there is water in it, and there is no doctor, and there is no medicine. What benefit is that to us? It doesn't benefit us. We need the word and the deed . . . When the date of independence and freedom came, our brothers, the Muslims, took the responsibility. They didn't complete

their mission. They failed. They will tell you, there is no money, there is no budget. Where is the budget we saw yesterday [in the colonial period]? The budget of yesterday, where is it, and that of today? It went. It was eaten. We need that budget to be present again.[7]

"If the minister were here, I would speak to him with this tongue," insisted one man, "the minister carries the responsibility before God. Before God on the Day of Judgment, what happened to that Muslim community (*umma*), those terrible things, God will give them their right." These men do not reject biomedicine in favor of traditional Sufi healing; on the contrary, they demand biomedicine as a citizen's political right. But they use an older, precolonial language of sovereignty and rights to describe the Muslim polity. God has given His *umma* the right to life and bodily health, and God will punish political leaders who fail in their duty to act as servants of His community. The failure of the state is experienced viscerally in the suffering body—the body is the base of protest and the location of political sovereignty.

The medical protest of the Lamtiyyin men thus suggests a political imaginary different from both French republican and Moroccan *salafi* conceptions of the Moroccan body politic. There is an embrace of biomedical technologies, knowledge, and doctors. The men remember the epidemics of the protectorate period—*tifus* (typhus), *jarba* (mange), *bu hamrun* ("redness," or measles), *jadri* (smallpox), and *qra' (tinea capitis*, a fungal infection of the scalp)—and they attribute disease to microbes: "The reason is negligence in childhood . . . He doesn't wash himself well, he doesn't clean himself, and that stays until it becomes 'microbe,' until that sickness climbs up to the head. It is cured with a machine, with medicine and a machine."

But the men assert the superiority of Moroccan sainthood over positive science. They recount the story of a Moroccan doctor who studied in Europe and returned to Morocco to practice medicine in a big office. One day he was struck by *bu zellum*, a shooting pain from the base of the spine down the leg. After "getting tired of curing himself with medicines," the Moroccan doctor traveled to France to have the leg amputated. One *madame* in the hospital [a French nurse] told him, "You see, there is no medicine for the illness that you have. But there are marabouts [saints] in Morocco who can cure that illness. I will make an appointment for you, and I will give you the paper, and you will go to Morocco, and you will look for the marabouts. They are the ones that will cure you." He went to Taounat mountain and found the descendant of a saintly family, an 'Azami *sharif*, who "cut" *bu zellum* for him: "And they cut that stem with a knife, and he was cured, by the permission of God."

Healing reveals a Moroccan Muslim body at the intersection of divine and temporal worlds, an entity transcending time, biology, and the man-made state. The young Moroccan doctor travels to France, acquires French learning, and brings it back to Morocco, only to discover that Western positive (*zahiri*) sciences are useless to heal the deepest pain of his own body. The doctor suffers Stefania Pandolfo's fragmented Moroccan subjectivity, "the epistemological 'cut,'" a double exclusion from culture, community, and from the present.[8] His pain flows from this cut, an amputation that is an alienation from the land, from God's community, and from God's immanence. His cure offers a glimpse into the living Moroccan polity that breathes beside the official Moroccan nation-state, a body that only Sufi sainthood can restore to health and wholeness.

Medical pluralism, or the mixing of traditional healing with biomedicine, has been interpreted as dissent from the state, a result of the costliness of biomedicine, or an alternate conception of illness and the body. The quest for therapy in Lamtiyyin neighborhood demonstrates all three aspects. 'Abd al-Haq ben Yahya had "an illness in his back" that "caused a water to flow" out of his spinal column: "It comes out in drops, when it flows on the flesh, the burning [*hariq*] and pain [*wuja'*] begins." The pain increased until he walked stooped-over with a cane: "I went to Fauque [a French doctor in the local hospital], and they did an X-ray for me, the picture came out, they looked in my blood [*qallabat fi dimi*]." After the doctors failed to cure him, he sat in front of the hospital where an 'Azami *sharifa* found him:

> She said, sir, why are you sitting here? I told her, I have "rheumatise."
> She said, the "rheumatise," its solution is easy. You will bring capers, you will crush them up, and then you will eat them. I bought capers, I crushed them, sifted them from the chaff, I mixed it with honey, with that *sharifa*, God bring her goodness. I began eating it, until [bad] blood started to flow from my belly [*hawwad dim min al-kirsh diyali*]. "Microbe" went out of me, from the anus. It was in my back and my leg, from here it seized me.

In this cure, there is a confrontation between ways of knowing. Galenic physiology is present in the water (Greek humor) lodged in the man's back and leg, a "bad blood" that flows out from the anus, bringing relief.[9] 'Abd al-Haq's therapy narrative shows the limitations of Western biomedical knowledge and technologies (positive knowledge); the doctor can see inside the body with *radio, scanner, les analyses*, but French medicine provides visibility, not relief, and cannot cure pain. The human body is cured only by God's mercy (*baraka*), a healing communicated to the body by one of His saints, the ('Azami) *sharifa*. Cure evokes a transcendent Islamic body and the higher authority of Moroccan saintly knowing.

Medical pluralism is also an effect of economic injustice, and traditional therapies have become the refuge of the poor. Economics inspired 'Abd al-Haq to try capers to treat his wife's diabetes, because he was "unemployed and could not afford the pills": "We covered her legs in it [the capers], all during the night, her legs itched her, she scratches, and something came out of her, like fever [*harara*], that sugar came out of her." But capers are not a permanent solution. "My wife, she has the gallbladder. And she has the large intestine. The doctors said, 'You don't do the operation here, you must go to France. For France, she has to have three million [30,000 dirhams] to do the operation.' What should I do? If you would like to see these things with your own eyes, I have the *visitat* [papers] and the picture [X-ray]."

Another patient with "pain in his kidneys and back" started his therapy by drinking water from the Sidi Harazem shrine because it was less expensive:

> They say I need tests. They are very expensive and it is hard to do them.
> My son brought me water from Sidi Harazem, I drank that. He brought
> me 5 liters, you can buy it at Bab Ftuh for 3 dirhams. I brought some
> herbs from Ben Shaqrun, he gave me *haris al-hajr* [the stone-breaker],
> and I ate that for three months. The pain returned, and Ben Shaqrun said,
> you can take *skum* [asparagus]. And I said no, I need to go to the doctor.
> He wanted me to take the herbs, but I said it was time to go to the doctor.
> I couldn't sleep with the pain.[10]

TOWARD A POSTCOLONIAL POLITICS OF THE ISLAMIC BODY

We consider what colonial medicine in Morocco reveals about the body and biopolitics, welfare states imperial and post-colonial, and individual subjectivity.

First, biomedicine and biomedical technologies have their own logics, which often operate independently of the state. In theory, French medical technologies in Morocco could extend the control of the protectorate over Muslim women's bodies by rendering them readable and transparent. But the transparency of the biological body does not necessarily create state power, for the X-ray enabled Muslim women's bones to speak the true causes of Muslim maternal and infant mortality. Medicalization in Morocco was a constellation of factors: a new scientific visibility of the body, a new state inscription of bodies-as-texts into law, a divorce of clinical data from colonial sociology, and the social interaction of French and Moroccan medical actors—social workers, grandmothers, nurses, doctors, mothers, and midwives.

As Moroccan medicine has transitioned from colonial to international public health, Foucault's theory of liberalism as modern governmentality sheds light on the operation of biopower in a postcolonial world. Neoliberal states now claim that health inequities and death in the non-West are natural, the inevitable results of a "natural" global marketplace that operates beyond the legitimate purview of Western states to intervene. Lyautey's protectorate Morocco foreshadowed a postcolonial world in which transnational global economic systems exploit foreign labor, a technocratic governance that affects life, health, and death from oceans away. However flawed the French imperial welfare state may have been, it assumed at least partial responsibility for the health and reproduction of colonized labor. Postcolonial global capital abdicates all responsibility for the welfare of its foreign workers, a global regime in which "the most basic right—the right to survive—is trampled in an age of great affluence."[11]

Finally, this book argues for a reading of politics in the Islamic world as embodied, for the body as a mode of political analysis. In December 2010, the Tunisian Muhammad Bu 'Azizi (Mohamed Bouazizi) publicly destroyed his own body, thus bringing down the regime of then-president Ben Ali. The falls of the regimes of Saddam Hussein in Iraq and Mu'mar Qaddafi in Libya were concretized by the pulling-down and dismemberment of their public statues, the tearing of their photographic images. In Egypt, citizens collectively seized the public through a corporeal occupation of Tahrir Square in 2011; social media are no substitute for an actual bodily occupation of the public, the assertion of individual subjectivity in public space. The Muslim body remains a space where politics and sovereignty are imagined and debated. As a *Philadelphia Inquirer* reporter found shortly after September 11, 2001, residents of Kabul, Afghanistan, walked outside the city to touch the graves of Al-Qaeda fighters. When asked why he did this, a Kabul mechanic replied, "Because I heard it cured sickness, and because this government is illegitimate. It was set up by the Americans."

These examples require us to think beyond biopolitics as inscribing the body to biopolitics as a dialogue between citizen and body politic through the body, the Muslim body itself as forum and signifier. If we see the body and the body politic as intertwined, if, as Jean Comaroff contends, the body individual and the body social are "mutually constituitive," then we open alternate perspectives. Sufi and positive epistemologies coexist in a human being striving for self-definition. Rather than seeing the post-colonial Islamic body as an incomplete or failed modernity, we find embodiment-as-process, the work of a subjectivity making itself.

NOTES

INTRODUCTION

1. Mauchamp to Legation, January 7, 1906, Archives des Affaires Étrangères, Nantes (hereafter cited as AAE Nantes), Tangier Legation Series, Carton 342.

2. Comaroff, *Body of Power, Spirit of Resistance: The Culture and History of a South African People*, 8.

3. Arnold, *Colonizing the Body: State Medicine and Epidemic Disease in Nineteenth-Century India.*

4. Prakash, "Body Politic in Colonial India." On the limits of Foucault in the colonies, see Vaughan, *Curing Their Ills: Colonial Power and African Illness*, x.

5. Taussig, *Colonialism, Shamanism, and the Wild Man: A Study in Terror and Healing*, 5.

6. White, *Speaking with Vampires: Rumor and History in Colonial Africa*; White, "'They Could Make Their Victims Dull': Gender and Genres, Fantasies and Cures in Colonial Southern Uganda."

7. Boddy, *Wombs and Alien Spirits: Women, Men and the Zar Cult in Northern Sudan.*

8. Comaroff and Comaroff, "The Madman and the Migrant: Work and Labor in the Historical Consciousness of a South African People."

9. I owe this interpretation to Kugle, *Sufis and Saints' Bodies: Mysticism, Corporeality, and Sacred Power in Islam*, 13.

10. Bourdieu, *Outline of a Theory of Practice*, 94.

11. Comaroff, *Body of Power*, 6.

12. Kugle, *Sufis and Saints' Bodies*, 13.

13. Ibid., 33.

14. Ibid., 29.

15. Ann Laura Stoler first called for extending biopolitics to colonial history; see her *Race and the Education of Desire: Foucault's History of Sexuality and the Colonial Order of Things.*

16. Foucault, *The Birth of Biopolitics: Lectures at the Collège de France, 1978–1979*, 15–16.

17. Of this large literature, I mention only a few examples of state and missionary campaigns against traditional healing in sub-Saharan Africa: Boddy, *Civilizing Women: British Crusades in Colonial Sudan*; Ranger, "Godly Medicine: The Ambiguities of Medical Mission in Southeast Tanzania."

18. Foucault, *The History of Sexuality: An Introduction*, 143.

19. Latour, *We Have Never Been Modern.*

20. Pandolfo, "The Thin Line of Modernity: Some Moroccan Debates on Subjectivity," 142.

21. Ibid.

22. Ibid., 118.

23. Latour, *We Have Never Been Modern*, 37.

24. Thus answering a question that Pandolfo poses ("The Thin Line of Modernity," 141).

25. Laroui, *Les Origines sociales et culturelles du nationalisme marocain*.

26. Geertz, *Islam Observed: Religious Development in Morocco and Indonesia*, 44.

27. Messick, *The Calligraphic State: Textual Domination and History in a Muslim Society*; Winichakul, *Siam Mapped: A History of the Geo-Body of the Nation*.

28. Combs-Schilling, *Sacred Performances: Islam, Sexuality, and Sacrifice*, 25.

29. Mohammed Lahbabi, cited in Pennell, *Morocco since 1830: A History*, 297–300; Waterbury, *North for the Trade: The Life and Times of a Berber Merchant*.

30. Hammoudi, *Master and Disciple: The Cultural Foundations of Moroccan Authoritarianism*.

31. Latour, *We Have Never Been Modern*, 15–16.

32. Bazzaz, *Forgotten Saints: History, Power and Politics in the Making of Modern Morocco*.

33. Of this literature, I mention only the classic Hourani, *Arabic Thought in the Liberal Age, 1798–1939*, and two recent works: El Shakry, *The Great Social Laboratory: Subjects of Knowledge in Colonial and Postcolonial Egypt*, and Schayegh, *Who Is Knowledgeable Is Strong: Science, Class, and the Formation of Modern Iranian Society, 1900–1950*.

34. Thus I argue that the anti-Sufism of *salafiyya* is a consequence of the Islamic internalization of Western epistemology, not Wahhabi influence. For an overview of the question, see Sirriyeh, *Sufis and Anti-Sufis: The Defence, Rethinking and Rejection of Sufism in the Modern World*.

35. Mauchamp, *La Sorcellerie au Maroc, oevure posthume*, 103.

36. Bhabha, "Of Mimicry and Man: The Ambivalence of Colonial Discourse," in *The Location of Culture*, 85–92.

37. Conklin, *A Mission to Civilize: The Republican Idea of Empire in France and West Africa, 1895–1930*, 1–6.

38. See Noiriel, *État, nation et immigration: Vers une histoire du pouvoir* and "République et exclusion en France à la fin du XIXe siècle."

39. Wilder, *The French Imperial Nation-State: Negritude and Colonial Humanism Between the Two World Wars*, 1–10.

40. Ibid., 52.

41. Abi-Mershed, *Apostles of Modernity: Saint-Simonians and the Civilizing Mission in Algeria*.

42. Trumbull, *An Empire of Facts: Colonial Power, Cultural Knowledge, and Islam in Algeria, 1870–1914*.

43. Segalla, *The Moroccan Soul: French Education, Colonial Ethnology, and Muslim Resistance, 1912–1956*, 74.

44. Foucault, *The Birth of the Clinic: An Archaeology of Medical Perception*; Ackerknecht, *Medicine at the Paris Hospital, 1794–1848*; Comaroff, "Medicine: Symbol and Ideology."

45. Ellis, *The Physician-Legislators of France: Medicine and Politics in the Early Third Republic, 1870–1914*.

46. Curtin, *Death by Migration: Europe's Encounter with the Tropical World in the Nineteenth Century*.

47. Keller, *Colonial Madness: Psychiatry in French North Africa*.

48. Mauchamp, *La Sorcellerie au Maroc*, 75.

49. Wilder, *The French Imperial Nation-State*, 46–74.

50. Robert Delavignette, cited in ibid., 69.

51. L.-H.-G. Lyautey, "Du rôle social de l'officier dans le service militaire universel" and "Du rôle colonial de l'armée."

52. Rabinow, *French Modern: Norms and Forms of the Social Environment.*

53. Boubrik, *Saints et société en Islam: La confrérie ouest-saharienne Fâdiliyya.*

54. Mauchamp to the French Legation, September 25, 1906, AAE Nantes, Tangier Legation Series, Carton 342.

55. Watenpaugh, *Being Modern in the Middle East: Revolution, Nationalism, Colonialism, and the Arab Middle Class.*

56. Latour, *We Have Never Been Modern*, 20.

57. Mitchell, introduction and "The Stage of Modernity" in *Questions of Modernity.*

58. Latour, *We Have Never Been Modern*, 30.

59. Ibid., 31.

60. Ibid., 99.

61. Merleau-Ponty, *The Phenomenology of Perception.*

62. Turner, "Chihamba the White Spirit: A Ritual Drama of the Ndembu," in *Revelation and Divination in Ndembu Ritual*, 37–179.

63. Crapanzano, *The Hamadsha: A Study in Moroccan Ethnopsychiatry*, 1–11.

64. Mitchell, introduction and "The Stage of Modernity" in *Questions of Modernity.*

CHAPTER 1

1. The author mentions that they adopted the "blameworthy" (*malamatiyya*) style affected by some Sufi saints (al-Ifrani, *Nuzhat al-hadi bi akhbar muluk al-qarn al-hadi*).

2. Ibid., 238.

3. Feierman, "Colonizers, Scholars, and the Creation of Invisible Histories," 187; see also Feierman, "Healing as Social Criticism in the Time of Colonial Conquest."

4. Fabian, *Remembering the Present: Painting and Popular History in Zaire*, 297–298.

5. Cornell, *Realm of the Saint: Power and Authority in Moroccan Sufism*, xxxiv.

6. Feierman, "Colonizers, Scholars, and Invisible Histories."

7. Cornell, *Realm of the Saint.*

8. Al-Jilani, *The Book of the Secret of Secrets and the Manifestation of Lights [Kitab Sirr al-Asrar wa Mazahar al-Anwar]*, 7.

9. Laroui, *Les Origines sociales et culturelles du nationalisme marocain*, 71.

10. The sultan was invested by a public oath of allegiance; in the *bay'a* of 1822, the people of Rabat "swear before God and His angels to hear and execute the orders of the imam within the licit and possible . . . We obey him as God commanded us, and he respects our rights and those of all his subjects as God has prescribed" (Laroui, *Les Origines sociales et culturelles du nationalisme marocain*, 76–77). The sultan as servant of the *umma* is thus quite different from the autocratic philosopher-king of al-Farabi's "City of Virtue" (*al-madina al-fadila*).

11. Ibn 'Arabi, *At-Tadbirat al-ilahiyyah fi islah al-mamalakat al-insaniyya*, 23–59.

12. Chodkiewicz, *Seal of the Saints: Prophethood and Sainthood in the Doctrine of Ibn 'Arabi*.

13. Consider Titus Burckhardt's classical formulation, "Authentic Sufism can never become a 'movement' for the very good reason that it appeals to what is most 'static' in man, to wit, contemplative intellect" (Burckhardt, *An Introduction to Sufism*, 20). Sufi politics have been viewed either as a utilitarian use of religion by states (Ottoman and Safavid empires) or a politicization of Sufi brotherhoods as social actors. An emerging literature moves beyond these dichotomies to consider a Sufi way of politics. For example, Ross, *Sufi City: Urban Design and Archetypes in Tuba*; Heck, *Sufism and Politics*.

14. Rosenthal, *Political Thought in Medieval Islam: An Introductory Outline*, 157.

15. Patricia Crone argues that the Sufi path seeks freedom from the body, "The answer was that as long as they had bodies, humans had to accept their enslavement to the law . . . since it was from the union of body and soul that evil inclinations stemmed . . . it was by obeying [God's law] that humans could hope to acquire immortality as disembodied souls" (Crone, *God's Rule: Government and Islam*, 327).

16. Gellner, *Saints of the Atlas*; Geertz, *Islam Observed*.

17. The historians Abdallah Laroui and Amira Bennison have suggested that the Morocco of 1912 was already a nation (Laroui, *Les Origines sociales et culturelles du nationalisme marocain*; Bennison, *Jihad and Its Interpretations in Pre-Colonial Morocco: State-Society Relations during the French Conquest of Algeria*). Edmund Burke has also traced nationalism to the pre-protectorate period (*Prelude to Protectorate in Morocco: Precolonial Protest and Resistance*, 209).

18. On the Idrisids, see also Hart, "Moroccan Dynastic *Shurfa'*-hood in Two Historical Contexts: Idrisid Cult and 'Alawid Power."

19. Cornell, *Realm of the Saint*, 203.

20. Ibid., 206.

21. "Know, may God preserve you, that the Perfect Human Being is the axis (*qutb*) around which revolve the manifestations of being (*aflak al-wujud*) from the beginning to the end" (al-Jili, quoted in ibid., 210).

22. Ibid., 215.

23. Al-Andalusi, a Jazulite *shaykh*, quoted in ibid., 218.

24. Cornell notes the practical aspect of local pilgrimage, for the Portuguese occupied a number of Moroccan port cities and thus blocked access to Mecca by sea (*Realm of the Saint*, 180).

25. See also Abun-Nasr, *A History of the Maghrib in the Islamic Period*, 207–208.

26. Quoted in Cornell, *Realm of the Saint*, 270–271.

27. Ibid., 221–222, 183. Jazulite ideas are at the root of Moroccan tribal claims to *baraka* (Hart, "Making Sense of Moroccan Tribal Sociology and History," 14; Pennell, "Lineage, Genealogy and Practical Politics: Thoughts on David Hart's Last Work."

28. The Moroccan jurist al-Tawadi called the *awliya'* "places of refuge for the slaves of God . . . a door among the doors of His mercy"; al-Kattani calls them "a refuge for those who fear and a place for the sinners and rebels to find peace, and the afflicted to find sanctuary" (*Kitab salwat al-anfas wa muhadathat al-akyas bi man uqbira min al-'ulama' wa al-sulaha bi Fas*, 37, 40; my translation).

29. Al-Jazuli, quoted in al-Kattani, *Salwat al-anfas*, 35 (my translation).

30. Eliade, *The Sacred and the Profane: The Nature of Religion*; Franke, "Khidr in Istanbul: Observations on the Symbolic Construction of Sacred Spaces in Traditional Islam."

31. On the Marinids, see Shatzmiller, *The Berbers and the Islamic State: The Marinid Experience in Pre-Protectorate Morocco*; Abun-Nasr, *A History of the Maghrib*, 103–118.

32. Al-Jazna'i (Djaznâi), *Zahrat El-As (La Fleur du myrte), Traitant de la fondation de la ville de Fès; Texte arabe et traduction par Alfred Bel*, 34–35.

33. The Berber dynasties immediately following the Idrisids let the original grave of Idris II fall into ruin (Salmon, "Le Culte de Moulay Idris et la Mosquée des Chorfa à Fès").

34. The Marinid sultan was nevertheless killed in 1465, but Scott Kugle notes that Idris II was so essential to political legitimacy that the Sa'adiyyan dynasty expanded his shrine "to rebind the body politic together" (Kugle, *Sufis and Saints' Bodies*, 60–77).

35. Elite patronage of shrines often transformed social memory; see Wolper, *Cities and Saints: Sufism and the Transformation of Urban Space in Medieval Anatolia*, and Beck, "Sultan Isma'il and the Veneration of Idris I at Mawlay Idris in the Djabal Zarhun."

36. Michaux-Bellaire, *Quelques tribus des montagnes de la region du Habt*, 64.

37. Mawlay 'Ali, interview by the author, March 13, 1999, Lamtiyyin Clinic, Fez.

38. F., interview by the author, March 13, 1999, Lamtiyyin Clinic, Fez.

39. P. Brown, *The Cult of the Saints: Its Rise and Function in Latin Christianity*.

40. Ross, *Sufi City*; see also Nasr, *Islamic Art and Spirituality*.

41. Quoted in al-Kattani, *Salwat al-anfas*, 39. Al-Harithi called visitation "a cure and a light for the hearts"; his student Muhammad ibn 'Atiya said, "God purifies the heart of the visitor, like a white cloth washed of dirt." Others agreed that it is a "cure for the hearts and a rest for the body" (35).

42. Ross, *Sufi City*, 18–20.

43. Al-Jazuli, quoted in Cornell, *Realm of the Saint*, 217.

44. "[The pilgrim] reaches God the Highest by means of [the *wali*]" (quoted in al-Kattani, *Salwat al-anfas*, 37).

45. Martin, "Description de la ville de Fès, Quartier de Keddan."

46. Ibid. In Tangier, ten years after a former slave population came to work in the city (1885), a new *wali* appeared at the grand Sokko Square, "Sidi Bou 'Abid at-Tanji" (the Father of Slaves). The new *wali* was said to be a descendant of the Sus *wali* Sidi Ahmad ibn Musa, and the community erected a mosque on the grave. A French observer noted that it had been one of several unmarked graves (Salmon, "Notes sur les superstitions populaires dans la region de Tanger").

47. Nora, "Between Memory and History: *Les Lieux de Mémoire*."

48. For an excellent overview of scholarship on the body in Islamic studies and a Sufi theory of corporeality, see Kugle, *Sufis and Saints' Bodies*, 1–41.

49. Also Qur'an 51:20–21: "*There are certainly Signs in the Earth for people of certainty, and in yourselves as well. Do you not then see?*" For God's hands, see Murata, "God's Two Hands," in *The Tao of Islam: A Sourcebook on Gender Relationships in Islamic Thought*, 81–114. For God's creation of Adam, see Murata, *The Tao of Islam*, 9–11, and Kugle, *Sufis and Saints' Bodies*, 29.

50. From the *Sahih* of al-Bukhari, quoted in Homerin, "Ibn Taimiya's *Al-Sufiya wa-al-Fuqara*."

51. Legey, *Essai de folklore marocain: Lettre-Préface du Maréchal Lyautey*, 21 (my translation). Another popular version of an emanationist universe: "Moroccans think the world is composed of seven oceans, seven earths, and seven skies. The first

sky is the one we see, composed of solidified water, the second is iron, the third copper, fourth silver, fifth gold, sixth rubies, seventh light, and all of them are inhabited" (1).

52. For an Orientalist view, see, for example, Marçais, *Manuel d'art musulman: L'architecture Tunisie, Algérie, Maroc, Espagne, Sicile*; and Marçais, *Tunis et Kairouan*.

53. "One of the best men said that he saw the Chosen One [Prophet Muhammad] standing in al-Qila mountain outside Bab Al-Guisa and he was reading the Sura al-Ilaq Quraysh and arrived at the end of it asking for protection from all that is feared by means of the *baraka* of that imam [Mawlay Idris]" (al-Kattani, *Salwat al-anfas*, 70–74). The quotation is on 75.

54. Ibid., 38, 27.

55. Ibid., 68.

56. Quotation from the *da'wa* of Idris II, which resembles that of Muhammad. The *Salwat al-anfas* describes a writing between Idris's shoulder blades with the pen of the Almighty, "This one is from the lineage of the Prophet of God Muhammad, the messenger of God." Idris also resembles the Prophet physically: "White color which has drunk of red, the blackest eyes, curly hair, soundness of body, a beautiful face, a long, aquiline nose, beautiful eyes, wide shoulders, small palms and feet, a small opening between his teeth, eyes of deep black" (ibid., 63–64).

57. Ibid., 65–66.

58. Mawlay 'Ali, interview by the author, March 13, 1999, Fez.

59. Secret, "Rites et coutumes de l'eau," in *Les Sept printemps de Fès: Des airs, des eaux, des lieux; Fès, capitale thermale*, 76.

60. He was buried in a mill, and his companions bought a neighboring house, added to it, and made it a *zawiya* with a library (al-Kattani, *Salwat al-anfas*, 108).

61. Quoted in al-Kattani, *Salwat al-anfas*, 44. Al-Kattani says much the same himself: "If the visitor acts in a place from true *niya* [faith/innocence], then he benefits from that place without question" (43).

62. Al-Kattani, *Salwat al-anfas*, 183.

63. Kugle describes Idris II's tomb as "a royal court of a saint, open to the public, through which the people reconfirm their allegiance to God, to the Prophet whose message they strive to follow, to the king who rules them, and to each other as citizens of the urban space of Fez" (*Sufis and Saints' Bodies*, 59).

64. Al-Kattani, *Salwat al-anfas*, 40.

65. In the Najjarin neighborhood, a well-known shop called Hanut an-Nabi was said by residents to levitate in the air, for a *wali* inside lifted the people by the hand into the Prophet's presence (ibid., 164).

66. Ibid., 30, 32. Many healing practices thus used earth from the graves of the saints, either for eating or for making into a paste.

67. Al-Kattani: "Mawlay Ahmad bin Muhammad al-Sqalli ... visited ... Mawlay al-Tayyib ibn Muhammad al-Wazzani in Wazzan and took *baraka* from him. He gave him one silver coin and told him that some of his friends [adepts of the Tayibiyya order] ... would have followers in the city of Fez, because in the cities are the people of paper and God brought this to pass" (*Salwat al-anfas*, 164). The scholar 'Umar al-Sharqawi (d. 1260) was said to have received a certificate (*ijaza*) from the *qadi* of the *jinn* Shamharush (285).

68. Ibid., 142. It is worth noting that most of the scholars of al-Kattani's text who achieve *walaya* do so through meeting a Sufi *shaykh*, rather than scientific study.

69. Recorded in al-Nasiri, *Kitab al-Istiqsa li-Akhbar Duwwal al-Maghrib al-Aqsa*. The French translation, *Kitab elistiqsa li akhbari doual elmaghrib elaqsa*, is edited by Eugène Fumey.

70. Geertz collected this tradition in the area of al-Yusi's tomb (*Islam Observed*, 31–35).

71. The scholars (*'ulama'*) were often simultaneously Sufis and *shurafa'* (Burke, "The Political Role of the Moroccan Ulema, 1860–1912").

72. Al-Tabrani, "Al-Kathir," citing 'Ubada bin al-Samit; quoted in al-Kattani, *Salwat al-anfas*, 38.

73. Al-Kattani, *Salwat al-anfas*, 242–248.

74. Ibid., 281.

75. Ibid., 157.

76. Ibid., 158.

77. His bizarre behavior so outraged the people that the *qadi* had him hung in chains in the insane asylum (*maristan*). The next morning the *qadi* saw the *majdhub* pass by, stamping the ground with his feet, as was his custom. The people rushed into his cell and found the *majdhub*'s manacles closed and empty. Sidi al-Waryaghli was installed in a room in al-Sagha neighborhood, where the people visited him to be healed from sickness (ibid., 199–200).

78. Organic illness: Dols, *Majnun: The Madman in Medieval Society*, 1–173; possession: Crapanzano, *The Hamadsha*; radical asceticism: Ahmet Karamustafa argues that the *majnun* creates a wilderness for himself in society through his antinomian behavior (*God's Unruly Friends: Dervish Groups in the Islamic Middle Period, 1200–1550*, 1–23).

79. My Khaddouj, interview by the author, March 22, 1999, Fez.

80. Mawlay Ali, interview by the author, March 22, 1999, Fez.

81. Ibid.

82. Al-Jazuli, quoted in Cornell, *Realm of the Saint*, 185.

83. Quoted in Cornell, *Realm of the Saint*, 90.

84. Al-Kattani, *Salwat al-anfas*, 151–152. A "hair pulled from dough" describes how the angels extract the soul from the body after death (Halevi, *Muhammad's Grave: Death Rites and the Making of Islamic Society*).

85. Al-Kattani, *Salwat al-anfas*, 152.

86. Murata, *The Tao of Islam*, 14.

87. Ibn 'Arabi, quoted in al-Kattani, *Salwat al-anfas*, 242–248.

88. For colonial-era studies of Mawlay Ya'qub, see Secret, "Moulay Yacoub: 12 ans de consultation thermale," in *Les Sept printemps de Fès*, 95–100; Meynadier, "Les eaux chloro-sulfurées-sodiques de Moulay-Yacoub"; "Stations climatiques et hydrothermales du Maroc."

89. The eponymous "Lalla Shafiya" (Secret, "Rites de magie thermale: La journée d'un berbère à Moulay Yacoub").

90. Muhammad ibn Ja'far al-Kattani, quoted in Michaux-Bellaire, "Description de la ville de Fès," 308. Pilgrims often radically transformed saints' biographies in popular memory (Renaud, "État de nos connaissances sur la médecine ancienne au Maroc: Programme d'études et sources d'investigations").

91. On Galenic medicine in Morocco, see Renaud, "État de nos connaissances"; Leclerc, *Histoire de la médecine arabe*; Faraj, *Relations médicales hispano-maghrébines au XIIe siècle*.

92. Maimonides was born in Cordova, Spain in 1135 and lived in Fez in 1160 (Kraemer, "Maimonides and the Spanish Aristotelian School").

93. Goodman, *Ibn Tufayl's Hayy ibn Yaqzan*, 115.

94. Ibid., 149.

95. Ibid., 103.

96. Lawrence Conrad has argued that remedies against *jinn* and the evil eye are relics of pre-Islamic animism (Conrad, "Arab-Islamic Medicine"). Dols argues that Muslims learned *zar* healing from African animists or from Christians (*Majnun*, 174–260, 274–310).

97. See Pandolfo, "Detours of Life: Space and Bodies in a Moroccan Village"; Ensel, *Saints and Servants in Southern Morocco*; Combs-Schilling, *Sacred Performances*.

98. Thus Vincent Crapanzano and Bernard Greenwood separate organic from spiritual disease (Greenwood, "Cold or Spirits? Ambiguity and Syncretism in Moroccan Therapeutics").

99. Byron and Mary-Jo DelVecchio Good describe Ibn Sina's cosmology: "The Ptolemaic conception of concentric spheres, the Aristotelian understanding of the elements fire, water, earth and air, and the Plotinian view of the emanations of pure intelligences and souls" (Good and Good, "The Comparative Study of Greco-Islamic Medicine: The Integration of Medical Knowledge into Local Symbolic Contexts," 259).

100. Kuhn, *The Structure of Scientific Revolutions*.

101. Although al-Antaki was not himself a Moroccan, there are more manuscript copies of his *Tadhkira* in the National Library of Rabat than of any other medical text, and the Moroccan physician ʿAbd as-Salam ibn Muhammad ibn Ahmad al-ʿAlami (d. 1905) wrote a popularization of Antaki in the Fez dialect, *Diya an-nibras fi hal mufradat al-antaki bi-lugha Fas* (Light of the Lamp in the Vocabulary of Antaki in the Language of Fez). Nineteenth-century North African medical authors wrote glosses of the *Tadhkira*, including the Algerian ʿAbd ar-Razzaq al-Jazaʾiri, and French physicians in Morocco mention the *Tadhkira* as the most-studied medical text; see Renaud and Colin, *Documents marocains pour servir à l'histoire du "Mal franc," textes arabes, publiés et traduits avec une introduction*.

102. Al-Antaki, *Tadhkira awla al-albab wa al-jamia' li'ajbi al-ʿajab*, Chapter One, 2.

103. "Indeed it is established that phlegm, as analogized to food, is not well-cooked, and blood is cooked to a perfect balance, and yellow bile is as exceeding the balance but not burned, and black bile is burned" (al-Antaki, *Tadhkira*, 9).

104. Ibid., 103.

105. Marginalia from ibid., 4–5.

106. "If he organizes only the visible things using evidence as a means, this is the sultanate" (ibid., 2).

107. Islamic scholars often use the verb *fada* to describe the action of the Prophet Muhammad receiving revelation of the Qur'an from the Angel Gabriel.

108. "In gnosis, knowledge and being coincide; it is there that science and faith find their harmony" (Nasr, *An Introduction to Islamic Cosmological Doctrines*).

109. In particular, the animals, plants, sun, moon, life processes, and man himself are referred to as signs; see Qur'an 88:17–20, 16:68–69, 10:5–6, 87:2–5, 45:3, 42:29, 80:24–29, 30:22. See also Murata, *The Tao of Islam*, 11.

110. This may be why these physicians included "magic" remedies in their medical works (Musallam, *Sex and Society in Islam*).

111. Al-Antaki, *Tadhkira*, Section 4, 5.

112. For example:

The letters: a, h, Ta, m, f, sh, dh, b, w, y, n, S, t, Dh
The part of the body: hair on the head
The astrological sign: Aries
The nature: like fire

113. "Another *khatim* (seal) to prevent hemorrhage and miscarriage, even for animals: write the writing you see here on a lead tablet [*louh*] on Saturday of any month and hang it by colored silk thread" (al-Antaki, *Tadhkira*, Section 4, 199).

114. Muhammad brought revelation to the *jinn* as well as mankind (46:29–32); see also Philips, *Ibn Taymeeyah's Essay on the Jinn (Demons)*, 33.

115. For non-Qur'anic discussion of the *jinn*, in law, see Philips, *Ibn Taymeeyah's Essay on the Jinn*, 31–32. Contemporary interviews confirm Ibn Taymiyya's claim: "Yes, as we hurt them with that hot water . . . Them too, they hurt us. And if we didn't pour it, they don't hurt us" (My Khaddouj interview, March 22, 1999).

116. Schimmel, "Aspects of Mystical Thought in Islam."

117. Philips, *Ibn Taymeeyah's Essay on the Jinn*, 17.

118. Al-Kattani, *Salwat al-anfas*, 23.

119. A *sharif* spit three times in the eyes of patients to cure chronic eye infections, trichiasis, corneal ulcers, and granular conjunctivitis; the 'Isawa spit in the throats of patients with sore throats; even Moroccan Jews collected the saliva of all men praying in the synagogue and used it to treat eye ailments (Legey, *Essai de folklore marocain*, 142). On saliva as a transfer of *baraka*, see Bakker, *The Lasting Virtue of Traditional Healing: An Ethnography of Healing and Prestige in the Middle Atlas of Morocco*, 179. There is precedent for this in the Sunna of the Prophet, for Muhammad cured his son-in-law 'Ali by spitting in his eyes; see Lings, *Muhammad: His Life Based on the Earliest Sources*. For the practice of dissolving verses in water, see Legey, *Essai de folklore marocain*, 83. Legey also finds that water retained the memory of death (165–166).

120. *'Ilm al harf* converts letters to numbers in order to unite the patient, his mother, his zodiacal sign, the Qur'an, the names of God, days of the week, and kings of the *jinn* into a single call (*da'wa*). But that science has always been viewed as marginal (Delphin, *L'Astronomie au Maroc*, 16).

121. "This custom, which was based on the Prophet's practice of cutting off the coiled locks of Arabs who converted to Islam from polytheism, was used by al-Jazuli as both a rite of passage and as a symbol of initiation into *At-Ta'ifa al-Jazuliyya* as an institution" (Cornell, *Realm of the Saint*, 180–181).

122. "Salafism was essentially a method that served all the schools of thought, all group interests, service of makhzenian centralization, bourgeois reformism, magisterial position of the ulama" (Laroui, *Les Origines sociales et culturelles du nationalisme marocain*, 429).

123. Ibid., 306.

124. For a history of Islamic modernist thought, none has surpassed the magisterial *Arabic Thought in the Liberal Age*, by Albert Hourani, 140–159.

125. For an overview of 'Abduh's influence, see Kurzman, *Modernist Islam, 1840–1940: A Sourcebook*.

126. Al-Afghani, cited in Keddie, *Sayyid Jamal ad-Din "Al-Afghani": A Political Biography*, 171–181.

127. "The Europeans have now put their hands on every part of the world . . . In reality this usurpation, aggression have not come from the French or the English. Rather it is science that everywhere manifests its greatness and power" (al-Afghani, "Lecture on Teaching and Learning," from Kurzman, *Modernist Islam, 1840–1940*, 104).

128. Muhammad Hajwi, quoted in Laroui, *Les Origines sociales et culturelles du nationalisme marocain*, 382).

129. See Landau-Tasseron, "The 'Cyclical Reform': A Study of the *Mujaddid* Tradition."

130. Kugle, *Rebel between Spirit and Law: Ahmad Zarruq, Sainthood, and Authority in Islam*, 132.

131. Radtke et al., *The Exoteric Ahmad ibn Idris: A Sufi's Critique of the Madhahib and the Wahhabis*, ix.

132. He described Satan as a jurist whose pure rationalism leads to error (Berque, *Al-Yousi: Problèmes de la culture marocaine au XVIIème siècle*, 100).

133. Knut, *Sufi and Scholar on the Desert Edge: Muhammad b. 'Ali al-Sanusi and His Brotherhood*.

134. Bazzaz, *Forgotten Saints*, 9.

135. Ibid., 91.

136. Ibid.

137. On Abu Himara, see Dunn, "Bu Himara's European Connexion: The Commercial Relations of a Moroccan Warlord"; Laroui, *Les Origines sociales et culturelles du nationalisme marocain*, 354–356.

138. Quoted in Bazzaz, *Forgotten Saints*, 52–53.

139. Bazzaz, *Forgotten Saints*, 52–53.

140. On al-Kattani's activism on behalf of 'Abd al-Hafiz, see Bazzaz, *Forgotten Saints*, 128–138, and Laroui, *Les Origines sociales et culturelles du nationalisme marocain*, 390–399.

141. For a French translation of the public destitution of 'Abd al-'Aziz in Fez, see *Revue du Monde Musulman* 5:424–435.

142. For the fourteen conditions of the first *bay'a*, see al-Manuni, *Madhahir yaqdha al-maghrib al-hadith*, 2:349–353.

143. 'Abduh condemned Sufi knowledge in *Risalat al-Tawhid* (The Theology of Unity), and he considered Sufism a "social illness." Reform (*islah*) had to remove such false beliefs and replace them with "authentic Islamic beliefs" and hard work, reason, and this-world effort ('Abduh, "Al-Islah al-Haqiqi wa al-Wajib lil-Azhar").

144. Quoted in Laroui, *Les Origines sociales et culturelles du nationalisme marocain*, 403. On the draft constitutions proposed for Morocco, see al-Manuni, *Madhahir yaqdha al-maghrib al-hadith*, 2:399–444.

145. He honored the Treaty of Algeciras; he received the *mission militaire français* headed by Émile Mangin on January 4, 1909; and the loan of 104 million francs he contracted in 1910 put Morocco into complete economic dependence on France (Laroui, *Les Origines sociales et culturelles du nationalisme marocain*, 399–402).

146. Bazzaz, *Forgotten Saints*, 138–142.

147. A supporter of Mawlay Muhammad suffered a similar punishment for seditious writing (Harris, *With Mulai Hafid at Fez: Behind the Scenes in Morocco*, 145).

148. Foucault, *The Birth of Biopolitics*, 45–46.

149. Cited in al-Kattani, *Salwat al-anfas*, 17.

150. Serels, "Aspects of the Effects of Jewish Philanthropic Societies in Morocco"; see also Semach, "Le Saint d'Ouezzan, Ribbi Amran ben Divan, et les saints juifs du Maroc," and Ben-Ami, *Haaretset Haqedoshim beqereb Yehudei Maroqo.*

151. Legey, *Essai de folklore marocain*, 4; see also Chrifi-Alaoui, "Typologie du récit légendaire du saint judéo-musulman au Maroc."

152. Kodesh, *Beyond the Royal Gaze: Clanship and Public Healing in Buganda.*

153. Al-Kattani, *Salwat al-anfas*, 26.

154. His sons led forces against the French at Marrakesh (1912), Tiznit (1917), Kerdous, and Wajjan (1934). On Sufi Islamic resistance to European invasion and its ultimate failure, see Dunn, *Resistance in the Desert: Moroccan Responses to French Imperialism, 1881–1912.*

CHAPTER 2

1. Renan, *L'Islamisme et la science: Conférence faite à la Sorbonne le 29 mars 1883.*

2. Wilder, *The French Imperial Nation-State*, 1–4.

3. Burke, "The Image of the Moroccan State in French Ethnographic Literature: A New Look at the Origin of Lyautey's Berber Policy" and "The Sociology of Islam: The French Tradition."

4. Rivet, *Lyautey et l'institution du protectorat français au Maroc, 1912–1925.*

5. This chair was a true collaboration of scientists and colonial interests. Senators campaigned for its creation, and the colonial governments of Algeria, Tunisia, and West Africa provided the funding. There was no allotment in the metropolitan budget for the conquest of Morocco before 1904; see Burke, "La mission scientifique au Maroc: Science sociale et politique dans l'âge d'impérialisme."

6. Trumbull, *An Empire of Facts*. The Muslim *mentalité* operated according to the "science of the concrete," what Claude Lévi-Strauss would later call *la pensée sauvage* (Lévi-Strauss, *The Savage Mind*).

7. Arnold, introduction to *Warm Climates and Western Medicine: The Emergence of Tropical Medicine, 1500–1900*, 4.

8. I thus reverse the argument of Patricia Lorcin, who argues in "Imperialism, Colonial Identity, and Race" that physicians were the agents of racial categorization in Algeria.

9. Boudin, *Essai de géographie médicale, ou Études sur les lois qui président à la distribution géographique des maladies, ainsi qu'à leur rapports topographiques entre elles, lois de coïncidence et d'antagonisme.* See also Périer, *Le Docteur Boudin: Notice historique sur sa vie et ses travaux, lue à la société d'anthropologie dans la séance solonnelle du 20 juin 1867, suivie d'un index bibliographique.*

10. Dr. Ernest Renard, médecin-major de 1ère classe en chef à l'Hôpital de Miliana, February 10, 1881, "De l'acclimatement en Algérie," Archives Historiques du Service de Santé Militaire, Val-de-Grâce Hospital, Paris (hereafter cited as Val-de-Grâce), Carton 68, dossier 12.

11. Goedorp, médecin en chef de l'Hôpital militaire d'Oran, "De l'acclimatement des Européens dans l'Algérie," *L'Echo d'Oran*, June 10, 1848.

12. Osborne, *Nature, the Exotic, and the Science of French Colonialism*.

13. Périer, *De l'Hygiène en Algérie, suivi d'un mémoire sur la peste en Algérie par A. Berbrugger* and *De l'Acclimatement en Algérie*.

14. Périer, *De l'Hygiène en Algérie*, 33, 6. Hippocratic climatology influenced French military hygiene, particularly during the expeditions to Egypt (1798–1801), Morea (1829–1831), and Algeria (1840–1842); see Osborne, "Resurrecting Hippocrates: Hygienic Sciences and the French Scientific Expeditions to Egypt, Morea, and Algeria."

15. Périer, *De l'Hygiène en Algérie*, 28–29, 165.

16. Ibid., 46.

17. Ibid., 67–68.

18. Osborne, "The Scientific Basis of Acclimatization in France," in *Nature, the Exotic, and the Science of French Colonialism*.

19. Abi-Mershed, *Apostles of Modernity*, 32.

20. Saint-Simonians in North Africa include Ferdinand de Lesseps and Prosper Enfantin. On Saint-Simonian physicians in Algeria, see Lorcin, *Imperial Identities: Stereotyping, Prejudice, and Race in Colonial Algeria*.

21. Worms, *Exposé des conditions de l'hygiène et de traitement propres à prévenir les maladies et à diminuer la mortalité dans l'armée en Afrique, et spécialement dans la province de Constantine, suivi d'une théorie nouvelle de l'intermittence, et de la nature ainsi que du siège des maladies des pays chauds*, v; the morbidity data is from Moulin, "Tropical without the Tropics: The Turning-Point of Pastorian Medicine in North Africa," 161.

22. Worms, *Exposé des conditions de l'hygiène*, v.

23. Ibid., v.

24. Ramsey, *Professional and Popular Medicine in France, 1770–1830: The Social World of Medical Practice*; Weiner, *The Citizen Patient in Revolutionary and Imperial Paris*; Foucault, *The Birth of the Clinic*.

25. Arnold, introduction to *Warm Climates and Western Medicine*, and Osborne, "Resurrecting Hippocrates." By the end of the century, North Africa had become the crucible of Pasteurian innovation; see Pelis, *Charles Nicolle: Pasteur's Imperial Missionary; Typhus and Tunisia*. For the quotation, see "Note, Algiers, July 13, 1839," Val-de-Grâce, Carton 68, dossier 26.

26. Ackerknecht, *Medicine at the Paris Hospital*.

27. Two graduates of the Qarawiyyin described the university in a manuscript, *Kitab al-akyas fi jawab 'ala asila' 'an hifat wa tadris bi Fas*. The French translation by Delphin was published as *Fas, son université et l'enseignement supérieur musulman* (1889).

28. The French claimed that the Qarawiyyin library was nearly empty, but evidence suggests that Moroccans hid the books, knowing that the French had pillaged Algerian libraries for the Bibliothèque Nationale; see Basset, *Les Manuscrits arabes de deux bibliothèques de Fas*. Evening courses in Fez included medicine, mathematics, astronomy, metaphysics (*kalam*), Sufism, lexicography, philology, history, geography, and the science of writing talismans; see Delphin, *Fas, son université et l'enseignement supérieur musulman*.

29. "The *ragaz* meter, which one joking calls *hmar at-tolba*, 'the donkey of the students' . . . These *urguza*, once learned, are engraved for life in the memory of the stu-

dent" (Renaud, "L'Enseignement des sciences exactes et l'édition d'ouvrages scientifiques au Maroc avant l'occupation européenne"). For a history of printing and the book trade, see Fawzi, *Kingdom of the Book: The History of Printing as an Agency of Change in Morocco between 1865 and 1912.* For Fez lithographs conserved at Harvard University, see Fawzi, *Fihris majmuʿat al-kutub wa-al-dawriyat al-ʿarabiyah fi Jamiʿat Harvard.*

30. Mathieu, "Notes sur les pratiques médicales indigènes à Figuig"; see, for example, Val-de-Grâce, Carton 71, dossier 56.

31. Renaud, "Un registre d'inventaire et de prêt de la bibliothèque de la mosquée ʿAli ben Youssef à Marrakech, date de 1111H./1700 J.C."

32. Berbrugger, *Voyages dans le sud de l'Algérie et des états barbaresques de l'ouest et de l'est, par El-'Aïachi et Moula-Ah'med. Traduits . . . Par Adrien Berbrugger,* 132–134.

33. Kahhak, "Un diplôme de médecin marocain à Fès en 1832." For another example, see Raynaud, *Étude sur l'hygiène et la médecine au Maroc, suivie d'une notice sur la climatologie des principales ville de l'Empire,* 120–121.

34. Henri Cenac, "De la médecine chez les Arabes: Une tournée dans le cercle de Batna 1865," Val-de-Grâce, Carton 68, dossier 31.

35. Ricque, "Du traitement spécial de certains affections chez les indigènes de l'Algérie," Val-de-Grâce, Carton 68, dossier 24.

36. Drs. Giscard and Arutin, "Notes de médecine arabe," 1832–1834, Val-de-Grâce, Carton 68, dossier 27.

37. "Deux ans à Tanger par M. Dulac, 1847–1849," Val-de-Grâce, Carton 71, dossier 56.

38. Ibid. The British surgeon William Lempriere also recorded examples of couching for the cataract in Morocco; see Lempriere, *Tour from Gibraltar to Tangier, Sallee, Mogodore, Santa Cruz . . . Including a Particular Account of the Royal Harem,* 29.

39. On Algerians fleeing those sick with cholera, see "Rapport Générale, Algérie: Populations Indigènes, Choléra de 1849–1850 et de 1850–1851," Val-de-Grâce, Carton 68, dossier 25. On the immediate burial of victims of cholera, see É.-L. Bertherand, *Médecine et hygiène des Arabes: Études sur l'exercice de la médecine et de la chirurgie chez les musulmans de l'Algérie . . . précédées de considérations sur l'état général de la médecine chez les principales nations mahométanes,* 254–255. Dr. Bertherand rejected direct human transmission of cholera (1855), and the Rapport Générale attributed cholera to population movements and changes in temperature or geography (Val-de-Grâce, Carton 71, dossier 54).

40. Vedrenes, "Relation médicale du 12e chasseurs à cheval, pendant la campagne du Maroc (1859)," Val-de-Grâce, Carton 71, dossier 54.

41. "Médecine des Arabes," Note communiquée par M. Arectin, chirurgien-aide au Val-de-Grâce, Octobre 1842, Val-de-Grâce, Carton 68, dossier 32. For the quotation, see Vedrenes, Val-de-Grâce, Carton 71, dossier 54.

42. Vedrenes, Val-de-Grâce, Carton 71, dossier 54.

43. Henri Cenac, "De la médecine chez les arabes: Une tournée dans le cercle de Batna 1865," Val-de-Grâce, Carton 68, dossier 31.

44. Philippe, "Des moyens à favoriser la propagation de la médecine française chez les arabes et l'emploi des Thébibs pour arriver à ce but, 1858," Val-de-Grâce, Carton 68, dossier 30.

45. "Rapport sur un nouveau mode de traitement de la syphilis chez les arabes," Val-de-Grâce, Carton 68, dossier 32.

46. Raynaud, *Étude sur l'hygiène*, 183.

47. On the political and scientific attacks on environmental monogenism, see Osborne, *Nature, the Exotic, and the Science of French Colonialism*, 89. Périer himself later developed racial theories of Kabyles and Arabs; see Lorcin, "Imperialism, Colonial Identity, and Race in Algeria, 1830–1870: The Role of the French Medical Corps." Bertherand became secretary general of the Société de Climatologie Algérienne, director of the *Journal de médecine et de pharmacie de l'Algérie*, and a member of the Conseil d'hygiène et de salubrité publiques d'Alger.

48. Bertherand's arguments were shared by his medical colleague Eugène Bodichon (1810–1885); see Lorcin, "Imperialism, Colonial Identity, and Race."

49. É.-L. Bertherand, *Les Orphelinats de colonisation, à propos du peuplement de l'Algérie: Sous les rapports ethnologique et hygiènique des immigrants*, 6.

50. Ibid., 8–20.

51. After founding the Société Protectrice de l'Enfance Algérienne, Bertherand experimented with using Jewish, Italian, Maltese, Muslim, and Spanish women as wet nurses for French infants; see É.-L. Bertherand, *L'Assistance et la mortalité enfantine en Algérie*. See also É.-L. Bertherand, "Enseignement préparatoire à la colonization."

52. É.-L. Bertherand, *Les Orphelinats de colonisation*, 26.

53. É.-L. Bertherand, *Médecine et hygiène des Arabes*, 294.

54. Bertherand wrote of Muslim women: "The clitoris is voluminous and very preeminent, the vagina very ample" (*Médecine et hygiène des Arabes*, 190). He claimed that syphilis was the basis of North African pathology (315).

55. Ibid., 201.

56. É.-L. Bertherand, *La médecine légale en Algérie* and "La synocope et la folie emotive des accouchées au point de vue médico-légal."

57. É.-L. Bertherand, "De la création des hopitaux arabes," 1–4.

58. "The Arabs have no idea of the general composition of simple drugs," yet "in combining metals, one is put in the form of an adjective, *rsass mkebret* (sulfurated lead) . . . and medicinal substances are generally characterized according to 1. customary usage . . . 2. according to color, calcium carbonate (*thine beidha*) . . . 3. according to the presumed origin—cobalt *hadjaret iokhedjou menha zeurniq*, stone from which one gets arsenic" (É.-L. Bertherand, *Médecine et hygiène des Arabes*, 123).

59. Ibid., 38, 191.

60. Ibid., 54.

61. Ruedy, *Modern Algeria: The Origins and Development of a Nation*, 76–88.

62. For a description of *la loi Warnier*, see Lorcin, "Imperialism, Colonial Identity, and Race."

63. From 1867 to 1872, European births exceeded deaths by 2,477, and the army's mortality rate approached that of the metropole; see A. Bertherand, *De l'Acclimatement en Algérie: Communication faite au congrès de l'association française pour l'avancement des sciences en 1881.*

64. Nicolet, "Jules Ferry et la tradition positiviste."

65. Ibid., 33.

66. Quoted in Rivet, *Lyautey et l'institution du protectorat*, 1:22–23.

67. Mary Pickering highlights the anti-imperialism of Comte, who sympathized

with racial intermarriage and African religions. By the end of his career, Comte rejected the hubris of unchecked reason and sought love in a "religion of Humanity"; see M. Pickering, "Auguste Comte."

68. Evans-Pritchard, *The Sociology of Comte: An Appreciation*, 3.

69. As J. S. Mill wrote of Comte, "Thus, the truths of number are true of all things, and depend only on their own laws; the science, therefore, of Number, consisting of Arithmetic and Algebra, may be studied without reference to any other science. The truths of Geometry presuppose the laws of Number, and a more special class of laws peculiar to extended bodies, but require no others: Geometry, therefore can be studied independently of all sciences except that of number . . . The phenomena of human society obey laws of their own, but do not depend solely upon these: they depend upon all the laws of organic and animal life, together with those of inorganic nature, these last influencing society not only through their influence on life, but by determining the physical conditions under which society has to be carried on" (*Auguste Comte and Positivism* [1865], quoted in Evans-Pritchard, *The Sociology of Comte*, 3).

70. Latour, *We Have Never Been Modern*, 15.

71. Comte, *Discours sur l'esprit positif.*

72. Ibid., 6, 45; M. Pickering, "Auguste Comte," 2.

73. Comte, *The Catechism of Positivism, or Summary Exposition of the Universal Religion*, 294.

74. Jean Robinet, "La Politique positive et la question tunisienne," quoted in Nicolet, "Jules Ferry et la tradition positiviste," 33.

75. Said, *Orientalism*, 130; on Renan's positivism, see Pitt, "The Cultural Impact of Science in France: Ernest Renan and the *Vie de Jésus.*"

76. Renan, quoted in Said, *Orientalism*, 132.

77. Jews were no longer Semites, because they had blended into European society, yet Renan developed his theory of the Semite by using the Hebrew Bible; see Renan, *Le Livre de Job, traduit de l'hébreu par Ernest Renan.*

78. Renan, *Système comparé et histoire générale des langues sémitiques*, 23.

79. Renan, "Nouvelles considérations sur le caractère général des peuples sémitiques et en particulier sur leur tendance au monothéisme"; Renan, *Système comparé et histoire générale*, 16.

80. Renan, *Système comparé et histoire générale*, 13.

81. Renan, "Mahomet et les origines de l'Islamisme."

82. Ibid.

83. Renan, *L'Islamisme et la science.*

84. Ibid., 20.

85. Nasr, *Science and Civilization in Islam*, 69.

86. For the scholastic method, see Makdisi, *The Rise of Colleges: Institutions of Learning in Islam and the West*. For the debt of European medical schools to Arab learning, see Siraisi, *Avicenna in Renaissance Italy: The Canon and Medical Teaching in Universities after 1500*. European scholars often preferred the Muslim philosophers to the original Greek texts after direct translation became available; see Campbell, *Arabian Medicine and Its Influence on the Middle Ages*, 1:167–168.

87. Renan, *Averroès et l'averroïsme, essai historique*, 7.

88. Ibid., from the preface of the 1867 edition (17), quoted in the preface to the 1997 edition (8).

89. The review was a survey of Islamic societies from the Philippines to Morocco; see Rivet, *Lyautey et l'institution du protectorat*, vol. 1, chs. 1 and 2.

90. Edmond Doutté likewise echoes Renan's arguments about science, poetry, and language as well; see Doutté, *Magie et religion dans l'Afrique du Nord*, 11–20. For Rabourdin's views, see his *Algérie and Sahara*, quoted in Trumbull, *An Empire of Facts*, 139.

91. Quoted in Trumbull, *An Empire of Facts*, 139.

92. Al-Afghani, "Religion versus Science."

93. On his rejection of materialists, see Hourani, *Arabic Thought in the Liberal Age*, 125–127, and Keddie, *An Islamic Response*, 171–181.

94. M. Pickering, "Auguste Comte," 42.

95. Durkheim adopted Comte's theory selectively. He rejected Comte's stage models of change and his unified notion of human evolution; see Durkheim, "La Sociologie en France."

96. Durkheim, from Lukes, *Emile Durkheim: His Life and Works, A Critical Study*, 436.

97. Lukes, *Emile Durkheim*, 441–442.

98. For religion as a "first philosophy of nature," see ibid., 438. For the differentiation of religion into other fields, see Durkheim, "On the Definition of Religious Phenomena," cited in ibid., 240–241.

99. "The history of scientific classification is, in the last analysis, the history of the stages by which [the] element of social affectivity has progressively weakened, leaving more and more room for the reflective thought of individuals" (Durkheim, quoted in Lukes, *Emile Durkheim*, 445).

100. For a discussion of the "Republican subject," see Conklin, *A Mission to Civilize*.

101. Samné, *De l'Assistance considérée comme un moyen de colonisation: L'assistance au Maroc . . . rapport présenté au congrès coloniale française, tenu à Paris le 29 mai 1904*, 17–23.

102. The Finnish sociologist Edward Westermarck (1862–1939) applied sociological methods to Morocco, but drew more from English anthropology and was less influential on the French colonial establishment. Doutté used Ignatius Goldziher, Ernest Renan, and English sociology eclectically, but his basic method was Durkheimian *sociologie*; see Doutté, *Magie et religion*, 1.

103. Doutté, *Magie et religion*, 5.

104. Durkheim wrote in 1897: "The principle of this method is that religious, legal, moral, economic facts must be treated . . . as social facts. To describe them or explain them, they must be attached to a determined social milieu, to a definite type of society" (Durkheim, "Préface").

105. J. G., "Edmond Doutté 1867–1926."

106. Pascon, "Le rapport 'secret' d'Edmond Doutté: Situation politique du Houz, 1er janvier 1907."

107. On Doutté's method and emergence from the Algerian ethnographic tradition, see Trumbull, *An Empire of Facts*, 30–48, 82–87, 147–180.

108. Samné, *De l'assistance considérée comme un moyen de colonisation*.

109. R. Millet, *La France au Maroc: Discours prononcé par M. René Millet, An-*

cien Resident Général à Tunis. Banquet du 30 novembre 1909 sous la présidence de M. Étienne, le Prince d'Arenberg (President du Comité de l'Afrique Française, et Guillain, député, President du Comité du Maroc), 22.

110. Le Chatelier proposed emulating British policy in Egypt and limiting metropolitan expenditure on Morocco to 125 million francs over ten years; see Le Chatelier, *Sud-Oranais et Maroc*, 46–49, and, *Lettre à un Algérien sur la politique saharienne*, 3.

111. Doutté, *Notes sur l'Islam maghribin: Les marabouts*, 102–118.

112. Le Chatelier, *Les Confréries musulmanes du Hedjaz* and *L'Islam au XIXe siècle*.

113. Le Chatelier, *L'Islam au XIXe siècle*, 97.

114. Le Chatelier, *Notes sur les villes et tribus du Maroc en 1890*. According to Le Chatelier: "The *scientific* study, in a word, of the native societies will greatly modify our ideas about them. When we know them better we will know better how to apply to each the procedures appropriate to it . . . The studies of ethnography and native sociology must be everywhere the first preoccupations of our governors" (*Questions d'économie coloniale: Lettres à M. Eugène Étienne, Vice-President de la Chambre des Députés*, 222–223).

115. Le Chatelier, *Sud-Oranais et Maroc*, 17–18.

116. Ferry was a member of the *mission militaire* of 1877; see Ferry, *La Réorganization marocaine (Rapport au Comité du Maroc)*, 10–11.

117. Doutté, "Notes sur l'Islam maghribin."

118. Doutté, *Les Tas de pierres sacrés et quelques pratiques connexes dans le Sud du Maroc*.

119. Ibid., 23.

120. Doutté, *Merrâkech*, 107.

121. Doutté, *Notes sur l'Islam maghribin*, 32.

122. Doutté, *Magie et religion*, 599.

123. Ibid., 112–113.

124. Ibid., 58.

125. Keller, *Colonial Madness*, 1–10.

126. Doutté, *Magie et religion*, 36–37.

127. Ibid., 8, 7.

128. Doutté, *L'Islam algérien en l'an 1900*, 37; Doutté, Préface to Gabriel-Rousseau, *La Mausolée des Princes Sa'adiens à Marrakech*.

129. Doutté, *Notes sur l'Islam maghribin*.

130. Doutté, *Merrâkech*, 26–32.

131. In 1859, the governor-general of Algeria hired the French magician Jean-Eugène Robert-Houdin (1805–1871) to show Muslim Algerians that the Sufi brotherhoods "could not represent miracles of a messenger of the Almighty . . . and we wanted to show that we are superior to them in all things, even in magic" (Doutté, *Les Aissaoua à Tlemcen*, 27–29). Robert-Houdin performed a show in Algiers, and the terrified Muslim crowd stampeded from the theater.

132. Doutté, *Magie et religion*, 26.

133. J. G., "Edmond Doutté," 533.

134. Le Chatelier, *Politique musulmane, I: Lettre au "Standard" par A. le Chatelier*, 12–13.

135. Segalla, *The Moroccan Soul*.

136. AAE Nantes, Maroc DAI, Carton 227. See also Houroro, *Sociologie politique coloniale au Maroc: Cas de Michaux-Bellaire*.

137. Lyautey, cited in Juin, introduction to *Lyautey et le médecin*; Weisgerber, *Au Seuil du Maroc moderne*, 7–8.

138. Lyautey to Ministère de la Guerre, February 19, 1921, Archives Nationales de France (hereafter AN), Carton 475 AP 172; Lyautey to Ministère de la Guerre, report, February 9, 1921, AN, Carton 475 AP 172.

139. Lyautey immediately opened infirmaries in the Chaouia, Fez, and Marrakesh after the conquest; see Lyautey to General Commandant la Region de Fez, November 12, 1912, Bibliothèque Générale de Rabat (hereafter BGR), Carton 1713. See also Colombani, "La pénétration pacifique au Maroc: Lyautey et le médecin (1912–1925)."

140. Brochier, *Livre d'Or du Maroc: Dictionnaire de personnalités passées et contemporaines du Maroc*.

141. Pierson, *Naissance d'une vocation: Colombani, disciple de Lyautey*.

142. Delorme, "Une inspection générale médicale au Maroc en 1908."

143. Thévenin, "Du climat de Mogador sous le rapport des affections pulmonaires"; Ollive, "Géographie médicale: Climat de Mogador et de son influence sur la phthisie."

144. "Relation d'une épidémie de cholera à Tanger, Maroc, 1860, par Dr. Castex, Médecin major à l'hôpital militaire, ex-attaché à la mission de France au Maroc," in Service Historique de l'Armée de Terre (hereafter SHAT), Carton 1 K 21, Lacau Papers, dossier 6.

145. Raynaud, *Étude sur l'hygiène*, 72–77.

146. Mauran, "Considérations sur la médecine indigène actuelle au Maroc."

147. Raynaud, *Étude sur l'hygiène*, 128.

148. Mauran, *La Société marocaine: Études sociales, impressions et souvenirs, avec une lettre-préface de M. Le Générale d'Amade, et une lettre de M. Guiot*, 214–218.

149. Comaroff, "Medicine: Symbol and Ideology."

150. Remlinger, "Essai de nosologie marocaine."

151. Lacapère, "La lutte contre la syphilis au Maroc."

152. Colombani, *L'Effort prophylactique au Maroc*, 5.

153. Marcovich, "French Colonial Medicine and Colonial Rule: Algeria and Indochina"; Pelis, *Charles Nicolle*.

154. Moulin, "Les instituts Pasteur de la méditerranée arabe: Une religion scientifique en pays d'Islam."

155. Vaughan, *Curing Their Ills*, 6.

156. Flaubert, *Flaubert in Egypt: A Sensibility on Tour*, 65; Raynaud, *Étude sur l'hygiène*, 70–72, 110, 135, 143; Jourdan, "Le rôle du médecin dans la société marocaine," 1292; Steiner, "Medizinisher Brief aus Marokko Tangier, August 1908."

157. Proschan, "Syphilis, Opiomania, and Pederasty: Colonial Constructions of Vietnamese (and French) Social Diseases"; Vaughan, "Syphilis in Colonial East and Central Africa: The Social Construction of an Epidemic"; Vaughan, "Syphilis and Sexuality: The Limits of Colonial Medical Power," in *Curing Their Ills*; Callahan, "Syphilis and Civilization: A Social and Cultural History of Sexually-Transmitted Disease in Colonial Zambia and Zimbabwe, 1890–1960."

158. Remlinger, "Les maladies vénériennes et la prostitution au Maroc."

159. Doutté, *Notes sur l'Islam maghribin*, 97–8.

160. On Fournier and syphilis, see Corbin, *Women for Hire: Prostitution and Sexuality in France after 1850*. The French scientific approach contrasts with the moralistic orientation of U.S. policies; see Brandt, *No Magic Bullet: A Social History of Venereal Disease in the United States since 1880*.

161. Lacapère, "La lutte contre la syphilis au Maroc."

162. Remlinger, "Essai de nosologie marocaine"; "Rapport du général commandant les troupes debarquées au sujet de l'organisation de l'assistance médicale aux indigènes de la Chaouia, annexe au journal politique d'Octobre 1908," in SHAT, Carton 3H 87; Lepinay, "La Lutte contre les maladies vénériennes au Maroc."

163. Crissey and Parish, *The Dermatology and Syphilology of the Nineteenth Century*.

164. Leredde, *Instructions complémentaires relatives au diagnostic et au traitement de la syphilis*. Such misdiagnosis greatly inflated syphilis statistics in Africa and France; see Vaughan, *Curing Their Ills*, and Crissey and Parish, *The Dermatology and Syphilology of the Nineteenth Century*.

165. Lacapère and Laurent, *Le Traitement de la syphilis par les composés arsenicaux*, 111–115. The complement-fixation antibody test developed by August von Wassermann in 1906 is not used today because it is not specific for syphilis.

166. Pharaon and Bertherand, *Vocabulaire français-arabe à l'usage des médecins, vétérinaires, sages-femmes, pharmaciens, herboristes*; Renaud and Colin, *Documents marocains pour servir à l'histoire du "Mal franc."*

167. Dr. A. Cassar found the rate of tabes among his Tunisian Muslim patients to be 0.055 per 100, approximately one-three hundredth of the rate Fournier recorded in Paris (16.9 per 100); see Cassar, *Influence de l'arsénotherapie sur la fréquence de la paralysie générale progressive et du tabès chez le Musulman tunisien*. Studies demonstrating that North Africans had neurological syphilis were ignored; see Salzes, "Quelques cas de syphilis nerveuse chez les indigènes de l'Afrique du Nord."

168. Lacapère, *La Syphilis arabe: Maroc, Algérie, Tunisie*.

169. On the cultural association of syphilis with genius, see Hayden, *Pox: Genius, Madness, and the Mysteries of Syphilis*, and Williams, *The Horror of Life*.

170. Cassar, *Influence de l'arsénotherapie*, 10–11.

171. Jeanselme, *Histoire de la syphilis, son origine, son expansion: Progrès realisés dans l'étude de cette maladie depuis la fin du XVe siècle jusqu'a l'époque contemporaine*, 406–409.

172. Cassar, *Influence de l'arsénotherapie*.

173. Remlinger, "Essai de nosologie marocaine," 132.

174. I am indebted to Dr. La'arbi Idrissi, toxicologist and former director of the National Institute of Hygiene in Morocco, for these observations.

175. Doctors, however, attributed the change to an "allergy" or a mutation of the spirochete, rather than to an improvement of the native mind; see Cassar, *Influence de l'arsénotherapie*, 17–19.

176. Foucault, *The Birth of the Clinic*.

177. Decrop and Salle, *Album de documents photographiques syphiligraphie et de dermatologie marocaines*.

178. Kuhn, *The Structure of Scientific Revolutions*; Fleck, *The Genesis and De-*

velopment of a Scientific Fact. See also van den Belt, "Spirochaetes, Serology, and Sal-varsan: Ludwik Fleck and the Construction of Medical Knowledge about Syphilis."

179. Lacapère, "La mortalité infantile au Maroc et ses rapports avec la syphilis."

180. Decrop and Salle, Album de documents photographiques.

181. A. Pickering, The Mangle of Practice: Time, Agency, and Science.

182. Fleck, The Genesis and Development of a Scientific Fact.

183. Wilder, The French Imperial Nation-State, 52.

184. See, for example, Salmon and Michaux-Bellaire, "Les tribus arabes de la val-lée du Lekkous."

185. 'Abduh, "Ikhtilaf al-qawanin bi-ikhtilaf ahwal al-umam."

186. 'Abduh, "Tafsir al-Quran al-Hakim."

187. 'Abduh, "Al-Islah al-Haqiqi."

CHAPTER 3

1. Quoted in Mauchamp, La Sorcellerie au Maroc, 33.

2. Jules Bois, "Émile Mauchamp et la sorcellerie au Maroc," in ibid., 44.

3. Mauchamp's diary, in Guillemin, Biographie du Docteur Émile Mauchamp, 52–53.

4. White, Speaking with Vampires.

5. Ibid., 5.

6. Here I evoke Lynn Hunt's "many bodies" of Marie Antoinette, which "repre-sented the threats, conscious and unconscious, that could be posed to the republic" (L. Hunt, The Family Romance of the French Revolution, 94).

7. Fahmy, All the Pasha's Men: Mehmed Ali, His Army, and the Making of Mod-ern Egypt.

8. For an eyewitness Moroccan account of this mission, see Miller, Disorienting Encounters: Travels of a Moroccan Scholar in France in 1845–1846; The Voyage of Muhammad As-Saffar.

9. The exception is the Moroccan historian Bahija Simou; see Les Réformes mili-taires au Maroc de 1844 à 1912.

10. Burke, "The Political Role of the Moroccan Ulema," 91–125.

11. SHAT, Carton 3H1.

12. Rousselle, Médecins, chirurgiens et apothicaires français au Maroc (1577–1907); see also McClellan and Regourd, "The Colonial Machine: French Science and Colonization in the Ancien Regime."

13. Nékrouf, Une Amitié orageuse: Moulay Ismaïl et Louis XIV; Bamford, Fight-ing Ships and Prisons: The Mediterranean Galleys of France in the Age of Louis XIV; Friedman, Spanish Captives in North Africa in the Early Modern Age; Bookin-Weiner, "Corsairing in the Economy and Politics of North Africa."

14. Penz, Les Captifs français du Maroc au XVIIe siècle (1577–1699). Slaves be-came a source of information about Morocco; see Ockley, An Account of South-West Barbary: Containing What Is Most Remarkable in the Territories of the King of Fez and Morocco. Written by a Person Who Had Been a Slave There a Considerable Time; and Published from His Authentick Manuscript. To Which Are Added Two Letters: One from the Present King of Morocco to Colonel Kirk; the Other to Sir Cloudesly Shovell: With Sir Cloudesly's Answer.

15. Friedman, Spanish Captives in North Africa, 102.

16. SHAT, Carton 3H1.

17. Burel report, from SHAT, Carton 3H1.

18. Ollive, "Géographie médicale," 372–374.

19. Feraud report, SHAT, Carton 3H1.

20. On music, see the letter of Bonelli, September 7, 1870, in SHAT, Carton 3H2; and Charmes, *Une Ambassade au Maroc*, 136.

21. Caille, *La Mission du Capitaine Burel au Maroc en 1808*, 9–11.

22. "The next day the Sultan was waiting for me, he served me tea which he poured into a cup, and having filled it with milk, he himself presented it to me. He then called for pen and ink, they brought him a scrap of paper, a small horn ink-stand and a pen of reed. He wrote a prayer, which he gave the *fakih* to read, then he gave it to me to read, and accompanied me as I read, with his finger pointing, word by word. He corrected my pronunciation when I made a mistake" (Badia y Leblich, *Voyages d'Ali Bey el Abbassi en Afrique et en Asie pendant les années 1803, 1804, 1805, 1806 et 1807*, 46).

23. Ibid.

24. Ibid., 48–49.

25. On the Moroccan translation of foreign technical manuals and scientific books into Arabic, see al-Manuni, *Madhahir yaqdha al-maghrib al-hadith*, 1:191–206; on Moroccan interest in astronomy and algebra, 1:206–236; on efforts to modernize the manufacture of sugar and cotton, 1:105–109; on the reorganization of the postal service, 1:123–134; on a Moroccan school for engineers established in Fez in 1844, 1:143–147.

26. SHAT, Carton 3H2.

27. On the physician 'Abd al-Salam al-'Alami, see Amster, "Abd al-Salam," and al-Manuni, *Madhahir yaqdha al-maghrib al-hadith*, 1:237–243. On the Qasr al-'Aini school, see Sonbol, *The Creation of a Medical Profession in Egypt, 1800–1922*.

28. "The named Si Ahmed Tenisamani, doctor in Fez, declares he studied medicine at the school instituted in Tangier by Mouley el Hassan . . . after receiving his diploma, he was designated by the *makhzen* as military doctor attached to the expedition of Moulay Abdesselam el Mrani, of Ben el Bagdadi and of Mahboub, where he fulfilled his role using European methods" (AAE Nantes, Maroc DACH, Carton 84). See also Raynaud, *Étude sur l'hygiène*, 60.

29. AAE Nantes, Maroc DI, Carton 614.

30. SHAT, Carton 1 K 21, Lacau papers.

31. Colonel Harry MacLean was the primary British agent on Gibraltar; see SHAT, Carton 3H1, Marois and Strohl reports. On the Italian technical mission of 1888 and the Bab al-Makina arsenal in Fez, see SHAT, Carton 3H2, and Simou, *Les Réformes militaires au Maroc*, 237–284.

32. SHAT, Carton 3H1, Marois and Strohl reports.

33. AAE Nantes, Tangier Legation, Carton 176, dossier 2.

34. Delphin, *L'Astronomie au Maroc*, 19–20.

35. Until 1894, the French had only a map by Beaudouin (from 1846) at 1: 1,500,000, and a derivative map at 1:500,000 of 1894. Larras took topographical measurements of all Moroccan cities except Tetuan and produced thirty-five maps (1899–1908), including two of Casablanca and Safi-Marrakesh at 1:250,000. The cartographer René de Flotte-Roquevaire also drafted maps from Larras's data; see SHAT, Carton 1 K 194, Larras Papers, Carton 1.

36. *Mahalla* was a mobile version of the sultan's court, the purpose of which was

to reinforce central authority, punish legal infractions, and collect taxes. Linarès published an account of the journey as "Voyage au Tafilalet avec S.M. le Sultan Moulay Hassan en 1893."

37. Legation to Linarès, June 28, 1892, and May 5, 1893; Linarès to Legation, June 9, 1892; all in AAE Nantes, Tangier Legation, Carton 201.

38. Val-de-Grâce, Linarès file.

39. Rivet, *Lyautey et l'institution du protectorat*. In addition to the Mission Scientifique du Maroc, the Ministry of Foreign Affairs approved forty-seven private scientific explorations of Morocco from 1900 to 1912; see AAE Nantes, Tangier Legation, Cartons 340, 341.

40. SHAT, Carton 3H63. In 1904, Larras proposed requiring roads, canals, railroads, the postal service, and the telegraph to have a French "technical counselor" who would take over as director of public works under a future protectorate; see SHAT, Larras Papers.

41. AN, Carton 475AP174.

42. *Al-ta'lif al-mubarak fi hukm sabun al-sharq wa sham al-buji wa sunduq an-nar al-majlub tilka min bilad al-kuffar la'anahum Allah wa hukm khiyata ahl al-dhimma qabbahahum Allah*. See also Laroui, *Les Origines sociales et culturelles du nationalisme marocain*, 321–329.

43. Kenbib, "Structures traditionnelles et protections étrangères au Maroc au XIXe siècle."

44. Quoted in Laroui, *Les Origines sociales et culturelles du nationalisme marocain*, 294–296.

45. Xicluna, "Le fetoua des 'oulama de Fès."

46. SHAT, Carton 1 K 194, Larras Papers.

47. Astrolabes were used to set them; see Badia y Leblich, *Voyages d'Ali Bey el Abbasi*, 107.

48. Miller, *Disorienting Encounters*.

49. Val-de-Grâce, Carton 71, dossier 53.

50. Ibid. And indeed, the Banu Snassen were the first casualties of Lyautey's military advance from Oujda in 1907; see Porch, *The Conquest of Morocco*. The artillery expert Jules Erckmann reported hearing, "the Christians come to study our country and prepare an imminent conquest" (SHAT, Carton 3H1). Larras found that his theodolite attracted much hostile attention in the countryside (SHAT, Carton 1 K 194, Larras Papers).

51. Ultimately, the council was successful, and the quarantine of ships from Morocco was abolished in 1845 (letter of January 19, 1839, AAE Nantes, Tangier Legation, Carton 201). Such hygiene councils existed elsewhere in North Africa; see Gallagher, *Medicine and Power in Tunisia, 1780–1900*.

52. Quarantine stations existed at Catihou, Malta, Gibraltar, Mahon, Alahon, Marseille, and the Isle of Mogador. Many pilgrims died in quarantine, revolted, or entered Morocco clandestinely (AAE Nantes, Tangier Legation, Carton 201); see El Bezzaz, "La Chronique scandaleuse du pèlerinage Marocain à la Mecque au XIXème siècle."

53. Raynaud, *Étude sur l'hygiène*.

54. AAE Nantes, Maroc CD, Carton 475.

55. SHAT, Carton 3H87, dossier 3.

56. The dispensaries were created at Mediouna, Ber Rechid, Boubeker, Settat, Oulad Said, Kasbah ben Ahmed, du Boucheron, Camp Boulhaut, Bou Znika (AAE Nantes, Tangier Legation, Carton 344).

57. Segonzac, *Au Coeur de l'Atlas: Mission au Maroc, 1904–1905.*

58. AAE Nantes, Tangier Legation, Carton 342.

59. Gallagher, *Medicine and Power in Tunisia.*

60. Val-de-Grâce, Carton 68, dossier 31.

61. Ibid.

62. AAE Nantes, Maroc DI, Carton 614.

63. The French authorities prosecuted Moroccan violators but had to tolerate native practitioners who had begun their practices before 1912 (letter of August 2, 1947, AAE Nantes, Maroc DI, Carton 614).

64. White, *Speaking with Vampires,* 5.

65. Burke, *Prelude to Protectorate in Morocco.*

66. Godard, *Description et histoire du Maroc: Comprenant la géographie et la statistique de ce pays, depuis le temps les plus anciens jusqu'à la paix de Tétouan en 1860,* 238–239. French doctors noted examples of variolation practiced in Mogador, Safi, Algeria, and the Middle Atlas; see Raynaud, *Étude sur l'hygiène,* 182, and Trolard report, AAE Nantes, Tangier Legation, Carton 342.

67. Lady Mary Wortley Montagu, the wife of the British ambassador to Turkey in the early eighteenth century, learned variolation in Constantinople and introduced the practice to England, inspiring Jenner to create a [safer] vaccine; see H. Bazin, *The Eradication of Smallpox: Edward Jenner and the First and Only Eradication of a Human Infectious Disease.* Variolation is practiced in China, India, and sub-Saharan Africa; see Arnold, *Colonizing the Body,* and White, *Speaking with Vampires,* 102.

68. É.-L. Bertherand, *Médecine et l'hygiène des Arabes.*

69. "A good rifleman will visit the shrine of Sidi Ali, in Tamegrout; he spends the night there with his rifle, to impregnate it with blessing . . . after the shot of initiation, the tattooing takes place" (Herber, "Tatouage et religion"). On the Nasiriyya, see Ensel, *Saints and Servants in Southern Morocco.*

70. Herber, "Tatouage et religion," 81–82.

71. *Jaysh* tribes were required to provide the sultan with soldiers in exchange for the usufruct of crown lands and exemption from taxes. For the tattooing of soldiers in the *jaysh,* see SHAT, Carton 1 K 194, Larras Papers, and letter, September 7, 1870, SHAT, Carton 3H2.

72. Marois and Feraud report, SHAT, Carton 3H1; SHAT, Carton 1 K 194, Larras Papers.

73. Feraud report, SHAT, Carton 3H1; see also Sebti, "Chroniques de la contestation citadine: Fès et la révolte des tanneurs (1873–1874)."

74. Trolard report, AAE Nantes, Tangier Legation, Carton 342.

75. Schroeter, *Merchants of Essaouira: Urban Society and Imperialism in Southwestern Morocco, 1844–1886.*

76. Burke, *Prelude to Protectorate,* 105–109.

77. Poisoning rumors circulated about Drs. Mauchamp and Trolard, (letter of October 12, 1907, AAE Nantes, Tangier Legation, Carton 342). During the French conquest of Algeria, a rumor spread in Boghar, Cherchell, Oran, Tlemcen, Nemours, Bone, and Orléansville that vaccination was a French method of marking Muslim chil-

dren for later abduction and conversion to Christianity (Val-de-Grâce, Carton 68, dossier 29).

78. Letter of de Campredon, AAE Nantes, Tangier Legation, Carton 343.

79. For his biography, see Katz, *Murder in Marrakesh: Émile Mauchamp and the French Colonial Adventure*; Guillemin, *Biographie du Docteur Émile Mauchamp*; and Katz, "The 1907 Mauchamp Affair and the French Civilising Mission in Morocco."

80. He occupied a *makhzan* residence without permission and disputed with his French colleagues, the French hospital in Tangier, French drug companies, and agents of foreign governments (AAE Nantes, Tangier Legation, Carton 342).

81. There were eight *médecins missionaires*, and General Amande opened nine native dispensaries in the Shawiya in 1907 at Mediouna, Ber Rechid, Boubeker, Settat, Oulad Said, Kasbah ben Ahmed, du Boucheron, Camp Boulhaut, and Bou Znika, which had more than 300 patients a day (letter of October 21, 1908, AAE Nantes, Tangier Legation, Carton 344).

82. Katz, "The 1907 Mauchamp Affair," 156.

83. According to the testimony of Mohammed Touggani: "The day of the murder of Dr. Mauchamp, one of the moqaddems of the quarter, named Djilali ben el Gueschte, went in the morning to tell me to arm myself to kill Mauchamp. It is, he told me, the order of the makhzen. He gave the same order to other inhabitants of the quarter . . . When the doctor arrived, the moqaddems gave the order to strike" (May 26, 1910, AAE Nantes, Tangier Legation, Carton 269).

84. Resistance to the French in Mauritania was conducted with arms provided largely by the sultan of Morocco.

85. On March 28, 1907, the French delivered the "Declaration of Justification of the Invasion of Oujda" and demanded the removal of Warzazi, the establishment of a new police force, and the creation of a French hospital in Marrakesh (AAE Nantes, Tangier Legation, Carton 269).

86. The testimony of 'Ali ben Brahim, a servant of Mauchamp, about the murder changed between 1907 and 1910. After first blaming the *makhzan* in a deposition of March 19, 1907, he then identified 'Abd al-Hafiz and al-Warzazi as the culprits: "In sum, said the witness, one tried to create agitation, trouble in the interests of Mawlay Hafiz. He was in agreement with the Warzazi. He . . . recommended to Warzazi to act. [They] had the *muqaddemin* act and the drama was accomplished. The complicity of Mawlay Hafiz and the Warzazi is certain. They prepared the murder together. Everyone in Marrakesh knows it" (Report of June 8, 1910, AAE Nantes, Tangier Legation, Carton 269).

87. Mauchamp's diary, in Guillemin, *Biographie du Docteur Émile Mauchamp*, 52–53.

88. Mauchamp to Legation, January 7, 1906, AAE Nantes, Tangier Legation, Carton 342.

89. Allouche, "Lettres chérifiennes inédites relatives à l'assassinat du Dr. Mauchamp et à l'occupation d'Oujda en 1907."

90. Bouvier, letter of March 31, 1907, in AAE Nantes, Tangier Legation, Carton 269, and in Katz, "The 1907 Mauchamp Affair," 155.

91. SHAT, Carton 3H63.

92. Burke, *Prelude to Protectorate*, 87–88.

93. On the Hafiziyya, see ibid., 99–127.

94. Depositions of Bouvier, Lennox, Gentil, and Benchimol, along with an anonymous letter dated March 23, 1907, AAE Nantes, Tangier Legation, Carton 269.

95. Letters written by Mauchamp to his family, in Guillemin, *Biographie du Docteur Émile Mauchamp*.

96. Burke, *Prelude to Protectorate*, 92–93.

97. AAE Nantes, Tangier Legation, Carton 269.

98. Deposition of ʿAli ben Brahim, AAE Nantes, Tangier Legation, Carton 269.

99. "Note au sujet des individus arrêtés," AAE Nantes, Tangier Legation, Carton 342.

100. European sources doubted these were the assailants; see Katz, "The 1907 Mauchamp Affair," 157–159.

101. Ibid., 157.

102. Their defiance implied a crisis of the authority of the sultan (ʿAbd al-ʿAziz). The Rahamna and Zamran tribes had collected taxes for the *makhzan* in the Sus and Dra regions until 1894; see Montagne, *Les Berbères et le makhzen dans le sud du Maroc: Essai sur la transformation politique des berbères sédentaires*, 137, 371.

103. The men may have been guilty. Warzazi arrested those suspects, yet the Rahamna defended Warzazi as well as the prisoners; see Burke, *Prelude to Protectorate*, 105.

104. The Glawa had tried unsuccessfully to conquer the Rahamna federation's tribal lands in 1886, but when the Glawa allied themselves with the French in 1913, they finally successfully subjected the Zamran and Masfiwa tribes to their authority; see Burke, *Prelude to Protectorate*, 340. The Hauz tribes also feared ʿAbd al-Hafiz's other ally, ʿAbd al-Malik al-Mtuggui, who occupied the land of another Hauz tribe, the Awlad Bu Sbaʿ, in 1905 (104).

105. Burke, *Prelude to Protectorate*, 113–116.

106. Bourqia, "Don et théâtralité: Réfléxion sur le rituel du don (hadiyya) offert au Sultan au XIXe siècle." The European powers also paid substantial annual *hadiyya*; see Burel report, SHAT, Carton 3H1.

107. On *mahalla*, see Capt. Verlet-Hanus, "Étude militaire sur la mehalla," SHAT, Carton 3H87, and Nordman, "Les expéditions de Moulay Hassan: Essai statistique."

108. SHAT, Carton 1 K 194, Larras Papers, Carton 1.

109. The French responded to this with a naval bombardment of the city of Larache; see the Caraman report of 1825, SHAT, Carton 1 K 194, Larras Papers, Carton 1.

110. SHAT, Carton 1 K 662, Ninard Papers, Carton 1.

111. Gentil report, AAE Nantes, Tangier Legation, Carton 269. Shlomo Deshen has argued that such attacks on urban Jews were a direct affront to the sultan's power; see Deshen, "Urban Jews in Sherifian Morocco," 213.

112. Burckhardt, letter of July 28, 1899, SHAT, Carton 1 K 194, Larras Papers, carton 1.

113. Mauchamp, *La Sorcellerie au Maroc*.

114. "P-V de constat," AAE Nantes, Tangier Legation, Carton 269.

115. The grass may have been an ironic reference to Muslim martyrdom; Leor Halevi, personal communication.

116. The tribes presented each of these pretenders with the same list of demands contained in the Fez *bayʾa* of 1908. Zayn received support from several tribes and was

presented the *bay'a* by the *'ulama'* of Meknes, and he constructed his own *makhzan*; see Burke, *Prelude to Protectorate*, 159–163.

117. Laroui, *Les Origines sociales et culturelles du nationalisme marocain*, 407–410.

118. The mellah was pillaged, Europeans were attacked, and the telegraph building was destroyed to prevent communication with the 1,500 French troops stationed four kilometers south of the city; see Simou, *Les Réformes militaires au Maroc*, 450.

119. Soldiers not involved in the mutiny were reintegrated into French-organized auxiliary troops under French command; see Gershovich, *French Military Rule in Morocco: Colonialism and Its Consequences*, 57.

120. Laroui, *Les Origines sociales et culturelles du nationalisme marocain*, 410.

121. Edmond Ferry described the sultan's state as a "chimera" (*La Réorganisation marocaine*, 10–11).

122. "Un régime régulier fondé sur l'ordre intérieur et la sécurité générale, qui permette l'introduction des réformes . . . administratives, judiciaries, scolaires, économiques, financières, et militaires" (A regular government founded upon internal order and general security, which permits the introduction of reforms . . . administrative, judicial, educational, financial, and military): Treaty of Fez, in Chastand, *Le protectorat français au Maroc*, 146–147.

123. As sultan, al-Hiba reversed non-Qur'anic taxes and announced the suppression of the *grands qaids*, allowed tribes to choose their *qaids*, and called for moral reform. He created ministries of war, justice, and foreign affairs before his "state" was destroyed by French troops; see Chef de Bataillon Verlet-Hanus, "Rapport sur les événements de Marrakech (août–sept 1912)," SHAT, Carton 3H90. Other Sufi-led revolts in the period May 1912–October 1913 included one by Muhammad al-Hajjami, a *sharif* and Sufi who called jihad among the Qashtala, Ghiyata, Hayaniyya and Jbala tribes; see al-Khalloufi, *Bouhmara du jihad à la compromission: Le Maroc oriental et le Rif de 1900 à 1909*, 116.

124. Kantorowicz, *The King's Two Bodies: A Study in Mediaeval Political Theology*, 9.

125. Comité d'Action Marocaine, *Plan de réformes marocaines*, 9–16.

126. "I carefully distanced from him all European promiscuities, the automobiles and the champagne dinners": Lyautey, letter of October 10, 1912, in L.-H.-G. Lyautey, *Choix de lettres*, 300.

127. "Ici la source de toute autorité est chez Sidna . . . Tout en représentant ici le Gouvernement de la France, je m'honore d'y être le premier serviteur de Sidna" (Lyautey, quoted in Bidwell, *Morocco under Colonial Rule: French Administration of Tribal Areas, 1912–1956*, 68).

128. On Mawlay Yusuf's interventions on behalf of the French Résidence, see Bidwell, *Morocco under Colonial Rule*, 63–69.

129. Lyautey, quoted in ibid., 68.

130. Combs-Schilling, *Sacred Performances*, 222–235.

131. Stacey Holden notes that after colonial rule, Fez residents showed their independence from the sultan by slaughtering the ram at home after a local prayer leader led a public sacrifice and before the sultan did; see Holden, *The Politics of Food in Modern Morocco*, 71.

132. Ibid., 222.

133. See Bourqia, "Don et théâtralité."

134. "En raison des circonstances actuelles et pour réparer la mauvaise impression produite sur le makhzen, sur la population indigène et sur les étrangers par le peu d'éclat qu'ont revêtu les cérémonies de la dernière fête de l'Aid el Kebir, il importe que toutes dispositions soient prises pour donner aux manifestations traditionnelles qui accompagneront la celebration de la prochaine fête du Mouloud, tout l'apparat et l'ampleur désirables" (In view of current circumstances and in order to repair the bad impression of the *makhzan* given to the native population and foreigners by the poor showing at the last festival of 'Aid al-Kabir, it is important that every effort be expended to ensure that the traditional ceremonies of the next Mouloud festival achieve all the desired magnitude and pomp): Lyautey, Circulaire au sujet de la fête du mouloud, January 29, 1914, AAE Nantes, Maroc DAI, Carton 12.

135. Fez was ordered to send 200 men, Meknes 125, Rabat 600, the Shawiya 200, Tadla Zaian 50, Marrakesh 200, the Doukkala 100, and the Haha 50 (Lyautey, circular letter to the regions, December 20, 1914). Their gifts were paid for by the Résidence; see note circulaire 317 SGC of 19 January 19, 1914, and of September 1, 1914, AAE Nantes, Maroc DAI, Carton 12.

136. Clancy-Smith, *Rebel and Saint: Muslim Notables, Populist Protest, Colonial Encounters (Algeria and Tunisia), 1800–1904*; Dunn, *Resistance in the Desert*. On the split within the Moroccan Fadiliyya, see Boubrik, *Saints et société en Islam*, 147–167.

137. Feraud, "Rapport Interprète Militaire Principale Feraud, 1877," SHAT, Carton 3H1, dossier 3; Ferry, *La Réorganisation marocaine*, 10–11; Salmon, "Essai sur l'histoire politique du nord-marocain." For a critical account of the Wazzani family, see Michaux-Bellaire, "La Maison d'Ouezzan." Alfred Le Chatelier had considered the *sharif* of Wazzan as a possible replacement for Sultan 'Abd al-'Aziz; see Le Chatelier, *Sud-Oranais et Maroc*, 32, and Le Chatelier, *Notes sur les villes*, 11–23.

138. Bidwell, *Morocco under Colonial Rule*, 130–137.

139. 'Abd al-Hay al-Kattani to Lyautey, 17 August 1914, AN, Carton 475, AP 314.

140. SHAT, Carton 3H90. The Ghiyata tribe had defied Mawlay Hasan and confiscated part of his artillery (SHAT, Carton 1 K 194, Larras Papers, Carton 1).

141. 'Abd al-Qadir had crushed the Darqawiyya brotherhood and lay siege to the Tijani leadership in Grand Kabylia. As a result, the Tijaniyya accepted French offers of protection; see Ruedy, *Modern Algeria*, 59–61, and Clancy-Smith, *Rebel and Saint*, 142, 194, 259.

142. Abu Himara also created a Sufi order of eclectic theology and notoriously staged phony "miracles"; see al-Khalloufi, *Bouhmara du jihad*, 47–57.

143. For Abu Himara's rise and fall, see Dunn, "Bu Himara's European Connexion," and Burke, *Prelude to Protectorate*, 63–65.

144. Dunn, *Resistance in the Desert*, 253.

145. Nurse, 'Umar Idrisi Hospital, interview by the author, March 22, 1999, Fez.

146. Women in Tangier visited the Wazzani to cure sterility; see Marois, "Relation d'un voyage au Maroc: Ambassade française, mars-avril 1877," SHAT, Carton 3H1; and Salmon, "El Qcar el Kebir: Une Ville de provence au Maroc septentrional."

147. For the quotation, see Rivet, *Lyautey et l'institution du protectorat*, 2:240.

148. Doutté, *Notes sur l'Islam maghribin*, 79–82. 'Abd as-Salam al-Wazzani married Emily Keene, a British governess in Tangier; see her autobiography, Emily, Shareefa of Wazan, *My Life Story*.

149. Doutté, *Notes sur l'Islam maghribin*, 292–293.

150. Nantes, Maroc DAI, Carton 65.

151. "Compte-rendu d'une tournée d'inspection, faite par médecin major 2e class *Cristiani* dans les infirmeries indigènes de la Region de Tadla," December 18, 1915, AN, Carton 475, AP 172, Dossier Santé publique.

152. Today the hospital staff jokingly calls them "Sidi Shuka" (Saint Shot) and "Mawlay Fanid" (Lord Pill); author's field notes, Fez, 1999.

153. Cornell, *Realm of the Saint*, 11. At the shrine of Sidi Bou Jida on the city outskirts, food and clothing were distributed to needy rural tribesmen. This tradition protected Fez from invasion by rural tribes in times of famine.

154. Author's field notes, January 9–11, 2006.

155. Décision du Resident Général no. 1870, 5 July 1913, AN, Carton 475, AP 172, dossier: Infirmeries Indigènes dans la Region de Fès: Projet d'organisation. For the patient population, see Cocard Hospital Archives, Intake Register, 1916.

156. The hospitals in Marrakesh and Mazagan together had 11,000 patient consults per month, and Safi had 4,000 per month; see Mauran, report to Lyautey, April 13, 1916, AN, Carton 475, AP 172.

157. Nurse, 'Umar Idrisi Hospital, interview.

158. Mawlay Ali, interview by the author, March 22, 1999.

159. BGR, Carton A836. The clinics of the Fez Madina had 14,991 consults in September 1918; see uncatalogued BGR carton, 1917–1921.

160. Author's field notes, 1999.

161. Interview R, March 12, 1999, Funduq al-Yuhudy clinic, Fez.

162. Dekester, *Utilisation du Marocain comme infirmier indigène*.

163. Headrick, *The Tentacles of Progress: Technology Transfer in the Age of Imperialism*; Adas, *Machines as the Measure of Men: Science, Technology, and Ideologies of Western Dominance*.

164. For example, see Mitchell, *Colonising Egypt*.

165. Pyenson, "Pure Learning and Political Economy: Science and European Imperialism in the Age of Imperialism."

166. Nasr, *An Introduction to Islamic Cosmological Doctrines*.

CHAPTER 4

1. "Procès-verbal du BMH de Mogador," October 6, 1924, BGR, Carton 633. "Procès-verbal" hereafter abbreviated "P-V."

2. "P-V du BMH de Mogador," August 27, 1925, BGR, Carton 634.

3. The *goutte de lait* (milk dispensary) also necessitated the formation of a "city dairy," where cows were screened by the city veterinarian for tuberculosis; see BGR, Cartons 647, 633. By 1926, the Mogador Goutte de Lait was distributing 18,000 bottles in a single month (Monthly Report, BMH de Mogador, August 1926, BGR, Carton A836).

4. "Extrait du P-V du BMH de Mogador," 15 December 1925, BGR, Carton A634.

5. On cholera and sewers in France, see Goubert, *The Conquest of Water: The Advent of Health in the Industrial Age*. On medicine and the French Revolution, see Weiner, *The Citizen Patient*. William Coleman dates the French welfare state from

1801; see Coleman, *Death Is a Social Disease: Public Health and Political Economy in Early Industrial France.*

6. Le Play, *La Réforme sociale* and *L'Organisation de la famille.* Le Play did not support the equality of social classes, however; see Shapiro, *Housing the Poor of Paris, 1850–1902.*

7. Lyautey is quoted in Wilder, *The French Imperial Nation-State,* 69. On Lyautey's interest in Le Play, see Rabinow, *French Modern: Norms and Forms of the Social Environment,* 86–110. On colonial hygiene in West Africa, see Conklin, *A Mission to Civilize,* Chapter 2.

8. Dr. Bouveret, "P-V du BMH de Mogador," December 22, 1926, BGR, Carton 632.

9. Wilder, *The French Imperial Nation-State,* 1–5. The approach in this chapter thus differs from that of historians of sub-Saharan Africa, who study the social conditions of colonial political economy as a source of epidemics; see Packard, *White Plague, Black Labor: Tuberculosis and the Political Economy of Health and Disease in South Africa*; Lyons, *The Colonial Disease: A Social History of Sleeping Sickness in Northern Zaire, 1900–1940*; Giblin, "Trypanosomiasis Control in African History: An Evaded Issue."

10. Lyautey's dictum comes from his "Discours sur la médecine coloniale," cited in Micouleau-Sicault, *Les Médecins français au Maroc: Combats en urgence (1912–1956),* 47. Lyautey on military doctors: "This role for the military physician with regard to the natives is an essential factor in the military mission itself, because there is no fact more firmly established than the efficacy of the physician as an agent of penetration, attraction and pacification" (Lyautey to minister of war, February 9, 1921, AN, Carton 475, AP 172). For the long quotation in the text, see Resident General Lyautey to General Commandant of Fez Region, November 12, 1912, BGR, Carton 1713.

11. Lyautey, "Discours sur la médecine coloniale," quoted in Micouleau-Sicault, *Les Médecins français au Maroc,* 47.

12. The *conseilleurs techniques* in 1919:

General medicine—Maute, chief of laboratory in Beaujoin Hospital
Syphilography—Lacapère, former chief of clinic at the faculty of medicine at St.
    Lazare Hospital
Scalp ailments and X-ray therapy—Noire, chief of laboratory at St. Louis Hospital
Bacteriology—Pinoy, Chef de Service at Institut Pasteur in Paris
Malaria—Paisseau, chief of clinic at the Paris faculty
Oto/rhino/laryngology—Guisez, Chief of surgical clinic at Hôtel-Dieu
Psychiatry—Clerambault, doctor of the infirmary at the Prefecture of Police in
    Paris and psychological expert at the Tribunal of the Seine

Lyautey, "Instruction relative à l'institution de conseilleurs techniques médicaux pour le Maroc à Paris," January 15, 1919, AN, Carton 475, AP 172. On his view of metropolitan medicine, see Lyautey, "Le Rôle néfaste des bureaux metropolitans," in *Lyautey et le médecin.*

13. Lyautey, letter, November 18, 1920, in BGR, unordered carton "1917–1921," folder "Ordre Général: Organisation Générale des Services (Divers, 1917–1921)."

14. Jourdan, "Le role du médecin dans la société marocaine."

15. "Accord entre la direction générale des services de santé et la direction des affaires civiles au sujet des formations municipals d'assistance et d'hygiène," BGR, unordered carton "1917–1921."

16. Lyautey, "Document Fondamental Feb. 9, 1921, Organisation du Service de Santé," AN, Carton 475, AP 172, folder 7.

17. In theory, an Arrêté Résidentiel (an order by the resident general) of May 24, 1918, created a Superior Council of Hygiene and Public Health for the protectorate. In reality, the regions were independent entities, each under a *médecin-chef*; see Jourdran, "Instruction pour les Médecins-Chefs de Service de la Zone des Villes et des Territoires Civils," BGR, unordered carton "1913–1920."

18. Municipalities became responsible for their health services after the separation of military and civilian health services; see "Rapport présénté par le Médecin-Inspecteur Oberlé, Directeur Général des Services de Santé du Maroc au Conseil Supérieur d'Hygiène," BGR, unordered carton "SP-Assistance Médicale aux Fonctionnaires." See also director of civil affairs to director general of finances, November 7, 1917, BGR, unordered folder "Hygiène." On the ballooning costs of health care, see Arrêté Résidentiel, November 6, 1920. Cities were soon in debt to the Pharmacie Centrale for medications; see Médecin Inspecteur Oberlé to director of civil affairs, BGR, unordered carton "1917–1921."

19. The *dahir* of 1913 invested the chief of municipal services (CMS) with this authority; see Lyautey, "Circulaire aux Commandants de Region," December 18, 1915, in BGR, unordered carton "Monthly Hygiene Reports, 1917."

20. René Martial, "Note au sujet du fonctionnement des services d'hygiène de la ville de Fès," AN, Carton 475, AP 172. Martial exchanged a number of letters first with the chief of municipal services, then with the Résidence, 1921–1923; see BGR, Carton 1395.

21. Jules Colombani, "La Place du médecin dans l'oeuvre de Lyautey," in *Lyautey et le médecin*.

22. "Les Hôpitaux indigènes du Maroc, Note du Dr. Laurent," AN, Carton 475, AP 172.

23. Sorbier de Pougnadoresse to chief of municipal services in Marrakesh, November 25, 1924, BGR, Carton 1447. A native with sufficient French culture could be hospitalized with Europeans; see AN, Carton 475, AP 172.

24. By 1922, only the card-carrying indigent among Europeans could have free care; see "Rapport presénté par Med inspecteur Oberlé, Directeur général des Services de Santé du Maroc au Conseil Supérieur d'Hygiène," 1922, AN, Carton 475, AP 172.

25. *Hubus*, or *waqf*, is a charitable trust in which proceeds from donated properties are spent for purposes designated by the benefactor, usually charitable and public. On *hubus* in Morocco, see also Bu Rugbah, *Dawr al-waqf al-hayah al-thaqafiyah bi al-Maghrib fi 'ahd al-dawla al-'Alawiya*; Britel and Rigaud, *Le Mécénat au Maroc*; and Stöber, *"Habous Public" in Marokko: Zur wirtschaftlichen Bedeutung religiöser Stiftungen im 20. Jahrhundert.*

26. Milliot, *Démembrements du Habous*. On intermediate forms of property in *hubus* water mills, see Holden, *The Politics of Food*, 44–45, 222–223.

27. For the French reforms, see the *dahirs* of February 27, 1914; June 2, 1915; July 3, 1913; July 21, 1913; and July 8, 1916, modifying article 8 of the *dahir* of Feb-

ruary 27, 1914, and July 8, 1916. In Fez, the ministry collected 1,870,000 francs from its *hubus* properties in 1913; that figure had quadrupled by 1917; see Holden, *The Politics of Food*, 96.

28. For the first two quotations, see Dumas, *Le Maroc*, 14, 35. For the third, see Chevrillon, *Visions du Maroc*, 20.

29. Richard Burton thus elucidated the French hygienist's view of Tangier; from his introduction to Leared, *Morocco and the Moors: Being an Account of Travels, With a General Description of the Country and Its People*, vii.

30. "Campagne Antipaludique," BGR, unordered carton "1913–1920."

31. Lyautey brought Dr. Edmond Sargent of the Algerian Institut Pasteur to Morocco after Sargent treated Lyautey's Armée de l'Orient for malaria in Macedonia in 1916; see Edmond Sargent, "Rencontres de Lyautey," in *Lyautey et le médecin*.

32. "Rapport Edmond Sargent, Paludisme dans la valée du Bas-Sebou, ville de Kenitra, June 21, 1919," AN, Carton 475, AP 172, "Dossier relatif aux infirmeries indigènes—groupes mobiles sanitaires et Assistance Publique."

33. "Attributions du Bureau d'Hygiène d'après le dahir du 15 mars 1920," BGR, Carton A837, folder "Marrakech."

34. Sargent, from "P-V de la conférence du 28 janvier 1924 tenue à l'occasion de la Mission au Maroc des Docteurs Sargent et Foley de l'Institut Pasteur d'Algérie," AN, Carton 475, AP 172. The Kenitra BMH distributed quinine to native children aged two to fifteen in order to "sterilize the reservoir of the virus"; see "P-V du BMH de Kenitra," December 22, 1925, BGR, Carton 632.

35. Abu-Lughod, *Rabat: Urban Apartheid in Morocco*, 146–147.

36. Prost admitted the military purposes of the cordon; see Wright, *The Politics of Design in French Colonial Urbanism*, 146; Abu-Lughod, *Rabat*, 147.

37. In Casablanca, Prost set aside twenty times the land area of the *madina* for the European city to expand, but set aside virtually none for future native housing; see Wright, *The Politics of Design*, 150–152.

38. Near Mogador, the Groupe Sanitaire Mobile vaccinated 100,000 tribesmen for smallpox in order to prevent an epidemic in the city; see "P-V du BMH de Mogador," 1925–1926, BGR, Carton 632.

39. Deschamps, *Souvenirs des premiers temps du Maroc français*, 231.

40. Chief of municipal services to Lyautey, November 13, 1913, BGR, Carton 1501.

41. General secretary of the protectorate to director of public health, February 4, 1914, BGR, Carton 1501.

42. General secretary of the protectorate to director of public health, February 4, 1914, BGR, Carton 1501. On the deportations, see "P-V du sous-commission municipale d'hygiène de Mogador," BGR, Carton 632. All buses from the Sus and Tafilelt regions were diverted to delousing stations; see "P-V du BMH de Mogador," February 1924, BGR, Carton 633, and "P-V du BMH de Marrakech," 1925, BGR, Carton A837.

43. "Rapport annuel du médecin-chef du BMH de Marrakech, 1925," BGR, Carton A837.

44. The *dahir* of February 19, 1914, made the reporting of contagious disease mandatory; the *dahir* of December 8, 1915, authorized the hygiene police to enter homes where contagious disease was suspected.

45. "P-V du BMH de Meknes," February 1927, BGR, Carton A1553; "P-V du BMH de Mogador," October 1924, BGR, Carton 633.

46. Yearly Report, Settat, 1929, BGR, Carton 1501.

47. Report of Dr. Fournial, "P-V du BMH de Marrakech," 1925, BGR, Carton A837.

48. "P-V du BMH de Settat," December 18, 1925, BGR, Carton 632.

49. Report of Dr. Fournial, "P-V du BMH de Marrakech," 1925.

50. Valeton, *Le Marabout de Sidi ben Achir (à Salé): Ses rapports avec l'assistance publique*. On the typhus alert at the shrine of Mawlay Idris in April 1916, see Rivet, *Lyautey et l'institution du protectorat*, 2:226. On Ben 'Isa, see BGR, Carton 649.

51. Allah ben Driss de Charaba escaped registration in Meknes when he stayed at the Funduq Tradji in 1927. After the BMH had located him, it rounded up all the *funduq* occupants for immediate delousing; see "P-V du BMH de Meknes," February 1927, BGR, Carton A1553.

52. For the prostitute and children, see "P-V du BMH de Marrakech," April 11, 1927, BGR, Carton A1553. For the quotation, see "P-V du BMH de Marrakech," 1925, BGR, Carton A837.

53. "P-V du BMH de Casablanca," July 6, 1914, BGR, Carton 641.

54. In Settat, the municipal authorities enlisted the *muqaddimin*, representatives of the *qaid*, and native police to visit cafés and *fanadiq*; see "P-V du BMH de Settat," December 19, 1925, BGR, Carton 632. For the quotation, see Monthly Municipal Report, Rabat, February 1938, BGR, Carton 1501. In Meknes, the *muqaddimin* did not report death; see Monthly Municipal Report, Meknes, 1935, BGR, Carton 649.

55. Annual health reports for Fez from 1912 to 1920 contained no native death data; see Fez Monthly Reports, BGR, Carton 1395. In March 1925, the chief of municipal services of Meknes wrote that the causes of indigenous deaths "cannot be indicated"; see Meknes Monthly Reports, BGR, Carton A836.

56. "Rapport sur le fonctionnement du bureau d'hygiène pendant l'année 1925," BGR, Carton 837.

57. "Attributions du bureau d'hygiène d'après le dahir du 15 mars 1920," BGR, Carton 837.

58. BGR, Carton A641.

59. Monthly Report, Meknes, March 1926, BGR, Carton A836.

60. The same measures were used at the weekly market in the city; see "Rapport annuel du médecin-chef du BMH de Marrakech, 1925," BGR, Carton A837.

61. *Contrôleur civil* of Salé to *intendant général*, representative of the Résidence, May 18, 1919, BGR, unordered carton "Hygiène."

62. Monthly Report, Bureau of Hygiene, Rabat, January 1938, BGR, Carton 1501 (emphasis in the original).

63. Ibid.

64. Ibid.

65. Martin, "Description de la ville de Fès."

66. "Rapport du CMS de Rabat (Capt. Riottot), Rabat January 16, 1914," BGR, Carton 1501. On the shelters at Bab-Teben and Bab al-Had, where 400 people were housed, see Rivet, *Lyautey et l'institution du protectorat*, 2:226.

67. Chief of municipal services of Casablanca, letter, January 17, 1917, BGR, Carton 1447.

68. Holden, *The Politics of Food*, 17–40, 101.

69. "Rapport du CMS de Rabat (Capt. Riottot), Rabat January 16, 1914," BGR, Carton 1501.

70. BGR, Carton 632; "P-V du BMH de Casablanca," March 19, 1927, BGR, Carton 1553.

71. "P-V du BMH de Casablanca," March 19, 1927, BGR, Carton 1553.

72. "P-V du BMH de Meknes," February 1927, BGR, Carton A1553.

73. Le Tourneau, *Fès avant le protectorat: Étude économique et sociale d'une ville de l'occident musulman*, 262; Martin, "Description de la ville de Fès," 628.

74. Many Muslim communities dedicated a tax collected on meat for charitable purposes; the Commission Municipale of Meknes approved a tax of 0.25 francs per kilogram of halal meat in 1934 for the Muslim Charity Society; see BGR, Carton 598, dossier "Contrôle des Municipalites." This was a continuation of the *"guerjouma* tax" imposed by the sultans; see Holden, *The Politics of Food*, 85.

75. "Exposition Coloniale 1922 à Marseille," BGR, unordered carton. In Salé, the *hubus* gave the Charity Society of Sidi Ben 'Ashir 13,000 francs in 1922, 1923, and 1924; see "Rapports trimestriels et mensuels, Instructions (BXII), Jan. Fev. Mars 1923," AAE Nantes, Maroc DACH, Carton 10, dossier "Bienfaisance."

76. "Rapport Secrétaire Générale du Protectorat à M. le Directeur de l'Administration municipale," June 5, 1931, BGR, Carton 1447.

77. Rivet, *Lyautey et l'institution du protectorat*, 2:239.

78. The Alliance Israélite Universelle, a French-Jewish organization, competed with the native *hebrot* to influence Moroccan Jewish communities; see Serels, "Jewish Philanthropic Societies in Morocco."

79. Secretary general of the protectorate to heads of *contrôle civil*, 12 June 1934, AAE Nantes, Maroc DI, Carton 622.

80. Resident general to president of the Rabat Section of the League of the Rights of Man, April 13, 1938, AAE Nantes, Maroc DI, Carton 625.

81. Letter, January 5, 1944, AAE Nantes, Maroc DI, Carton 625.

82. "P-V du BMH de Rabat," June 23, 1924, BGR, Carton 633; "P-V du BMH de Mogador," May 10, 1922, BGR, Carton 646.

83. "P-V du BMH de Mogador," September 13, 1926, BGR, Carton 632.

84. "P-V du BMH de Mogador," August 27, 1925, BGR, Carton 634.

85. The same occurred in other cities; see "P-V de Safi BMH," March 6, 1923, BGR, Carton 647; and "Projet d'arrêté municipal réglementant le commerce du lait de chèvre et des derivés du lait de chèvre," in "P-V du BMH de Meknes," April 10, 1923, BGR, Carton 633A. For Lyautey's instructions, see his letter, September 1913, BGR, Carton A1504, folder I: "Ordre Général: Organization (1914–1920)."

86. "P-V du BMH de Rabat," June 23, 1924, BGR, Carton 633; "P-V du BMH de Mogador," May 10, 1922, BGR, Carton 646.

87. Coleman, *Death Is a Social Disease*; Shapiro, *Housing the Poor of Paris, 1850–1902*.

88. Massignon, "Enquête sur les corporations d'artisans et de commerçants au Maroc (1923–1924), d'après les réponses au questionnaire transmis par circulaire du 15 novembre 1923 sous le timbre de la direction des Affaires Indigènes et du Service des Renseignements," 82.

89. On the artisan councils, see Yakhlef, "La Municipalité de Fès à l'époque du Protectorat, 1912–1956," 409.

90. On the municipal laws and craft guilds, see Lyautey, letter, September 1913, BGR, Carton A1504, and Yakhlef, "La Municipalité de Fès," 408–409. The regulations could also provide a space for negotiation; Stacy Holden's nuanced history (*The*

Politics of Food) illustrates how water millers and native Jewish and Muslim butchers used protectorate hygiene to their advantage. Another factor in the decline of the guilds was the protectorate's open-door economic policy. Japanese textiles and slippers bankrupted Moroccan silk weavers and slipper makers; see the Archives Municipales de Fès (hereafter cited as AMF), dossier "Artisanat." For the weavers, see Barbault, "Artisanat et proletariat traditionnels à Fès." Muslim members of the Meknes municipal council tried to create a tariff on Japanese goods; see "P-V du Commission Municipale de Meknes," April 19, 1934, BGR, Carton 598.

91. Sorbier de Pougnadoresse, letter, June 1916, BGR, Carton A641.

92. "P-V du BMH de Oujda," 1924, BGR, Carton A837.

93. "P-V du BMH de Rabat," July 31, 1923, BGR, Carton A647.

94. "P-V du BMH de Mogador," March 1926, BGR, Carton 632.

95. "P-V du BMH de Mogador," several sessions, BGR, Carton 632.

96. "P-V du BMH de Casablanca," February 3, 1927, BGR, Carton A1553; "P-V du BMH de Meknes," April 10, 1923, BGR, Carton 633A; "P-V du BMH de Mogador," March 1926 BGR, Carton 632; "P-V du BMH de Oujda," April 2, 1925, BGR, Carton A837.

97. See "P-V du BMH de Mogador," March 1926, BGR, Carton 632; and "P-V du BMH de Oujda," April 2, 1925, BGR, Carton A837.

98. In the municipal meetings, there were several mentions of overcrowding in the Jewish quarters and of attempts by both the leaders of the Jewish community and members of the Alliance Israélite Universelle to obtain new housing for Jews from the municipalities; see "P-V du BMH de Rabat," June 25, 1913, BGR, Carton A641. In Mogador, Dr. Bouveret found ten people to a room in the mellah; see "P-V du BMH de Mogador," January 6, 1922, BGR, Carton 646.

99. Report of Dr. Jacques in "P-V du BMH de Mazagan," 1922, BGR, Carton 646; Municipal Report of Rabat, February 1938, BGR, Carton 1501.

100. "P-V du BMH de Rabat," September 18, 1923, BGR, Carton 647.

101. Yakhlef, "La Municipalité de Fès," 2:573–4.

102. Report of Dr. Fournial, "P-V du BMH de Marrakech," 1925, BGR, Carton A837.

103. On prison labor in municipalities, see "P-V du BMH de Mogador," March 1924, BGR, Carton 633; "P-V du BMH de Settat," December 18, 1925, and "P-V du BMH de Rabat," 1914, both in BGR, Carton A641; "P-V du BMH de Rabat," 1931, BGR, Carton A654. In Kenitra in 1918, the municipal labor force consisted of sixty to seventy prisoners, twenty to thirty train station workers, and fifty to sixty military men.

104. Holden, *The Politics of Food,* 102.

105. "P-V du BMH de Casablanca," November 23, 1922, BGR, Carton 647.

106. Holden, *The Politics of Food,* 154–55.

107. David Attar to chief of municipal services of Fez, August 3, 1919, AMF, dossier "David Attar, Aide aux familles militaires."

108. Wright, *The Politics of Design.*

109. Quoted in Abu-Lughod, *Rabat,* 150.

110. Aline de Lens, unpublished journals, BGR archives.

111. "Une année d'assistance publique (6 juin 1913–6 juin 1914) adressé à M. Lyautey de Pean, Médecin Chef du Dispensaire de Rabat," AN, Carton 475, AP 172.

112. Pean, "P-V du BMH de Rabat," October 29, 1913, BGR, Carton A641.

113. Rabat Monthly Municipal Report, February 1938, BGR, Carton 1501.

114. Perrogon, "Rapport sur la prophylaxie de la peste et sur les measures à prendre pour son eradication" and "Note sur les propositions formulées par le Chef des Services Municipaux de Rabat au sujet d'un rapport du Dr. Perrogon sur la peste, 1917," BGR, Carton 1501.

115. Perrogon, "Rapport sur la prophylaxie de la peste," BGR, Carton 1501.

116. "The cases of plague were found almost exclusively in wooden constructions, the insalubrious housing near the workshop of Lepaire and Gosset and the Spanish area near Maison Benaim" (BGR, Carton 641). The first two victims of the epidemic of 1913 were a Spanish couple.

117. Companies like the Société des Constructions Mixtes rented wooden shacks at exorbitant prices to European immigrants and maintained them in defiance of municipal ordinances; see "Note sur les propositions formulées par le Chef des Services Municipaux de Rabat au sujet d'un rapport du Dr. Perrogon sur la peste, 1917," BGR, Carton 1501.

118. Report of BMH Rabat, November 8, 1916, BGR, Carton A641.

119. Abu-Lughod, *Rabat*, 150–152.

120. Chief of municipal services of Rabat, to resident general, report, February 3, 1917, BGR, Carton 1501.

121. Monthly report, Rabat Municipality, January 8, 1917, BGR, Carton 641; "Ville de Rabat, Rapport de fin d'année 1926," BGR, Carton 632.

122. Municipal Services of Rabat, report, October 1919, BGR, uncatalogued carton "1917–1921."

123. Letter, December 12, 1918, BGR, Carton 1501.

124. "P-V du BMH de Meknes," April 10, 1923, BGR, Carton 633.

125. "P-V du BMH de Rabat," November 8, 1916, BGR, Carton A641.

126. The *dahirs* of 1915 and 1918 allowed for the destruction of housing in cases of epidemic and municipal laws strengthened the push to demolish wooden shacks; see "P-V du BMH de Rabat," March 10, 1922, BGR, Carton 646. These efforts were focused in the Petite Sicile and Catalan neighborhoods; see Rabat BMH monthly report, August 1917, BGR, uncatalogued carton 1917–1921. A *sous-commission* (subcommission) of hygiene visited individual homes and condemned them, mostly properties inhabited by Spaniards; see "Commission d'hygiène et de salubrité urbaines, P-V de 19 Fevrier 1924," BGR, Carton 633. Plans for new housing began in 1919; see "Rapport Jan, Feb, Mars 1919, Services Municipaux de la ville de Rabat," BGR, Carton A701.

127. Perrogon, "Rapport sur la prophylaxie de la peste," BGR, Carton 1501.

128. Rabat Monthly Municipal Report, February 1938, BGR, Carton 1501.

129. Remlinger, "Un cas de nodosités juxta-articulaires observé au Maroc chez un Européen."

130. The BMH enlisted the Spanish consulate to encourage the reporting of disease; see BGR, Carton A11001, and "P-V du BMH de Rabat," BGR, Carton 1501. See also "Rapport mensuel du mois de September 1917, Hygiène Générale de Rabat," BGR, unordered carton.

131. Rabat, Monthly Questionnaire, Rabat, September 1917, BGR, unordered carton, "Monthly Hygiene Reports, 1917"; see also BGR, Carton Rabat A11001.

132. For the plague of 1911–1912, see Garcin and Sacquépée, "La peste des Ouled

Fredj (Maroc), La peste des animaux domestiques: Remarques sur la contagion de la peste et sur sa prophylaxie." For the quotation, see Morr, AN, Carton 649.

133. The Société Française de Secours au Blessés militaires, one of the three branches of the French Red Cross, sent nurses with the 1907 campaign; see SFSBM to minister of war, October 31, 1907, SHAT, Carton 3H63.

134. Lyautey and Huguet, "La Goutte de lait de Rabat."

135. Thirty-five percent of Italian and Spanish infants died in Meknes in 1924, compared with 21 percent of French infants; see M. Gaud, "La Mortalité infantile à Meknes."

136. On Mme. Lyautey, see Colombani, "Une grande figure de la croix rouge française, La Maréchale Lyautey"; Chaumont, "L'Oeuvre de madame la maréchale Lyautey au Maroc"; "Mort de la maréchale Lyautey—Elle sera inhumée jeudi à Rabat dans la mausolée où repose le Maréchal—La vie et l'oeuvre d'une grande française"; "En terre qu'ils ont tant aimée (décès de madame la maréchale Lyautey)"; "La maréchale n'est plus."

137. "Note au sujet des oeuvres de Mme. Lyautey, January 1, 1921," AN, Carton 475, AP 172.

138. The president of the republic issued a decree on January 14, 1918, creating sanatoria in the colonies of French West Africa and French Equatorial Africa for native soldiers with tuberculosis. Mme. Lyautey raised the funds; see "Mise au point de la question des sanatoria antituberculeux au 1 nov 1918," AN, Carton 475, AP 172. In 1922, the Fez tuberculosis clinic had 1,505 consultations in May alone; see BGR, Carton 1395.

139. "Réunion du Conseil Supérieur de l'Assistance, Projet de Budget pour l'Année 1929," BGR, Carton 1447.

140. Monthly Reports, Rabat, "P-V du BMH de Rabat," January–November 1927, BGR, Carton A1553.

141. Bouveret and Vallery-Radot, "Éléments de puériculture à l'usage des jeunes filles des écoles du Maroc."

142. French positive eugenics stood in contrast to German and British "negative" eugenics; see Pedersen, *Family, Dependence, and the Origins of the Welfare State: Britain and France, 1914–1945*, and Schneider, *Quality and Quantity: The Quest for Biological Regeneration in Twentieth-Century France.*

143. Bouveret and Vallery-Radot, "Éléments de puériculture," 13–14.

144. Ibid., 60.

145. Ibid., 46–48.

146. See Pedersen, *Family, Dependence, and the Origins of the Welfare State*; Elwitt, *The Third Republic Defended: Bourgeois Reform in France, 1880–1914*; Donzelot, *The Policing of Families.*

147. The league had committees in Oujda, Fez, Meknes, Kenitra, Rabat, Mazagan, Safi, Mogador, and Marrakesh; see "Ligue Marocaine d'hygiène scolaire, autorisée par arrêté viziriel du 14 octobre, 1921," BGR unordered carton "Exposition Coloniale 1922."

148. Dr. Lalande, the director of the BMH, and Dr. Roques, the medical inspector of Rabat schools, to director of the Public Health and Hygiene Service, December 13, 1926, BGR, Carton A1101.

149. By 1900, three-fourths of all single mothers in the Prefecture of the Seine re-

ceived aid from Public Assistance; see Fuchs, *Poor and Pregnant in Paris: Strategies for Survival in the Nineteenth Century.*

150. The boards were composed of the chief of municipal services, three French members of the municipal council, a representative of the local French charity society, and a municipal functionary who served as secretary; see "Note pour M. le Résident Géneral de R. Mangot," BGR, Carton 1447.

151. The *dahir* of May 24, 1914, required workers to obtain authorization from the secretary general of the protectorate before creating a union; see Ayache, *Le Mouvement syndical au Maroc*, 11–21.

152. "Un embryon d'assistance publique à Casablanca," *La Vigie marocaine*, Friday, December 7, 1923.

153. Ayache, *Le Mouvement syndical*, 22–26.

154. "Exposition coloniale de 1922 à Marseille, Sociétés ou oeuvres privées de bienfaisance du Maroc," BGR, unordered carton.

155. BGR, Carton 1447, folder "Réunion du conseil supérieur de l'assistance."

156. Eulogio Henche to chief of municipal services, Rabat, BGR, Carton 1447.

157. On the *hebrot*, see Laskier, *The Alliance Israelite Universelle and the Jewish Communities of Morocco, 1862–1962*, and Serels, "Aspects of the Effects of Jewish Philanthropic Societies in Morocco." Founded during World War II, the Moroccan branch of the Oeuvre de Secours aux Enfants operated from Casablanca with an annual budget of 11,000,000 francs; see M.C., "Une visite à l'O.S.E oeuvre de secours pour l'enfant juive."

158. Although the Alliance Israélite Universelle and the *hebrot* were hostile to Zionism until World War II, the French education and welfare they offered prepared Moroccan Jews for life in Europe, Canada, and Israel; see Laskier, *The Alliance Israelite Universelle.*

159. On the water system of Fez, see Allouche, "Un plan des canalisations de Fès au temps de Mawlay Isma'il d'après un texte inédit, avec une étude succincte sur la corporation des Kwadisiyya."

160. Colin, "La noria marocaine et les machines hydrauliques dans le monde arabe"; Mazières, "La situation economique du Maroc."

161. Le Tourneau describes the water distribution to the palace, Fes Jdid (97), and the Andalus quarter (113–114, 232–240) in *Fès avant le protectorat.* Moroccans used human waste to enhance agricultural productivity. In Marrakesh, guilds dried and collected waste from night-soil pits and transported it to fields outside the city for use as fertilizer; see "Inspection de la salubrité des maisons en construction et casier sanitaire des immeubles," in "Rapport annuel du médecin-chef du BMH de Marrakech, 1925," BGR, Carton A837.

162. Costeaud, cited in Le Tourneau, *Fès avant le protectorat*, 238.

163. "Mémoire militaire, sur l'empire de Maroc par Capt. 1ère classe au corps impérial du génie Burel, 1810," SHAT, Carton 3H1. However, the Marinid sultans canalized water from the spring of Omair rather than touch the River Fez, because "to touch the water of the Fassis would be to push them to eternal rebellion" (Le Tourneau, *Fès avant le protectorat*, 63).

164. Mawlay Hasan convened a committee in 1884 in response to accusations by Fez residents that millers and garden owners had taken water belonging to the Mawlay Idris mosque. The committee made the following report: "The Commission has gone

to the place called Sebaa Akdam across from the garden called Saidi, in Boujeloud, where there is a canal called the *kadus* of Moulay Idriss. Contestations were raised on the subject of the distribution of water of this canalization . . . if this construction existed in its current form since the time of Sultan Moulay Ismael, as the copy of an authentic testimony by Sidi Muhammad ben Larbi ben Abdesselam ben Brahim ed Doukkali dated month of April in Rejeb 1127, or if it is recently constructed . . . People from the quarters called Al-Lamtiyne and quarter Al-Andalous were present at the debates," Massignon, "Enquête sur les corporations d'artisans et de commerçants au Maroc," 226–228. See also Le Tourneau, *Fès avant le protectorat*, 237.

165. Strohl report, 1877, SHAT, Carton 3H1.

166. Marrakesh never had abundant water; the mellah and Badia quarters received only the overflow of the palace reservoirs. In 1922, Jews had to pay water carriers to bring water from 2.5 kilometers away; see "P-V de la sous-commission d'hygiène, BMH de Marrakech," May 12, 1922, BGR, Carton A646.

167. From one home, "during rainstorms, torrents of sewage invade all neighboring terrain and flood the rue d'Agadir"; see "P-V du BMH de Rabat," January 6, 1916, BGR, Carton A641. For the quotation, see "Document: Hotels, Rapport, Direction du Service de Santé, Troupes d'Occupation du Maroc, Rapport du Médecin Principal 1ère classe Eymeri, sur l'inspection sanitaire des hôtels du Maroc," BGR, unordered carton.

168. "P-V du BMH de Meknes," March 1, 1923, BGR, Carton A647.

169. "Bureaux Municipaux d'Hygiène, rapports annuels 1922–1926, Safi report 1925," BGR, Carton A837.

170. "P-V du BMH de Mazagan," November 4, 1925, BGR, Carton 634.

171. For the conjecture that Moroccans were immune to typhoid, see Bouveret and Pouponneau, *Le Médecin d'assistance au Maroc: Conseils pratiques au jeune médecin du service de la santé et de l'Hygiène publiques, Préface du Médecin-Inspecteur Oberlé*, 67; "P-V du BMH de Casablanca," March 20, 1923, BGR, Carton 647. For the doctor's report, see "Bureaux Municipaux d'hygiène, rapports annuels 1922–1926, Safi report 1925," BGR, Carton A837. On March 18, 1914, twenty-six Europeans in Casablanca met at a tavern to demand potable water and sewers from the Résidence; see "Casablanca: Attroupements et réunions publics, 1914," BGR, Carton A1504, folder II: "Police dans les villes: Ordre public (1912–1919)."

172. Lacour, Varanguien de Villepin, and Rebreyend, "La Rénovation de l'institution des habous."

173. "P-V du BMH de Casablanca," July 6, 1914, BGR, Carton A641. On water in Casablanca, see "Conseil supérieur de la santé et de l'hygiène publiques, P-V of March 15, 1922," BGR, Carton A1101.

174. "P-V du BMH de Rabat," October 29, 1913, BGR, Carton A641. That supply was augmented by several wells with pumps on the Zaers road; see "P-V du BMH de Rabat," September 18, 1923, BGR, Carton A647. The Aït Attig spring, which could have been used to supply the Kabibat quarter, was judged "too polluted" to drink from and not worth purifying; see "P-V du BMH de Rabat," July 31, 1923, BGR, Carton A647.

175. "Ville de Meknes, Bureau Municipal d'Hygiène, Rapport Annuel 1923," BGR, Carton 837.

176. "P-V du BMH de Rabat," July 10, 1916, and August 7 1916, BGR, Carton

A641; President of the Committee of the Israelite Community to Secretary General of the Protectorate, September 19, 1924, BGR, Carton 1142.

177. "Ville de Rabat, rapport fin d'année 1926 du Bureau d'hygiène et des formations sanitaires municipals de la ville de Rabat," BGR, Carton 632.

178. "P-V du BMH de Meknes," December 3, 1934, BGR, Carton 598.

179. "P-V du BMH de Rabat," September 16, 1924, BGR, Carton 633.

180. "P-V du BMH de Rabat," December 12, 1927, BGR, Carton A1553. For new native housing, the developer was expected to pay for the sewer network and then recover the cost by charging each homeowner for his sewer; see "Commission d'hygiène et de salubrité urbaines, Séance du 16 Septembre 1924," BGR, Carton 633.

181. "Bureau Municipal d'Hygiène de Rabat, Rapport Juillet 1938," BGR, Carton A1542.

182. In 1923, eighty-nine European cases of typhoid were declared; in 1924, only thirty-five to forty; see "P-V du BMH de Casablanca," November 20, 1924, BGR, Carton 633.

183. "P-V du BMH de Mogador," December 1926, BGR, Carton 632; "P-V du BMH de Casablanca," 17 December 1925, BGR, Carton 632; "P-V du BMH de Kenitra," 15 December 1923, BGR, Carton 647.

184. "Ville de Meknes, Bureau Municipal d'Hygiène, Rapport Annuel 1923," BGR, Carton 837.

185. "Bureau Municipal d'Hygiène et de Salubrité publique de Meknes: Rapport annuel 1935," BGR, Carton 649.

186. "Extrait du registre des procès-verbaux des séances de la commission d'hygiène et de salubrité urbaines de la ville de Rabat (Séance du 16 Septembre 1924), Abreuvoir Akari à Kebibat," BGR, Carton 633.

187. Rosenberg, *The Cholera Years: The United States in 1832, 1849, and 1866*; Evans, *Death in Hamburg: Society and Politics in the Cholera Years, 1830–1910*.

188. Huot to Commander of the Fez region, August 9, 1929, BGR, Carton 1501.

189. The voting districts were Lamtiyyin, 'Adwa, Andalus, and Fez Jdid, which included the palace and the Mawlay Abdallah quarter; see Yakhlef, "La Municipalité de Fès," 1:68.

190. General Gourand to Resident General Lyautey, October 21, 1912, quoted in Yakhlef, "La Municipalité de Fès," 70.

191. Holden, *The Politics of Food*, 100.

192. Quoted in Yakhlef, "La Municipalité de Fès," 84.

193. "Note sur l'usine d'équarrissage appartenant à la société industrielle 'El Fassia,'" Général Gueval to chief of municipal services, Fez, AAE Nantes, Maroc DAI, Carton 331A.

194. Ibid.

195. The quarters included R'mila, Keddan, Sidi Boujida, Bayn al-Mudun, Blida, Derb Tawil, and Saba' Luyat; see letter, February 22, 1923, AAE Nantes, Maroc DAI, Carton 331A.

196. "P-V du BMH de Fès," July 16, 1923, in BGR, Carton 647; see also Monthly Reports, BMH, January 1924, in BGR, Carton 1395.

197. Holden, *The Politics of Food*, 119–125; Yakhlef, "La Municipalité de Fès," 2:281–284.

198. Yakhlef, "La Municipalité de Fès," 2:298.

199. "Procès-verbal du Mejliss al-Baladi Musulman, Séance de 11.12.1926," cited in Yakhlef, "La Municipalité de Fès," 2:316.

200. Yakhlef, "La Municipalité de Fès," Volume 3, Appendix 5, "L'Oued Fès."

201. Yakhlef, "La Municipalité de Fès," 2:285.

202. Holden, *The Politics of Food*, 174–178.

203. Ibid., 177.

204. Mosques, schools, and *zawiyat* would be granted free access to potable drinking water; see LeMaire to secretary general of the protectorate, March 18, 1935, AMF, folder "L'Eau à Fès."

205. "Note relative aux débits d'été de l'Oued Fès à M. le CMS, Fès le 28 Octobre 1932, L'Ingenieur-Adjoint des T. P. Karst," AMF, folder "L'Eau à Fès."

206. "Réponse à Note de Service date 11 mai 1946 rélative à la repartition des eaux de l'Oued et l'adduction au Medina," AMF, folder "L'eau à Fès."

207. "D'autres fléaux en perspective," copied in Note to M. Artozoul, chief of municipal services, Fez, May 11, 1946, AMF, folder "L'eau à Fès."

208. Quoted in Segalla, *The Moroccan Soul*, 201–212.

209. The protectorate arrested the delegation members Muhammad Lahlou, 'Allal al-Fasi, and Muhammad al-Wazzani; see Halstead, *Rebirth of a Nation: The Origins and Rise of Moroccan Nationalism, 1912–1944*, 183.

210. Comité d'Action Marocaine, *Plan de réformes marocaines*, xiv, 27.

211. Ibid., xiii.

212. Ibid., 96–100.

213. Halstead, *Rebirth of a Nation*, 247–250.

214. Reprinted in "Meknès proteste et pousse un cri d'alarme," *L'Action du peuple*, June 17, 1937.

215. Ibid.

216. Al-Wazzani had previously complained that mosques and the population were deprived of water; see "L'eau de Boufekrane et son angoissant problème," *L'Action du peuple*, June 3, 1937.

217. "La grande tragédie de Meknès; La journée sanglante de Meknès, Le 2 septembre 1947," *L'Action du peuple*, September 17, 1937.

218. Wilder, *The French Imperial Nation-State*, 33.

219. Chénébeaux, "Le Bureau Marocain du Travail," 9.

220. Halsted, *Rebirth of a Nation*, 213–217; Segalla, *The Moroccan Soul*, 203–235.

221. Comité d'Action Marocaine, *Plan de réformes marocaines*, 47–48.

222. Ibid., 50.

223. Yakhlef, "La Municipalité de Fès," 1:86–87.

224. Abdessalam Benjelloun, "Les municipalités," *Al Hayat*, June 6, 1935, SHAT, Carton 3H1423.

CHAPTER 5

1. Lepinay and Speder, introduction to de Lens, *Pratiques des harems marocains: Sorcellerie, médecine, beauté*, vii–viii.

2. De Lens, *Pratiques des harems marocains*, 29. On de Lens, see Amster, "'The

Harem Revealed' and the Islamic-French Family: Aline de Lens and a French Woman's Orient in Lyautey's Morocco."

3. Foucault, *The Birth of Biopolitics*, 35.

4. Wilson, *Women and Medicine in the French Enlightenment: The Debate over "Maladies des Femmes"*; Léonard, "Women, Religion, and Medicine"; Schneider, *Quality and Quantity*; Barnes, *The Making of a Social Disease: Tuberculosis in Nineteenth-Century France*.

5. Donzelot, *The Policing of Families*.

6. Martin, "Description de la ville de Fès."

7. Badia y Leblich, *Voyages d'Ali Bey el Abbassi*, 143–144.

8. "L'Anonyme de Fès," cited in Lévi-Provençal, *Les Historiens des Chorfa: Essai sur la littérature historique et biographique au Maroc du XVIe au XXe siècle*, 139.

9. SHAT, Carton 1 K 662, Ninard Papers, Carton 1, Linarès file.

10. *La Revue marocaine de droit*, "Juridictions chérifiennes, Tribunal d'Appel du Chrâa, Audience du 24 Qaada 1368, Répudiation—répudiation par le tamlik—irrevocabilité—Vocation héréditaire des ex-conjoints (non)—Dernière maladie—Maladie accidentale—affection chronique—Capacité juridique—Mention Adoulaire—Preuve du contraire—Certificat Médical—Médecin non-musulman—Témoignage ou expertise: Caractère d'information de la science—Déclarations devant l'adoul—Attestation de l'identité du malade" (17 September, 1949).

11. É.-L. Bertherand, *Médecine et l'hygiène des Arabes*, 88–90.

12. Hamida, "Les modes de preuve dans la coutume de la tribu des Aid Izdeq."

13. Ibn Khaldun, quoted in Mathieu and Maneville, *Les Accoucheuses musulmanes traditionelles de Casablanca*, 89–91.

14. Mawlay Ali, interview by the author, March 15, 1999, Fez.

15. R., interview by the author, March 8, 1999, Funduq al-Yuhudy Clinic, Fez.

16. Nurse, 'Umar Idrisi Hospital, interview, March 22, 1999, Fez.

17. J., interview by the author, March 12, 1999, Lamtiyyin Clinic, Fez.

18. Mr. N., interview by the author, February 2, 1999, Fez.

19. Mawlay Ali, interview by the author, March 12, 1999, Fez.

20. On the absence of fixed fees: "Yes, people gave what they had, there was no fixed price, each one according to his own. She went to their homes. She delivered my mother-in-law," W., interview by the author, March 9, 1999, Funduq al-Yuhudy, Fez. For the quotation, see Bahia, interview by the author, February 13, 1999, Fez.

21. My Khaddouj, interview by the author, March 22, 1999, Fez.

22. Ibid.

23. Mauran, "Considerations sur la médecine."

24. Perho, *The Prophet's Medicine: A Creation of the Muslim Traditionalist Scholars*.

25. For biographical information on al-Qurtubi, see Ullmann, *Die Medizin im Islam*, and Leclerc, *Histoire de la médecine arabe*, 1:432.

26. Meyerhof and Joannides, *La Gynécologie et l'obstétrique chez Avicenne (Ibn Sina) et leur rapports avec celles des Grecs*; see also Musallam, *Sex and Society in Islam*, 66–68.

27. É.-L. Bertherand, "Contribution des arabes au propos des sciences médicales." For az-Zahrawi's gynecology and surgery, see Spink, "Arabian Gynaecological, Ob-

stetrical, and Genito-Urinary Practice, Illustrated from Abulcasis," and Schahien, "Die Geburtshilflich-gynäkologischen Kapitel aus der Chirurgie des Abulkasim, ins Deutsche übersetzt und kommentiert."

28. Weisser, *Zeugung, Vererbung und Pränatale Entwicklung in der Medizin des Arabisch-Islamischen Mittelalters*. See also Jahier and Noureddine, "De l'Obstetrique et de la pédiatrie en Espagne musulmane aux Xème siècle."

29. Al-Qurtubi gives glancing attention to *shariʿa* cases of prolonged gestation, but he considers the Greek sources superior; see al-Qurtubi, *Le Livre de la génération du foetus et le traitement des femmes enceintes et des nouveau-nés, publié, traduit et annoté par Henri Jahier et Abdelkader Noureddine*, 41.

30. Ibid., 23–24.

31. Ibid., 36–37.

32. For example, al-Qurtubi argues that a child born in the seventh or ninth month will live, but that a child born in the eighth month will die because of the pernicious effect of Saturn: "In the first month, when the fetus is still a formless drop, it stands under the sway of Saturn, whose nature is cold and dry. Because of this, the drop has no sense perception and no movement. In the second month it stands under the sway of Jupiter, whose nature is hot and wet. Now it begins to grow and form into a lump of flesh. If it is a boy, its color is white and its shape round; if it is a girl, its color is red and its shape like that of a banana. In the third month Mars, which is hot and dry, holds sway. At this stage nerves and blood appear in the lump of flesh. The sun, which is likewise hot and dry, determines the fourth month when the fetus begins to move. When in the fifth month cold Venus holds sway, the brain, the bones and the skin form. Mercury, relatively hot and dry, influences development in the sixth month, when the tongue and the hearing develop. In the seventh month the fetus stands under the sway of the moon, whose attributes are swift movements. By now the child is fully formed and thrusts outwards. If it is actually born this month, it can live, and grow, because it has experienced the influences of the seven planets in their entirety. However, if it remains in the womb, it again comes under the sway of Saturn in the eighth month, which is cold and dry. This quiets it, even makes it ill, so that if born now it cannot live. But in the ninth month, Jupiter rules again, bringer of life and growth. If the child is born now, it will live" (al-Qurtubi, quoted in Ullmann, *Islamic Medicine*, 112–113).

33. Al-Qurtubi, *Le Livre de la génération du foetus*, 52.

34. Islamic physicians did sometimes resent midwives as competitors; see Savage-Smith and Pormann, *Medieval Islamic Medicine*.

35. See, for example, Obermeyer, "Pluralism and Pragmatism: Knowledge and Practice of Birth in Morocco." Mary-Jo DelVecchio Good shows the pervasiveness of Galenic physiology in the Islamic world; see "Of Blood and Babies: The Relationship of Popular Islamic Physiology to Fertility."

36. Bahia, interview by the author, February 13, 1999, Fez.

37. My Khaddouj, interview by the author, March 22, 1999, Fez.

38. M.-J. Good, "Of Blood and Babies," 149.

39. Al-Qurtubi, *Le Livre de la génération du foetus*, 36.

40. Bahia interview; see also Slomka, "Medicine and Reproduction in Urban Morocco," 50–52.

41. Al-Qurtubi, *Le Livre de la génération du foetus*, 49.

42. Bahia interview.

43. According to a popular Moroccan belief, if the pregnant woman desires a food and does not receive it, her child will be born with a birthmark (*tawhima*) shaped like the desired food.

44. Mathieu and Maneville, *Les Accoucheuses musulmanes traditionelles*, 56–57.

45. Doumato, *Women, Islam, and Healing in Saudi Arabia and the Gulf*; Good and Good, "The Comparative Study of Greco-Islamic Medicine," and B. Good, "The Heart of What's the Matter: The Structure of Medical Discourse in a Provincial Iranian Town"; Delaney, *The Seed and the Soil: Gender and Cosmology in Turkish Village Society*.

46. The *Kitab al-rahma fi al-tibb wa al-hikma* was erroneously attributed to Jalal al-Din ʿAbd al-Rahman al-Siyuti; the true author was Muhammad al-Mahdawi ibn ʿAli ibn Ibrahim al-Sanabari al-Yamani al-Hindi (d. 1412). The book was first translated into French in French colonial Algeria in 1856; see Pharaon and A. Bertherand, *Livre de la miséricorde dans l'art de guérir les maladies et de conserver la santé*.

47. Abi ʿAbd Allah Muhammad ibn Yusuf al-Sanusi, "Sharh ʿala qula s [Prophet Muhammad] al-maʿda bayna al-daʾwa al-hamiya raʾs al-duwaʾ wa asl kul daʿ al-buruda" (1886), MS 4091, BGR, Maghribi script; ʿAbd Allah ibn Ahmad Adarraq, "Qasida fi munafiaʿ al-naʿnaʿ," MS 4094, BGR, Maghribi script; "Taqiyyid fi munafiaʿ al-safufat," MS 4101, BGR, author unknown, date unknown, Maghribi script.

48. ʿAbd Allah Sidi Muhammad ibn Yusuf ibn Khalsun, "Qalaʾid al-ʿafiyan fi siha badn al-insan," MS 4096, BGR.

49. "Tuhfa al-ʿaraws wa nuzha al-nafaws," Bibliothèque Nationale de France (hereafter BNF), MSS Orientales 3061, though al-Tijani may not be the author. Scandalous texts were often falsely attributed to respectable authors, to make them more acceptable. For example, no author is given for "Rajuʿa al-shaykh ila subaha" (The Return of the Old Man to Boyhood), MSS Orientales 3056, 3057, 3058, 3059, BNF.

50. Conserved in Rabat, the manuscript includes two texts. The first is a partial copy of "Zad al-Musafir" (Provision of the Traveler), by the Tunisian physician Abu Jaʿfar Ahmad ibn Ibrahim ibn Abu Khalid, called Ibn al-Jazzar. Although the copyist is unknown and the text is not dated, the paper, binding, and leather resemble manuscripts in the Qarawiyyin library from the sixteenth century. The copy has letters without points, misspellings, and dialectical spellings, which suggest that the copyist may have been a prison inmate.

51. The "reverse wind" is *al-rih al-maqloub*. In Moroccan colloquial, "*Al mar-a, kirsh-ha maqlouba*," or "The woman, her belly is reversed."

52. *Sufa* is literally translated as "wool tampon" and refers to a small wool ball treated with herbs or solutions that is inserted into the vagina.

53. *ʿArq aykar* is a Berber word, referring to a root. Traditional apothecaries in Fez were unable to identify the plant called "*khalal*" in the manuscript.

54. Specifically, purification here refers to a woman going to the *hammam* and washing herself once her menstrual period is over.

55. "Risala ʿilm amrad an-nisaʾ wa tawiqhunna ʿan al-habl," MS D1718/2758, BGR. For traditional pharmacology in Morocco, see Bellakhdar, *La Pharmacopée marocaine traditionnelle: Médecine arabe ancienne et savoirs populaires*.

56. At the end of the section there is a "Chapter Mentioning Remedies Which Bring Pregnancy" and "Medicine Which Completely Prevents Pregnancy"; see al-Antaki, *Tadhkira*, Section 3, 145–146 (my translation).

57. J., interview by the author, March 12, 1999, Lamtiyyin Clinic, Fez; Mawlay Ali interview, March 12, 1999, Lamtiyyin Clinic, Fez; Mawlay Ali and My Khaddouj, interviews by the author, March 15, 1999, Fez.

58. See Musallam, *Sex and Society in Islam*, especially Chapter 3. The *idda* is the time period a woman must wait after divorce or her husband's death before her remarriage, in order to ensure that she is not pregnant with a child by the first husband.

59. Quoted in Musallam, *Sex and Society in Islam*, 53–54.

60. Ibid., Chapter 3, "Conception Theory in Islamic Thought."

61. Giladi, *Infants, Parents, and Wet Nurses: Medieval Islamic Views on Breastfeeding and Their Social Implications*, 60.

62. "When a woman is pregnant and when a woman is suckling, her monthly period ceases. When pregnant, the best part of the blood turns to food, that is, it becomes the nourishment of the fetus, and the rest—and it is the corrupt part—passes to the breasts. Similarly, when suckling, all the menstrual blood passes to the breasts and is converted into milk for the nourishment of the child. And that is why the Prophet said: Do not kill your children secretly. For the practice of *al-ghayla* throws down the child . . . the effect of the corrupt food continues with a man until puberty and manhood. And should he be challenged to a test of strength by a duel, he will be overwhelmed in the fight, being weaker than the other" (Elgood, "Tibb-Ul-Nabbi or Medicine of the Prophet: Being a Translation of Two Works of the Same Name").

63. Legey, *Essai de folklore marocain*, 110.

64. Cited in Mathieu and Maneville, *Les Accoucheuses musulmanes traditionnelles*, 59.

65. Legey, *Essai de folklore marocain*, 106–107.

66. Ibid., 107–108.

67. Mawlay Ali interview, March 22, 1999.

68. M.A., interview by the author, May 18, 1999, Fez.

69. Anonymous, interview by the author, April 1, 1999, Tamgrout.

70. "*Shebba* and *harmel* are from the Prophet of God. Right? Lalla Fatima Zahra [the Prophet's daughter], went to her father, said to him, Father, have affection for me. Hasan and Hussein are sick. He said to her *shebba* and *harmel*, O Prophet of God" (My Khadddouj interview, March 22, 1999).

71. Philips gives numerous examples of hadith in which the Prophet and his companions used the Ayat al-Kursy against evil *jinn*. Ibn Taymiyya himself performed exorcisms, according to his student Ibn al-Qayyim; see Philips, *Ibn Taymeeyah's Essay on the Jinn*, 88–89.

72. My Khaddouj interview, March 22, 1999.

73. Mawlay Ali interview, March 22, 1999.

74. Legey, *Essai de folklore marocain*, 100–103.

75. Ibid., 132.

76. Ibid., 219.

77. Ibid., 110.

78. Ibid., 64. Legey notes that fortune-tellers (*shuwwafat*) drank the blood of the sheep from 'Aid al-Kabir ('Aid al-Adha) to give them the ability to see the future (64).

79. Bahia's husband, interview by the author, February 13, 1999, Fez.

80. Doutté, *Magie et religion*, 54–55, 33.

81. Mauchamp, *La Sorcellerie au Maroc*, 255–256.

82. A *bézoar* (bezoar) is a ball of indigestible materials, hair, and calcium formed in the gullets of large birds or in the digestive systems of animals, particularly cows and other ruminants. The bezoar was long believed to be an antidote to poison; see Arnaud, "L'oeuf de faon, ou la survivance inattendue du Bézoard."

83. De Lens, *Pratiques des harems marocains*, xiii.

84. Brett, "Legislating for Inequality in Algeria: The Sénatus-Consulte of 14 July 1865," 455.

85. Morand, *Introduction à l'étude du droit musulman algérien*.

86. On views of Muslim women in the Algiers School, see Mercier, *La Condition de la femme musulmane dans l'afrique septentrionale*; Milliot, *Étude sur la condition de la femme musulmane au Maghreb (Maroc, Algérie, Tunisie)*; Morand, *La Famille Musulmane*. Octave Depont is quoted in Clancy-Smith, "Islam, Gender, and Identities in the Making of French Algeria, 1830–1962."

87. Charles de Foucauld, quoted in R. Bazin, *Charles de Foucauld, explorateur du Maroc, eremite au Sahara*, 221, 319.

88. Samné, *De l'Assistance considérée comme un moyen de colonisation*, 29.

89. Léonard, "Women, Religion and Medicine," 41–43.

90. Mme. Lyautey, "Les oeuvres de l'enfance au Maroc."

91. Marmey and Marmey, "Contribution à l'étude de l'obstetrique au Maroc: Travail de la Maternité 'Maréchale Lyautey' à Rabat"; Huguet, "La goutte de laït de Rabat."

92. Lapin, "La lutte contre la tuberculose."

93. "P-V de réunion de commission municipale d'hygiène, February 26, 1926," BGR, Carton 632.

94. Oujda, Monthly Reports for 1922–1925, BGR, Carton 641; Bienvenue, "La Mortalité estivale infantile à Rabat et à Casablanca"; Herber, "La Mortalité estivale infantile de 0 à 1 an, à Rabat."

95. "P-V du BMH de Mogador," August 3, 1922, BGR, Carton 646.

96. Mauran, *La Société marocaine: Études sociales, impressions et souvenirs, avec une lettre-préface de M. Le Générale d'Amade, et une lettre de M. Guiot*.

97. Lal, "The Politics of Gender and Medicine in Colonial India: The Countess of Dufferin's Fund, 1885–1888"; Burton, "The White Woman's Burden: British Feminists and 'The Indian Woman,' 1865–1915."

98. Male contemporaries attested to her abilities: "She knows how to make the natives accept coercive measures they abhor and rise in their esteem. Her qualities as a woman help her to penetrate everywhere and obtain information which a man would not get . . . Mlle. Langlais does not know obstacles in accomplishing her mission" (quoted in Péraud, *La Femme médecin en Afrique du Nord: Son role d'éducatrice*, 46).

99. Mme. Eugénie Delanoë, Mlle. Sarah Broido, and Mme. Pokitonow were born in Russia; Mme. Marie Petresco-Burnol in Romania; Mlle. Gertrude Loeser in Prussia; and Mme. Wecke in Copenhagen; see BGR, unordered carton "Service de Santé, 1913–1920."

100. Françoise Legey, cited in Péraud, *La Femme médecin en Afrique du Nord*, 36–37; see also, *L'Afrique Française*, "Une française du Maroc (Mme. la Doctoresse Legey)."

101. Delanoë, "Protection de la femme et de l'enfant indigènes: Quelques questions de médecine sociale indigène à l'occasion du Ve Congrès de la Mutualité Coloniale et des Pays de Protectorat."

102. Broido, "Abolition de la réglementation de la prostitution: Conférence faite à l'Union française pour le Suffrage des Femmes de Casablanca."

103. Delanoë, "La prophylaxie antitrachomateuse exercée dans le milieu indigène marocain d'une façon suivie et energique depuis 10 ans fait baisser de moitié le nombre des trachomateux, elle diminue aussi et surtout la gravité des cas."

104. Delanoë, "Protection de la femme et de l'enfant indigènes," 71–72.

105. For the milk dispensary, see "Document: Les Hôpitaux Indigènes du Maroc, Note du Dr. Laurent, demobilisé du Maroc de Paris, 1918," AN, Carton 475AP172. A case of maternal death due to "hemorrhage resulting from uterine inversion by pulling on the cord" inspired the decision by the Jewish community in Meknes; see "P-V du Commission d'hygiène et de salubrité urbaine de Meknes," September 1933, BGR, Carton A1623.

106. Grand Vizier Moqri to Mohtasseb of Rabat, 23 djoumada 1, 1338 (February 14, 1920), AAE Nantes, Maroc DACH, Carton 84.

107. Legey, "Un centre de puériculture à Marrakech," 583–585.

108. Legey and Décor, "L'Assistance aux femmes en couches à la maternité indigène de Marrakech."

109. Ibid. Legey's monitoring system for native midwives inspired Dr. Bouveret to propose the same regulation in Mogador; see "P-V du BMH de Mogador," 25 February 1931, BGR, Carton A1623.

110. Legey and Décor, "L'Assistance aux femmes en couches."

111. "P-V du BMH de Mogador," December 14, 1922, and August 27, 1925, BGR, Carton 646; "P-V du BMH de Mogador," December 15, 1925, Monthly Report for Mogador, May 1927, and "P-V du BMH de Mogador," December 9, 1927, BGR, Carton A1553.

112. For French Algeria and French Indochina, see Stoler, "Rethinking Colonial Categories: European Communities and the Boundaries of Rule" and "Carnal Knowledge and Imperial Power: Gender, Race, and Morality in Colonial Asia."

113. Hardy and Brunot, *L'Enfant marocaine: Essai d'ethnographie scolaire . . . Avec la collaboration de Mlle Burtey, Mme Driss-Amor, Mme De Pressigny.*

114. Lepinay, from de Lens, *Pratiques des harems marocains*, vii.

115. Ibid., 140–141. The most dangerous *ta'am* is that prepared by the *jinn* themselves (141).

116. The Prophet Muhammad said: "A Jinn missionary came to me so I went with him and recited the Qur'an to them. Then [the Jinn] took me and showed me their tracks and remnants of their fires and they asked me to specify food for them, so I said, 'You may have as meat every bone on which Allah's name has been mentioned which falls in your hand, and every animal dropping for your animals.' The Prophet then said, 'So do not clean yourselves with them as they are the provisions of your brothers'" (a hadith quoted in Philips, *Ibn Taymeeyah's Essay on the Jinn*, 24).

117. M.A., interview by the author, August 21, 1999, Fez.

118. Legey, *Essai de folklore marocain*, 12.

119. Ibid., 14.

120. Ibid., 148.

121. De Lens, *Pratiques des harems marocains*, 57–58.

122. Raynaud, *Étude sur l'hygiène*, 111. "A woman who performed this in El Qsar died of fright, because the swollen cadaver cracked in her arms" (Michaux-Bellaire and Salmon, "El-Qcar El-Kebir").

123. Schiebinger, *Plants and Empire: Colonial Bioprospecting in the Atlantic World*, 11.

124. Ball, *Spicilegium Florae maroccanae*, cited in Jahandiez and Maire, *Catalogue des Plantes du Maroc*; Camus, *Contribution à la connaissance de la flore du Maroc: Actes du 1er congrès international de botanique tenu à Paris, à l'occasion de l'exposition universelle de 1900*; Perrot, *Les Matières premières usuelles d'origine végétale indigènes et exotiques.*

125. In India, an officer of the District of Chindwin recorded a native legend about the discovery of chaulmoogra oil: Rama, the king of Benares, was forced to abdicate and live in exile when he became infected with leprosy. He lived in a tree and cured himself by consuming its fruits. In the forest, he met a princess who was also a leper. He fed her the fruits, leaves, and roots of the "Kalaw" tree. She was cured and she married her savior; see Perrot, *Les Matières premières usuelles d'origine végétale indigènes et exotiques*, 50–59. In India, the chaulmoogra tree (*Taraktogenos kurzi*) was used; in Sierra Leone, the gorli tree (*Oncoba echinata*); in Brazil, *Carpotroche brasiliensis*; in Cambodia, the chong-bao tree (*Hydnocarpus anthelminthica*), in Siam, the ta-fung-chi tree (also *Hydnocarpus anthelminthica*); see Perrot, *Chaulmoogra et autres graines utilisables contre la lèpre*, 4.

126. Gentil and Perrot, *Sur les productions végétales du Maroc—Notice 10 De l'Office national des matières premières végétales—Contient en outre: (Maire, Dr. R.) Coup d'oeil sur la végétation du Maroc; (Gattefossé, J.) Les Plantes dans la thérapeutique indigène au Maroc; (Dufougeré Mme.), Sur les matières colorantes végétales employées au Maroc.*

127. Perrot, *Plantes médicinales et plantes à parfum au Maroc (Action du Comité Marocain, 1920–25).* On Perrot, see Bonnemain, "Le Professeur Émile Perrot: Sept ans de collaboration avec la Quinzaine coloniale (1907–1914)."

128. Mauran, *La Société marocaine*, 157–158; Massy, "Contribution à l'étude des produits susceptibles d'être fournis à l'industrie et à la matière médicale par les forêts du Maroc."

129. Fourment and Roques, "Contribution à l'étude des drogues indigènes nord-africaines—Le 'souak' ou 'Djouz' (juglans regia L.)."

130. *Bulletin d'Information du Maroc*, "L'Industrie pharmaceutique au Maroc."

131. *Bulletin de l'Institut d'Hygiène du Maroc*, "L'Institute d'Hygiène du Maroc."

132. Montagne, *Un Magasin collectif de l'Anti-Atlas: L'Agadir des Ikounka*, 6–7.

133. "Étude sur l'organisation des Tribunaux Coutumiers," 1930, SHAT, Carton 3H1418, dossier 1.

134. Poincaré, cited in Article 1 of the Protectorate Agreement of March 30, 1912, quoted in Chastand, *Le Protectorat français au Maroc*, 152.

135. The *dahir* of September 11, 1914, guaranteed "the right of Berber tribes to live under their customary laws"; quoted in Luccioni, "L'Élaboration du dahir berbère du 16 mai 1930."

136. Surdon, *Esquisses de droit coutumier berbère marocain: Conférences données au cours préparatoire au service des affaires indigènes pendant l'année 1927–*

1928, 212–213; see also Surdon, *Institutions et coutumes des berbères du Maghreb (Maroc-Algérie-Tunisie-Sahara), Leçons de droit coutumier berbère.*

137. Guerin, "Racial Myth, Colonial Reform, and the Invention of Customary Law in Colonial Morocco."

138. Denat, "Droit coutumier berbère Ichkern: Coutume de l'enfant endormi."

139. Aspinion, "Case 22, 1er Rebia I 1354 (3 juin 1935), Jugement du Tribunal coutumier des Aït Harkat de Guelmous, Bureau de Khénifra, déclarant la paternité d'un enfant né d'une femme mariée quatre fois et admettant la croyance de l'enfant endormi en pays Zaïan."

140. On divorce, see Zeys, "Case 7, 11 Août 1924 (10 moharrem 1343), Jugement du Tribunal coutumier des Aït Seghrouchen d'Immouzer pronoçant le divorce par consentement mutual," 17. On discreetly taking a paramour, see Denat, "Coutumes berbères Ichkern: Dissolution du mariage."

141. Aspinion, *Contribution à l'étude du droit coutumier berbère marocain (Étude sur les coutumes des tribus Zayanes)*, 163. Only a few tribes influenced by Arab *shurafa'* gave women the right to inherit: the Aït Ammou Aïssa, Aït Taskert, Aït Tameskourt, Aït El Herri, Aït Nouh, Aït Arrouggou, Aït Sidi Bou Abbed, Aït Bou Hemmad and Aït Lahssen. On women and inheritance under Berber law, see also Surdon, *Esquisses de droit coutumier berbère marocain*, 17.

142. *La Revue marocaine de droit*, "Jurisprudence chérifienne, Tribunaux du chrâa, Mariage (nullité)—Prohibition d'une cinquième co-épouse. Filiation—Filiation putative—conditions."

143. In a *shari'a* court, a husband had to prove that he could not be the father; see *La Revue marocaine de droit*, "Jurisprudence chérifienne, Tribunal d'Appel du Chrâa, Arrêté du 29 rabia I 1368 (29 janvier 1949), Désaveu de paternité—serments d'anathème (lican)—Conditions d'admission."

144. Denat, "Droit coutumier berbère Ichkern: Coutume de l'enfant endormi," 158; Hamida, "Les modes de preuve dans la coutume de la tribu des Aid Izdeq."

145. Aspinion, "Case 22, 1er Rebia I 1354 (3 juin 1935), Jugement du Tribunal coutumier des Aït Harkat de Guelmous." In other cases, if the woman's family swore to her pregnancy, the court supported her position.

146. Aspinion, *Contribution à l'étude du droit coutumier berbère marocain.*

147. The word may also be *raqqad*. In a hagiography conserved by the Regagda tribe and recorded by Edouard Michaux-Bellaire, the tribe's saintly ancestor himself had a prolonged gestation. His mother was a postmenopausal woman who suddenly bore a son; she explained that the miraculous child had been "sleeping." The child was nicknamed "Raggad" (sleeping one), and the tribe is thus named Regagda; see Michaux-Bellaire, "Les tribus arabes de la vallée du Lekkous." See also Amor, "Essai médico-légal—Les gestations à long terme et le droit musulman."

148. Miller, "Sleeping Fetus."

149. Russell and Suhrawardy, *A Manual of the Law of Marriage from the Mukhtasar of Sidi Khalil*, Khalil's "Chapter on Repudiation," 134n4. The Qur'an is explicit about breastfeeding, "*The repudiated mothers will nurse their children for two complete years, if the father wishes the time to be complete*" (2:233) and "*His mother carries him in her breast and endures hardship upon hardship, he is not weaned until after two years*" (31:13).

150. The companions of the Prophet agreed with this opinion, according to a Ma-

liki *qadi* in Cairo cited in Mathieu and Maneville, *Les Accoucheuses musulmanes traditionnelles*, 42–43.

151. "Omar accorded a delay of four years to the wife of a man who had disappeared . . . The same delay was given by Othman and Ali" (Khalil, from the *Mukhtasar*, quoted in Mathieu and Maneville, *Les Accoucheuses musulmanes traditionnelles*, 44). Khalil thus required a widow who believed herself pregnant to observe an *idda* of four to five years (Chapter 15, translated in Russell and Suhrawardy, *A Manual of the Law of Marriage*, 261–262).

152. Malik, *Al-Muwatta*, quoted in Mathieu and Maneville, *Les Accoucheuses musulmanes traditionnelles*, 43.

153. See Powers, *Law, Society, and Culture in the Maghrib, 1300–1500*.

154. Al-Wansharisi, *Kitab al-Mi'yar*, quoted in Mathieu and Maneville, *Les Accoucheuses musulmanes traditionnelles*, 44.

155. Marcel Morand argued that Islamic jurists adopted the concept of the *raqid* to give all children a father and to avoid applying the punishment for adultery; see Champagne, "Le mythe de l'enfant qui dort chez la femme marocaine."

156. Delanoë, "Considerations générales sur le fonctionnement du service des femmes et enfants à l'hôpital regional de Mazagan pendant l'année 1925," 872, and "Les croyances indigènes sur la grossesse."

157. Denat, "Droit coutumier berbère Ichkern." The *raqid* was a widespread belief; Dr. Legey found it in Marrakesh in 1926, de Lens recorded it in Meknes in 1925, Dr. Jahier and the legal expert Bousquet found it in female patients in Algeria, and Native Affairs officers reported it in the Berber countryside; see Jahier and Bousquet, "L'enfant endormi: Notes juridiques, ethnographiques et obstétricales." On the *raqid* in Algeria, see Gaudry, *La Femme chaouia de l'Aurès: Étude de sociologie berbère*, 110.

158. Mathieu and Maneville, *Les Accoucheuses musulmanes traditionnelles*, 48.

159. Ibid., 45–6. Legey found that Jewish women in Marrakesh also believed in the *raqid* and ate the heart of an onion flavored with saffron to awaken the sleeping child; see Legey, *Essai de folklore marocain*, 70.

160. Remlinger and Bailly, "Le diagnostic biologique de la grossesse en médecine indigène et devant les tribunaux musulmans."

161. Ibid.

162. AAE Nantes, Maroc DI, Carton 733, folder 1: "Justice coutumière, rapports annuels, 1930–1949."

163. *La Revue marocaine de droit*, "Juridictions chérifiennes, Tribunal d'Appel du Chrâa, Audience du 24 Qaada 1368, Répudiation—répudiation par le tamlik—irrevocabilité—Vocation héréditaire des ex-conjoints (non)—Dernière maladie—Maladie accidentale—affection chronique—Capacité juridique—Mention Adoulaire—Preuve du contraire—Certificat Médical—Médecin non-musulman—Témoignage ou expertise: Caractère d'information de la science—Déclarations devant l'adoul—Attestation de l'identité du malade" (17 September, 1949).

164. *La Revue marocaine de droit*, "Jurisprudence chérifienne, Tribunal d'Appel du Chrâa (Arrêt du 8 Joumada I 1368—8 mars 1949), Filiation—Durée de la conception, Partage—Survenance d'héritier—Rescision."

165. Remlinger and Bailly, "Cent réactions de Friedman pour le diagnostic biologique de la grossesse."

166. Ibid.

167. Fischbacher, "Aspects de la médecine au Maroc-certificats."

168. Champagne, "Le mythe de l'enfant qui dort."

169. Jahier and Bousquet, "L'enfant endormi," 25; Remlinger and Bailly, "Cent réactions de Friedman," 264.

170. Bousquet and Jahier, "Les vices redhibitoires de la femme en droit musulman: Remarques juridico-médicales"; al-Qarawani, *Risala ou traité abrégé de droit malékite et morale musulmane, traduction avec commentaire et index analytique par E. Fagnan*, 126.

171. Charnot, *La Toxicologie au Maroc: Mémoires de la société des sciences naturelles du Maroc*, 31–32.

172. Ibid., 14.

173. Ibid., 60.

174. Ibid., 61.

175. "The natives of Tizi n Test use principally a mix of ginger, mandrake and melted rancid butter. The paste obtained is used to make cakes, but is often incorporated into 'maajoun.' According to Moroccans, this brings extreme depression and death after one year" (ibid., 66).

176. Ibid., 65–66.

177. Ibid., 618–621.

178. For this and other extensive assistance with Moroccan toxicology, I am indebted to Dr. Laʿarbi Idrisi, former director of the National Institute of Hygiene in Rabat.

179. If he found a black liquid in the stomach and added sulfuric acid, the resulting violet color revealed the presence of *"addad"* (Charnot, *La Toxicologie au Maroc*, 578–579). Charnot drew on the work of his predecessors, notably the French Algerian pharmacist Lefranc.

180. Institut National d'Hygiène du Maroc (INHM), unclassified toxicology records.

181. Report #42, November 27, 1947, INHM, toxicology records.

182. Chastand, *Le Protectorat français au Maroc*, 147.

183. Lauren Benton has argued that colonial legal regimes "facilitated conquest and colonization in most places—not by producing order, exactly, but by generating a framework for conflict" (Benton, *Law and Colonial Cultures: Legal Regimes in World History, 1400–1900*, 27).

CHAPTER 6

1. Mathieu and Maneville, *Les Accoucheuses musulmanes traditionelles*.

2. Monica Green argues that medical encroachment on midwives in Europe began in the premodern period (*Making Women's Medicine Masculine: The Rise of Male Authority in Pre-Modern Gynaecology*).

3. Mathieu and Maneville, *Les Accoucheuses musulmanes traditionelles*, 9–10.

4. Ibid., 182.

5. On Moroccans' apparent immunity to tuberculosis, see Thévenin, "Du climat de Mogador," and Ollive, "Géographie médicale." For the cases in Fez, see "P-V du BMH de Fès," May 1922, BGR, Carton 1395. In Oujda, the BMH physician wrote, "As dis-

ease is impossible to track among the natives, the number of persons with this illness must be much higher (than the thirteen declared cases) and the danger of propagation considerable"; see "P-V du BMH de Oujda," 1925, BGR, Carton A837.

6. "P-V du BMH de Rabat," 1934, BGR, Carton A1182.

7. Colombani, "À propos de l'état sanitaire du Maroc et de son prétendu caractère infecteur."

8. Montagne, "Note sur la Kasbah de Mehdiya."

9. Dahane, "Itinéraire ethnographique de Montagne dans les années vingt."

10. Montagne, *Les Berbères et le makhzen dans le sud du Maroc: Essai sur la transformation politique des berbères sédentaires.*

11. Ray, "Quelques aspects economiques et sociaux de l'émigration nord-africaine en France."

12. Quoted in Montagne, *Naissance du prolétariat marocain, enquête collective 1948–1950,* 104–105. The Sus imported 47,945 tons in 1950, 13,444 of grain and 6,625 of sugar (103).

13. Pasquier-Bronde, "La vie économique et l'organisation du travail."

14. Created by the *dahir* of February 1, 1928, the goal of the Sociétés Indigènes de Prévoyance was "maintenance and development of cultivation and plantations, improvement and growth of animal husbandry, mutual aid, insurance, creation of cooperatives, battle against usury" (Coliac, "Intervention des sociétés indigènes de prévoyance dans la lutte contre la formation d'un prolétariat indigène"); see also Swearingen, *Moroccan Mirages: Agrarian Dreams and Deceptions, 1912–1986.*

15. Montagne, "L'évolution moderne des pays arabes."

16. Ibid.

17. Montagne, "Un plan d'enquêtes sociologiques—Démographie et questions sociales marocaines."

18. Ecochard, "Problèmes d'urbanisme au Maroc."

19. Célérier, "Les mouvements migratoires des indigènes au Maroc"; emphasis in the original.

20. Baron, Huot, and Paye, "Condition économique et niveaux de vie des travailleurs indigènes au douar Doum."

21. Baron, Huot, and Paye, "Logements et loyers des travailleurs indigènes à Rabat-Salé." Some could not even afford this housing; see Baron and Mathieu, "Quelques budgets de travailleurs indigènes."

22. Adam, "Le prolétarisation de l'habitat dans l'ancienne medina de Casablanca."

23. Ibid.

24. *Bulletin économique du Maroc,* "Résultats provisoires du recensement du 8 mars 1936."

25. The protectorate contributed 150 million francs to the cost of the food program, and Muslim charity societies provided most of the balance; see Pinta, "La lutte contre la misère au Maroc en 1945."

26. Gouvernement chérifien secrétariat général du protectorat, service de statistiques, "Dénombrement général de la population de la zone française de l'empire chérifien, effectué le 1er mars 1947, fasc. 3, ensemble de la population," SHAT, Carton 1418.

27. Breil, "Quelques aspects de la situation démographique au Maroc"; see also

Chevalier, *Le Problème démographique nord-africain.* A 1938 Rabat study found that the Jewish population had more than doubled in fifteen years; see Baron, Lummau, and Mathieu, "Notes démographiques sur la population israélite de Rabat."

28. Ecochard, "Problèmes d'urbanisme au Maroc."

29. Gauthronet to resident general of Morocco, March 7, 1916, and Gauthronet to minister of war, February 6, 1916, AAE Nantes Maroc DAI, Carton 332.

30. Devillars, "L'immigration marocaine en France."

31. Roger Maneville, "De l'évolution sociale et politique des marocains en France," 1946, SHAT, Carton 1418, dossier 5: affaires sociales. Maneville estimated the Moroccan population in France at 20,000 in 1946.

32. Remlinger, "La main d'oeuvre marocain en France et la propagation de la tuberculose au Maroc."

33. "P-V du BMH de Mogador," 22 December 1926, BGR, Carton 632. With no protectorate support, Bouveret created his own tuberculosis dispensary in 1927 with private funds; see "P-V du BMH de Mogador," May 1927, BGR, Carton A1553.

34. For the claim by the Ministry of War, see Lefrançois, "Les travailleurs marocains en France pendant la guerre." For the quotation, see Catrice and Buchet, "Les musulmans en France: Enquête à Gennevilliers."

35. Ben Salem, *La Tuberculose chez les ouvriers musulmans nord-africains en France.*

36. As late as 1936, native child health was still measured by studying the elite male students at *collèges musulmans*; see M. Gaud, "Développement de l'enfant indigène au Maroc." The pioneer in accurate reporting of native child nutrition may be Mathieu, "Contrôle de l'état de nutrition des indigènes musulmans d'un douar marocain suburban, 'bidonville' de Port-Lyautey."

37. Chenebault, "Contribution à l'étude de la tuberculose pulmonaire de l'enfant marocaine en milieu citadin."

38. Sanguy, "Remarques sur la mortalité infantile musulmane: Ses causes et ses remèdes," 206.

39. Mage-Humbert, "Aspects de la tuberculose pulmonaire chez l'enfant marocaine."

40. The children could be saved if treated early and fed meat, raw milk, proteins, and B vitamins; see Delon, "À propos du Kwashiorkor."

41. Houel, "La campagne de vaccination antituberculeuse."

42. In a study in Khouribga and Louis-Gentil (Sidi Qasim) in 1951, only 9.3 percent of children up to four years old, and 41 percent of children ten to fifteen years old, were found to have been exposed to tuberculosis; see Gaud, Houel, and Fayveley, "Indices tuberculiniques au Maroc."

43. Massonnaud, "L'évolution des corporations depuis notre installation au Maroc: Ses repercussions économiques et politiques."

44. For the *dahirs*, see Chénébeaux, "Le Bureau Marocain de Travail," 3. For the SFIO actions, see Yakhlef, "La Municipalité de Fès," 707–708. For the strike, see Hoisington, *The Casablanca Connection: French Colonial Policy, 1936–1943,* 99; see also Ayache, *Le Mouvement syndical.* A report of 1929 warned of connections between North Africans and communists; see Catrice and Buchet, "Les musulmans en France."

45. Maneville, "De l'évolution sociale et politique des marocains en France." Among Maneville's unpublished works, see "En suivant les travailleurs marocains en

France," October 1939, October 1940, "La situation des travailleurs marocains en France à la fin de l'année 1941," Rabat 1942, SHAT, Carton 3H1418.

46. Maneville, "De l'évolution sociale et politique des marocains en France."

47. Kenbib, "Les années de guerre de Robert Montagne (1939–1944)."

48. Montagne, *Naissance du prolétariat marocain*, 248.

49. Ibid., 21–22.

50. Ibid., 251.

51. Ibid., 239; Montagne, *Révolution au Maroc*, 269–271. On Moroccan street children, see also Anfreville de la Salle, "Une oeuvre d'humanité et de patriotisme: Les enfants marocains abandonnés"; Zeys, "Répression du vagabondage des jeunes marocains: Redressement et sauvetage de l'enfance indigène en danger moral." Anfreville de la Salle thought the protectorate made a poor patriarchal authority, however, and recommended recruiting private individuals to parent abandoned native children.

52. Montagne, *Révolution au Maroc*, 307–308.

53. Montagne, *Naissance du prolétariat marocain*, 259–260.

54. Sicault, "La protection médico-social de l'enfance au Maroc."

55. Abu-Lughod, *Rabat*, 227.

56. Crinson, *Modern Architecture and the End of Empire*. See also von Osten, "Architecture without Architects: An Anarchist Approach" and her museum exhibit "In the Desert of Modernity: Colonial Planning and After," August 29–November 2, 2008 at House of World Cultures, Berlin.

57. Morand, *La Famille musulmane*, 55.

58. Mauran, *La Société marocaine*, 149–150.

59. Hardy and Brunot, *L'Enfant marocaine*, 53.

60. Bey-Rozet, "Le Service social de la Santé Publique au Maroc: Son adaptation au monde musulman."

61. Legey, *Essai de folklore marocain*, 109.

62. Ibid., 130–132; Legey, "Un centre de puériculture."

63. Cismigiu, "Facteurs de mortinatalité et dystocie en milieu marocain."

64. Mage-Humbert, "Aspects de la tuberculose pulmonaire chez l'enfant marocaine." On the link of syphilis, tuberculosis, and the Muslim family, see also Chenebault, "Contribution à l'étude de la tuberculose pulmonaire de l'enfant marocaine en milieu citadin"; Imbert, "La tuberculose pulmonaire de primo infection chez l'enfant"; Gaud and Mage-Humbert, "La tuberculose pulmonaire au Maroc en milieu musulman."

65. Sanguy, "Remarques sur la mortalité infantile musulmane." Of the large literature on Moroccan congenital/hereditary syphilis, see Marmey and Marmey, "Contribution à l'étude de l'obstetrique au Maroc." Dr. Eugénie Delanoë was also prolific on the subject; see "Note sur le traitement de la syphilis chez les femmes enceintes."

66. Bonjean, "L'oeuvre de la France dans la protection de l'enfance au Maroc"; Lacapère and Laurent, *Le Traitement de la syphilis par les composés arsenicaux*, 169, 186–189.

67. Legey, "Un centre de puériculture"; Legey and Décor, "L'Assistance aux femmes en couches."

68. Counillon, "Les écoles franco-musulmans de fillettes au Maroc."

69. Hardy and Brunot, *L'Enfant marocain*, 9–14.

70. Letellier, "La famille indigène devant les problèmes sociaux modernes."

71. Counillon, "Les écoles franco-musulmans de fillettes au Maroc." Compare with the 42,014 total Moroccan students in 1945; see *Bulletin économique et social du Maroc*, "L'effort du Maroc pour l'instruction publique."

72. On the Rabat smallpox epidemic and Desgeorges, see "Ville de Rabat, Rapport de fin d'année 1926 du Bureau d'hygiène et des formations sanitaires municipales de la ville de Rabat, 7 March 1926," BGR, Carton 632; see also, BGR, Carton A11001, folder "Settat." For Desgeorges's experiences, "Rapport de Mademoiselle Desgeorges Infirmière-Visiteuse des écoles de Rabat, Decembre 1927," in BGR, unordered folder "Bienfaisance, l'oeuvre de Mme. Saint au Maroc." Desgeorges presented her plan to recruit female political agents: "The conquest of souls and evolution toward us can be possible only through the family—for this is made by women—mothers, sisters or wives. The evolution of the Moroccan will be through women or not at all" (Desgeorges, "Note sur la pénétration dans les milieux féminins musulmans," February 1930, BGR, unordered folder "Bienfaisance, l'oeuvre de Mme. Saint au Maroc").

73. Justice chérifienne, Tribunal du Pacha, to Benoit, November 20, 1930, in BGR, unordered folder "Bienfaisance, l'oeuvre de Mme. Saint au Maroc."

74. Direction des Affaires Indigènes [Native Affairs] to Contrôleur Civil, Chef de Region de Chaouia, March 27, 1931; Direction des Affaires Indigènes to General Commandant la Region de Fès, November 23, 1933, AAE Nantes, Maroc DI, Carton 622.

75. Lyazidi to Contrôleur Civil, July 28, 1932, AAE Nantes, Maroc DI, Carton 622.

76. Charbonneau, "L'Assistance et la prévoyance sociale au Maroc."

77. After the "Semaines Sociales" in Algiers (1933), Cardinal Leynaud called upon North African Catholics to address native social problems.

78. Suzanne Renard, "L'Aide aux mères."

79. AAE Nantes, Carton 613A.

80. M. Gaud, "La Fête des mères." Scouting camps (*les éclaireurs*) were opened to Moroccan boys, but because Arabs in Egypt and Syria had used scouting to create paramilitaries, efforts in Morocco were modest. Petain's "Chantiers de Jeunesse," which were intended to "remake the soul" of "overly individualist" young men through hard physical labor, were also introduced. A *chantier* was created in Boulhaut in 1941.

81. Bonjean, "L'Oeuvre de la France dans la protection de l'enfance au Maroc."

82. Funding came from Muslim charities, the French Red Cross, and the protectorate, which contributed 150 million francs; see Pinta, "La Lutte contre la misère au Maroc en 1945."

83. Bonjean, "L'Oeuvre de la France dans la protection de l'enfance au Maroc."

84. Bey-Rozet, "Le Service social en milieu musulman."

85. Rabat (Sidi-Fatah, Mechouar, Douar Doum, Douar Debbagh), Casablanca (Carrières Centrales, Aïn-Chock, Ben M'sick, Rue Lecatelet), Fez (Adoua, Douh Bou Ayad, Dokkarat, Funduq Yuhudi), Meknes (Borj Mawlay Umar, Sidi El Harichi, Derb Driba, Beni M'Hamed, Souika), Marrakesh (Bab el Khemis, Doukkala), Agadir (Cité Industrielle, Medina Talborj, Douar Anza), Oujda (Maison du Cadi); see *Maroc médical*, "Tableau des Formations d'Accouchement, de Gynécologie, de Consultations prénatales, Centres d'education sanitaire, organisés par la Direction de la Santé Publique et de la Famille au Maroc."

86. In 1951, 6,903 pregnant women visited PMI clinics; see Cauvin, "La protection de la femme enceinte au Maroc."

87. Le Coeur, "Les Rites de passage d'Azemmour."

88. Yegenoglu, *Colonial Fantasies: Towards a Feminist Reading of Orientalism*, 39–67.

89. Mathieu and Maneville, *Les Accoucheuses musulmanes traditionnelles*, 97, 122.

90. *Maroc médical*, "Les muwallidat: Leur rôle dans l'assistance obstétricale au Maroc."

91. Scheper-Hughes and Lock, "The Mindful Body: A Prolegomenon to Future Work in Medical Anthropology"; Van Hollen, *Birth on the Threshold: Childbirth and Modernity in South India*, 11.

92. Lacascade, *Puériculture et colonisation: Étude sur la puériculture au Maroc (Aperçu du role colonisateur que peut jouer la femme médecin dans les pays d'occupation)*.

93. Ibid., 21. Dr. Decrop reported that Muslim women came to European maternities only with dystocia; see "Où en est la syphilis marocaine?"

94. Lacascade, *Puériculture et colonisation*, 48.

95. Decrop, "Où en est la syphilis marocaine?"

96. At Maurice Gaud Hospital in 1951–1952; see Cismigiu, "Facteurs de mortinatalité et dystocie en milieu marocain."

97. Data from 4,977 Muslim births, 5,579 Jewish births, and 579 Europeans; see Décor, "Vingt années d'activité d'une maternité en milieu marocain urbain." Muslim women did not enter the European maternities in great numbers when they were opened to them (Mme. Lyautey's Rabat maternity [1922], Andrée Saint's Fez maternity [1931]).

98. Cismigiu, "Facteurs de mortnatalité et dystocie en milieu marocain."

99. Ibid.; J. Marmey and Lacroix, "Indications de la symphyséotomie de Zarate dans la pratique obstétricale marocaine d'après 56 observations"; J. Marmey, "Avenir obstétrical des femmes symphyséotomisées (suivant la technique de Zarate)."

100. Chaperon, "Ostéopathies à tendance ostéomalacique en milieu marocain."

101. Ibid., 217.

102. J. Marmey, "Du choix de l'incision uterine au cours des césariennes abdominales, d'après 263 interventions pratiquées à la maternité de Rabat."

103. After the obstetrician Jean-Louis Baudelocque (1745–1810) rejected symphysiotomy, most French physicians opposed the procedure; see Dumont, "The Long and Difficult Birth of Symphyseotomy from Séverin Pineau to Jean-René Sigault."

104. Laffont, "Problèmes obstétricaux et gynécologiques en Afrique du Nord."

105. Décor, "Vingt années d'activité d'une maternité en milieu marocain urbain," 30.

106. J. Marmey, "Du choix de l'incision uterine au cours des césariennes abdominales."

107. Zarate modified the operation to respect the upper ligament of the symphysis and only partially bisect the lower ligament.

108. Infant mortality was 3 of 55 births for symphysiotomy (5 percent) and 19 of 171 for cesareans (11 percent) in Rabat during the period 1949–1952; see J. Marmey and Lacroix, "Indications de la symphyséotomie de Zarate."

109. Lacascade, *Puériculture et colonisation*, 13; Mathieu and Maneville, *Les Accoucheuses musulmanes traditionnelles*, 60.

110. Nobécort, Preface to Bouveret and Vallery-Radot, "Éléments de puériculture."

111. Cauvin, "La Protection de la femme enceinte au Maroc."

112. Examples of French housewives and social workers modeling the household arts: Belpeer, "Femmes musulmanes—[document relatant une experience d'action sociale dont l'initiative revient à Madame Belpeer, directrice de l'Action Sociale à A.T.O.M. à Marseille, qui a crée un centre d'Education Menagère pour les Femmes Musulmanes]," 5; L'Echo d'Oran, "Un témoignage de la grande oeuvre française au Maroc: L'éducation de la femme marocaine, plus importante que l'action médicale pour les assistantes sociales," 6.

113. Adolphe Pinard (1844–1934), an obstetrician, a prenatal advocate, and the founding father of French puériculture; quoted in Trillat, "Evolution de l'obstétrique au XXe siècle."

114. Bonjean, "Causes d'incompréhension entre l'Islam et l'Occident."

115. Mathieu and Maneville, Les Accoucheuses musulmanes traditionnelles; Bouveret and Vallery-Radot, "Éléments de puériculture," 47, 50, 55.

116. Bouveret and Vallery-Radot, "Éléments de puériculture," 47.

117. "She is the guardian of a mysterious science . . . The end of the qablat will be a sign that Moroccans have arrived at a superior degree of civilization by abandoning the old myths" (Mathieu and Maneville, Les Accoucheuses musulmanes traditionnelles, 181).

118. Ibid., 170.

119. Ibid., 179.

120. Maroc médical, "Les muwallidat."

121. Mathieu and Maneville, Les Accoucheuses musulmanes traditionnelles, 36.

122. Ibid., 102.

123. Even the "most evolved" students told their professors, "Your savants, who are great savants, believe pregnancy cannot be longer than nine months . . . but they are wrong because the Companions of the Prophet have affirmed the contrary, and God knows better" (ibid., 41–42).

124. Ibid., 88–89.

125. Ibid., 137.

126. Ibid., 126.

127. Noëlle Courtecuisse, interview by the author, December 13, 1999, Paris.

128. For the funeral, see Bulletin Spécial de Renseignments, October 5 1949, AAE Nantes, Maroc DI, Carton 622.

129. Noëlle Courtecuisse, personal archives.

130. World Health Organization, New Trends and Approaches in the Delivery of Maternal and Child Care in Health Services.

131. Fatima Mernissi, preface to Ech-Channa, Miseria: Témoignages, 17.

132. "Lettre ouverte à Mohamed Allal el Fassi, déporté au Gabon," L'Action tunisienne (Tunis), December 4, 1937.

133. The congress began September 6, 1935, and was described in Al Umma (Algiers), September 1935, and Nahda (Tunis), September 1935, SHAT, Carton 3H1423.

134. Hammoudi, "Construction de l'ordre et usage de la science coloniale: Robert Montagne, penseur de la tribu et de la civilisation."

135. 'Allal al-Fasi, The Independence Movements in North Africa, Al-Harakat al-Istiqlaliya, 1–8.

136. Ouazzani (Al-Wazzani), "Notre nationalisme."

137. Ouazzani (Al-Wazzani), *Combats d'un nationaliste marocain*, 1:143, 181.

138. Comité d'Action Marocaine, *Plan de réformes marocaines*, 30.

139. Bazzaz, "Reading Reform beyond the State: Salwat al-Anfas, Islamic Revival, and Moroccan National History."

140. Cornell, *Realm of the Saint*, 332.

141. 'Allal al-Fasi in *Al Maghrib*, April 16, 1937, SHAT, Carton 3H1423.

142. 'Umar 'Abdaljalil, "Tribune du fellah," *La Volonté du peuple*, March 1934, SHAT, Carton 3H1423; al-Wazzani, "Le problème de la misère."

143. "La misère au Maroc," *Al Atlas*, March 12, 1937, SHAT, Carton 3H1323.

144. Abdelqadir Tazi, "Un comité central de bienfaisance," *Majallat al-Maghrib*, February 1934, SHAT, Carton 3H1423, dossier "Analyse de la presse et des affaires musulmanes."

145. "La Bienfaisance et les habous," *Majallat al-Maghrib*, April 1934. Several Moroccan nationalists criticized the urban Muslim charity societies for corruption and for helping their own local populations.

146. *Al Hayat*, April 11, 1935, SHAT, Carton 3H1423.

147. *Majallat al-Maghrib*, December 1933, and Comité d'Action Marocaine, *Plan de réformes marocaines*, 86.

148. Comité d'Action Marocaine, *Plan de réformes marocaines*, 97–99.

149. Tract distributed by Muhammad Hasan al-Wazzani to the Congrès socialiste in Paris, May 1936; in Ouazzani, *Combats d'un nationaliste marocain*, 1:57; Comité d'Action Marocaine, *Plan de réformes marocaines*, 103–104.

150. Moroccan Ministry of Health Archives, Rabat (hereafter MMH), unordered carton, D1 Series, 1955–1956.

151. *L'Action du peuple* also reported that a delegation from Meknes presented the sultan with a petition asking him to forbid "processions and ceremonies contrary to Islam" on the occasion of the *mussems* of Ben 'Isa and Ben Hamdush; see "Une petition de la population musulmane de Meknes," *L'Action du peuple*, May 6, 1937.

152. "L'Interdiction des Aissaouas et des confréries similaires: Une grande réforme sociale," *L'Action du peuple* 2 (1933), cited in Spadola, "The Scandal of Ecstasy: Communication, Sufi Rites, and Social Reform in 1930s Morocco."

153. Ibid., in Spadola, "The Scandal of Ecstasy," 132.

154. Abdalkarim Ghallab, in *Al Alam*, January 5, 1955, MMH, unordered carton, D1 Series, 1955–1956.

155. Spadola, "The Scandal of Ecstasy."

156. A. Bouhlal, "The Camera within our Walls," al-Wazzani from *L'Action du peuple*, quoted in Spadola, "The Scandal of Ecstasy," 135.

157. Al-Fasi, cited in Baker, *Voices of Resistance: Oral Histories of Moroccan Women*, 20.

158. Al-Fasi authored this article under the pseudonym "Al-Maghribi," in *Al Umma* (Algiers), February 5, 1935, SHAT, Carton 3H1423. The president of the Association of North African Students in France also called these marriages "odious"; see "Les mariages avec les étrangères en Afrique du Nord," *Najah* (Constantine), May 22, 1935.

159. "La dernière visite de Madame Ponsot à Salé," *Al Akhbar* (Tetouan), March 29, 1936.

160. For al-Fasi, see "Third Congress of Muslim North-African Students, 1934," SHAT, Carton 3H1423.

161. "La femme marocaine et l'enseignement des filles," *Majallat al-Maghrib*, August–September 1935, SHAT, Carton 3H1423.

162. Muhammad Hasan al-Wazzani, "Les aspirations du <<Maghreb>>."

163. Sfrioui, "Les rites de naissance à Fès."

164. Ibid.

165. Ibid.

166. Foucault, *The Birth of Biopolitics*, 39.

167. Bargach, *Orphans of Islam: Family, Abandonment, and Secret Adoption in Morocco.*

168. Latour, *We Have Never Been Modern.*

169. Tazi et al., "Genetic Diversity and Population Structure of *Mycobacterium tuberculosis* in Casablanca, a Moroccan City with High Incidence of Tuberculosis."

170. In 1981–1984, King Hassan II was persuaded by the International Monetary Fund to eliminate food subsidies, which caused wheat flour prices in Morocco to rise by 40 percent; see Holden, *The Politics of Food.*

EPILOGUE

1. The water of Sidi Harazem is considered beneficial to the bladder, kidneys, and blood; anonymous interview by the author, Lamtiyyin clinic, March 12, 1999, Fez.

2. Fouad Bouchareb, interview by the author, February 26, 1999, Fez.

3. Capelli, "Risk and Safety in Context: Medical Pluralism and Agency in Childbirth in an Eastern Moroccan Oasis."

4. Nasr, *An Introduction to Islamic Cosmological Doctrines.*

5. Obermeyer, "Pluralism and Pragmatism."

6. Hunt, *A Colonial Lexicon of Birth Ritual, Medicalization, and Mobility in the Congo,* 1–11.

7. Anonymous interview by the author, Lamtiyyin, March 13, 1999, Fez.

8. Pandolfo, "The Thin Line of Modernity," 142.

9. Another patient described his tuberculosis in Galenic terms, as a corrupted humor created by the psychological influence of emotion on blood: "I never had a shot until a problem happened to me with *fqsa* [deep worry]. With that, the swollen glands came to me, those glands had in them *tilkuloz* [tuberculosis]."

10. Anonymous interview by the author, Funduq al-Yuhudy, March 12, 1999, Fez. Many Fez residents drink water from Sidi Harazem to clean the bladder, intestines, and kidneys.

11. Consider Farmer, *Pathologies of Power: Health, Human Rights, and the New War on the Poor,* 6.

BIBLIOGRAPHY

MANUSCRIPT SOURCES, ARABIC

Adarraq, ʿAbd Allah ibn Ahmad. "Qasida fi munafiaʿ al-naʿnaʿ." MS 4094, Bibliothèque Générale de Rabat.

Ibn Khalsun, ʿAbd Allah Sidi Muhammad ibn Yusuf. "Qalaʾid al-ʿafiyan fi siha badn al-insan." MS 4096, Bibliothèque Générale de Rabat.

MS 6462. Untitled. Includes the dictionary of medicines from Antaki beginning with r. Bibliothèque Nationale de France.

"Rajuʿa al-shaykh ila subaha." MSS Orientales 3056, 3057, 3058, 3059, 3060, Bibliothèque Nationale de France.

"Risala ʿilm amrad an-nisaʾ wa tawiqhunna ʿan al-habl." MS D1718/2758, Bibliothèque Générale de Rabat.

Sanusi, Abi ʿAbd Allah Muhammad ibn Yusuf al-. "Sharh ʿala qula s [Muhammad] al-maʿda bayna al-daʾwa al-hamiya raʾs al-duwaʾ wa asl kul daʿ al-buruda" (1886). MS 4091, Bibliothèque Générale de Rabat.

Siyuti, Jalal ad-Din al-. "Aydhah fi ʿilm al-nikah." MSS Orientales 3060, Bibliothèque Nationale de France.

"Taqiyyid fi munafiaʿ al-safufat." MS 4101, Bibliothèque Générale de Rabat.

Tijani, ʿAbd Allah ibn Muhammad al-. "Tuhfa al-ʿaraws wa nuzha al-nafaws." MSS Orientales 3061, Bibliothèque Nationale de France.

ARCHIVAL SOURCES, MOROCCO

Archives of the Municipality of Fez
    Folders:
        Artisanat
        David Attar
        Dispensaire Bab Boujat
        Dispensaire de l'Adoua
        L'eau à Fès/Oued Fès
        Fraternité franco-marocaine
        Sous-Commission d'Hygiène
        Secours de Naissance
Bibliothèque Générale de Rabat (BGR), Protectorate archives
    Series:
        Hygiène, procès-verbaux des réunions
        Rapports "Hygiène," by region
        Municipalité de Fès: Arrêtés municipaux
        Commissions municipales: procès-verbaux des réunions
        Services municipaux: rapports mensuels, trimestriels et semestriels
        Travaux publics municipaux
        Contentieux: plaintes et reclamations

Unordered cartons and documents
Aline de Lens Papers
Cocard Hospital Archives, Fez
Hospital Intake Registers, 1912–1945
Maternity Intake Registers, 1945–1952
Institut National d'Hygiène du Maroc, Rabat
Toxicology Records, 1931–1956
Moroccan Ministry of Health, Rabat

ARCHIVAL SOURCES, FRANCE

Archives des Affaires Étrangères, Nantes
Series:
Tangier Legation
Maroc CD
Maroc CDRG
Maroc DACH
Maroc DAI
Maroc DI
Maroc DIP
Carton: Maroc, Bureaux territoriaux, Fès 2
Archives Historiques du Service de Santé Militaire, Val-de-Grâce Hospital, Paris
Carton 68
Carton 71
Carton 170
Carton 204
Carton 829
Carton 830
Carton 3089
Linares personnel dossier, C2054
Archives Nationales de France, Paris (AN)
Series: Fonds Lyautey
Archives d'Outre Mer, Aix-en-Provence
Fonds Kniebiehler
Service Historique de l'Armée de Terre (SHAT)
Series:
3H1, Archives Maroc
3H2, Archives Maroc
Cartons:
1 K 21, Lacau Papers
1 K 194, Larras Papers
1 K 367, La Chapelle Papers
1 K 662, Ninard Papers
17 S 292
17 S 331
17 S 332
17 S 333

INTERVIEWS

Abbes Kabbaj, June 17, 1995, Fez.
Bahia, October 8, 1998, Fez.
N., February 2, 1999, Fez.
Bahia, February 13, 1999, Fez.
Fouad Boucharib, February 26, 1999, Fez.
Four anonymous interviewees, March 12, 1999, Funduq al-Yuhudy Clinic, Fez.
F., Mawlay Ali, A., and S., March 13, 1999, Lamtiyyin Clinic, Fez.
A., March 13, 1999, Lamtiyyin Clinic, Fez.
Mawlay Ali, March 15, 1999, Fez.
My Khaddouj, March 15, 1999, Fez.
My Khaddouj and Mawlay Ali, March 22, 1999, Fez.
Nurse, 'Umar Idrisi Hospital, March 22, 1999, Fez.
Anonymous interviewee, April 1, 1999, Tamgrout.
M.A., May 18, 1999, Fez.
Noëlle Courtecuisse, December 13, 1999, Paris, France.
Aicha Ech-Channa, January 13, 2012, Casablanca.

PERIODICALS

L'Action du peuple
Afrique française
Al Atlas [cited in Chapter 6, Note 143]
Archives marocaines
Archives de l'Institut Pasteur d'Algérie
Archives de l'Institut Pasteur de Maroc
Archives de médecine et de pharmacie militares
Bulletin de l'Institut d'Hygiène du Maroc
Bulletin économique du Maroc (becomes *Bulletin économique et social du Maroc*)
Bulletin de l'enseignement public au Maroc
Bulletin de l'Institut des Hautes Études Marocaines (becomes *Hésperis*)
Bulletin d'information du Maroc
Bulletin officiel du Protectorat de la République Française au Maroc
Bulletin officiel de l'Union Médicale (Organe des Unions Médicales du Maroc)
Bulletin de la Société de Géographie
Bulletin de la Société de Pathologie Exotique
Bulletin de la Société d'Histoire Naturelle de l'Afrique du Nord
Bulletin de la Société des Sciences Naturelles du Maroc
France-Maroc
Jeunesse
Majallat al-Maghrib [cited in Chapter 6, Notes, 144, 145, 147]
Maroc médical
Marseille médical
Presse médicale
Questions nord-africains: Revue des problèmes sociaux de l'Algérie, de la Tunisie, et du Maroc

Revue algérienne, tunisienne et marocaine de législation et jurisprudence
Revue générale de médecine et de chirurgie de L'Afrique du Nord
La Revue marocaine de droit
Revue marocaine de législation, doctrine, jurisprudence chérifiennes (Droit musul-man malékite, coutumes berbères, lois israélites)
Revue du monde musulman
La Vigie marocaine [cited in Chapter 4, Note 152]

PRIMARY PRINTED SOURCES, BOOKS AND ARTICLES

ʿAbduh, Muhammad. "Ikhtilaf al-qawanin bi-ikhtilaf ahwal al-umam." In Muham-mad ʿImara, ed., *Al-ʿAmal al-Kamila*, 309–315. Beirut: Muʾassasat alʿArabiyya li al-Dirasat wa al-Nashr, 1972.

———. "Al-Islah al-Haqiqi wa al-Wajib lil-Azhar" (True Reform and the Duty of the Azhar). *Al Manar* 10, no. 28 (February 1906): 921–930.

———. "Tafsir al-Quran al-Hakim." *Al Manar* 8, no. 24: 921–930.

L'Action tunisienne (Tunis). "Lettre ouverte à Mohamed Allal el Fassi, déporté au Ga-bon." December 4, 1937.

Adam, André. "Le prolétarisation de l'habitat dans l'ancienne medina de Casablanca." *Bulletin économique et social du Maroc* 13, no. 46 (1950): 44–50.

Afghani, Jamal al-Din al-. "Religion versus Science." In Nikki R. Keddie, ed., *An Is-lamic Response to Imperialism: Political and Religious Writings of Sayyid Jamal al-Din al-Afghani*, 181–187. Berkeley and Los Angeles: Univ. of California Press, 1968.

L'Afrique française. "Une française du Maroc (Mme. la Doctoresse Legey)." Septem-ber 1928: 361–362.

Albinet, Urbain. "Contribution à l'étude de la dystocie au Maroc." Thesis in medicine, Université de Toulouse—Faculté Mixte de Médecine et de Pharmacie, 1953.

Amor, Abdallah ben Caid. "Essai médico-légal—Les gestations à long terme et le droit musulman." *Union Islamique* 1 (1897–1898): 14–19.

Anfreville de la Salle. "La conquête sanitaire de nos colonies." *Revue des deux mondes* 22 (1914): 174–192.

———. "La lutte contre les principales maladies contagieuses à Casablanca." *Annales d'hygiène publique, industrielle et sociale* (1923): 712–725.

———. "Une oeuvre d'humanité et de patriotisme: Les enfants marocains abandon-nés." *L'Afrique française* (December 1927): 517–519.

Annuaire médical marocain 1934 établi par les soins du lien médical franco-marocain. Casablanca: Éditions de la Société Parisienne d'Expansion Chimique, 1934.

Antaki, Dawud ibn ʿUmar al-. *Tadhkira awla al-albab wa al-jamiaʿ liʿajbi al-ʿajab.* Lebanon: Al-Maktaba al-thaqafia, n.d.

Arnaud, D. "L'oeuf de faon, ou la survivance inattendue du Bézoard." *Maroc médical* 58 (November 15, 1926): 305–311.

Aspinion, Robert. "Case 22, 1er Rebia I 1354 (3 juin 1935), Jugement du Tribunal cou-tumier des Aït Harkat de Guelmous, Bureau de Khénifra, déclarant la paternité d'un enfant né d'une femme mariée quatre fois et admettant la croyance de l'enfant endormi en pays Zaïan." *Revue marocaine de législation, doctrine, jurisprudence chérifiennes* 3 (1935–1936): 54–61.

————. *Contribution à l'étude du droit coutumier berbère marocain (Étude sur les coutumes des tribus Zayanes)*. Casablanca: Editions A. Moynier, 1937.

Badia y Leblich, Domingo. *Voyages d'Ali Bey el Abbassi en Afrique et en Asie pendant les années 1803, 1804, 1805, 1806 et 1807*. Paris: Imprimerie de P. Didot l'aîné, 1814.

Barbault, Roger. "Artisanat et proletariat traditionnels à Fès." CHEAM [Centre des Hautes Études Administratives sur l'Afrique et l'Asie Modernes] mémoire no. 3139.

Barbet, Charles. *Questions sociales et ethnographiques—France, Algérie, Maroc*. Algiers: Carbonel, 1921.

Baron, R., Huot, and Paye. "Condition économique et niveaux de vie des travailleurs indigènes au douar Doum." *Bulletin économique du Maroc* 3, no. 13 (July 1936): 175–184.

————. "Logements et loyers des travailleurs indigènes à Rabat-Salé." *Bulletin économique du Maroc* 4, no. 15 (January 1937): 3–19.

Baron, R., Lummau, and J. Mathieu. "Notes démographiques sur la population israélite de Rabat." *Bulletin économique du Maroc* 5, no. 22 (October 1938): 271–274.

Baron, R., and J. Mathieu. "Quelques budgets de travailleurs indigènes." *Bulletin économique du Maroc* 4, no. 17 (July 1937): 208–215.

Basset, René. *Les Manuscrits arabes de deux bibliothèques de Fas*. Algiers: P. Fontana, 1883.

Bazin, René. *Charles de Foucauld, explorateur du Maroc, eremite au Sahara*. Paris: Plon, 1921.

Belpeer, M. "Femmes musulmanes—[document relatant une experience d'action sociale dont l'initiative revient à Madame Belpeer, directrice de l'Action Sociale à A.T.O.M. à Marseille, qui a crée un centre d'Education Menagère pour les Femmes Musulmanes]." *Documents nord-africains* 59 (June 16, 1952): 5.

Ben Salem, Mohammed. *La Tuberculose chez les ouvriers musulmans nord-africains en France*. Paris: Vigné, 1942.

Berbrugger, Adrien. *Voyages dans le sud de l'Algérie et des états barbaresques de l'ouest et de l'est, par El-'Aïachi et Moula-Ah'med. Traduits . . . Par Adrien Berbrugger*. Paris: Imprimerie Royale, 1846.

Bertherand, Alphonse. *De l'Acclimatement en Algérie: Communication faite au congrès de l'association française pour l'avancement des sciences en 1881*. Paris: Baillière, 1881.

Bertherand, Émile-Louis. *L'Assistance et la mortalité enfantine en Algérie*. Paris: Malteste, 1877.

————. "Contribution des arabes au propos des sciences médicales." *Paris médical* 17, 18, 19 (1883).

————. "De la création des hopitaux arabes." In *Nouveau projet d'organisation du corps des officiers de santé militaire basé sur une série de modifications apportées à l'ordonnance royale du 12 août 1836*, edited by Liandon, 1–4. Marseille: Barile, 1840.

————. "Enseignement préparatoire à la colonisation." *Bulletin de la société des sciences physiques, naturelles et climatologiques d'Alger*, 1882: 18–19.

————. *Hygiène de l'enfance algérienne, décès, naissances, maladies et modes d'allaitement comparés au point de vue des nationalités*. Algiers: Imprimerie de l'association ouvrière, 1889.

————. *Médecine et hygiène des Arabes: Études sur l'exercice de la médecine et de la chirurgie chez les musulmans de l'Algérie . . . précédées de considérations sur l'état général de la médecine chez les principales nations mahométanes.* Paris: Baillière, 1855.

————. *La Médecine légale en Algérie.* Algiers: Aillaud, 1868.

————. *Les Orphelinats de colonisation, à propos du peuplement de l'Algérie: Sous les rapports ethnologique et hygiènique des immigrants.* Algiers: Aillaud, 1877.

————. "La synocope et la folie emotive des accouchées au point de vue médico-légal." *Médecine hygiènique et médecine légale* 8, no. 7 (1872).

Bey-Rozet, Suzanne. "Le service social de la Santé Publique au Maroc: Son adaptation au monde musulman." *Maroc médical* (1953): 727–730.

————. "Le service social en milieu musulman." *Maroc médical,* no. 296 (1950): 158–160.

Bienvenue. "La mortalité estivale infantile à Rabat et à Casablanca." *Maroc médical* 31 (July 15, 1924): 217–218.

Blanchard, Maurice. *Précis d'épidémiologie—Médecine préventive et hygiène coloniales.* Paris: Vigot, 1934.

B.O. "Ordre des médecins du Maroc: Code de déontologie." *Bulletin Officiel du Protectorat de la République Française au Maroc,* no. 2121 (June 19, 1913): 828–834.

Boisboissel, Yves de. "Le meilleur collaborateur de Lyautey: La Maréchale." *Cahiers Charles de Foucauld* 33 (1954): 226–243.

Bonjean, Maurice. "Causes d'incompréhension entre l'Islam et l'Occident." *Cahiers du Sud,* 1947.

————. "L'oeuvre de la France dans la protection de l'enfance au Maroc." *Bulletin de l'Institut d'Hygiène du Maroc* 5 (1945): 6–22.

Bonsal, Stephen, Jr. *Morocco as It Is: With an Account of Sir Charles Euan Smith's Recent Mission to Fez.* London: Allen, 1893.

Boudin, Jean Christian. *Essai de géographie médicale, ou Études sur les lois qui président à la distribution géographique des maladies, ainsi qu'à leur rapports topographiques entre elles, lois de coïncidence et d'antagonisme.* Paris: Baillière, 1843.

Bourgin, Dr. "À propos du marabout de Sidi Belgacem. Étude sur la prophylaxie de la lèpre." Paper presented at the Exposition coloniale de Marseille, Marseille 1922.

Bousquet, G.-H., and Henri Jahier. "Les vices redhibitoires de la femme en droit musulman: Remarques juridico-médicales." *Revue d'Alger, Tunis, et Maroc de législation et jurisprudence* (March–April 1951): 52–58.

Bouveret, Charles, and A. Pouponneau. *Le Médecin d'assistance au Maroc: Conseils pratiques au jeune médecin du service de la santé et de l'hygiène publiques,* Préface du Médecin-Inspecteur Oberlé. Paris: Maloine, 1922.

Bouveret, Charles, and P. Vallery-Radot. "Éléments de puériculture à l'usage des jeunes filles des écoles du Maroc." *Bulletin de l'enseignement publique du Maroc,* February 1922: 1–110.

Bouyon, Marcel. "Ancienne résidence des Sultans Alaouites, La Casbah des Cherardas abrite maintenant L'Hôpital Cocard à Fès." *L'Echo d'Oran,* February 12, 1948: 4.

Breil, J. "Quelques aspects de la situation démographique au Maroc." *Bulletin économique et social du Maroc* 9, no. 35 (October 1947): 133–147.

Brochier, A. *Livre d'or du Maroc: Dictionnaire de personnalités passées et contemporaines du Maroc.* Casablanca: Imprimerie du Maghreb, 1934.

Broido, Sarah. "Abolition de la réglementation de la prostitution: Conférence faite à l'Union française pour le Suffrage des Femmes de Casablanca." *Maroc médical* 147 (September 15, 1934): 461–466, 496–503.

Brunel, René. *Essai sur la confrérie religieuse des 'Aissaoua au Maroc.* Paris: Geuthner, 1926.

Brunot, Louis. *Au Seuil de la vie marocaine.* Casablanca: Librairie Farairre, 1950.

Bulletin d'information du Maroc. "L'Industrie pharmaceutique au Maroc." Vol. 1, no. 3 (November 5, 1949): 44–45.

Bulletin de l'Institut d'Hygiène du Maroc. "L'Institut d'Hygiène du Maroc." Vol. 1 (January–March 1931).

Bulletin économique du Maroc. "Résultats provisoires du recensement du 8 mars 1936." Vol. 3, no. 13 (July 1936): 255–257.

Bulletin économique et social du Maroc. "L'effort du Maroc pour l'instruction publique." Vol. 15, no. 52 (1951): 168–174.

Butavand, Arlette. *Les Femmes médecins—missionaires.* Paris-Louvain: Édition de l'Aucam, 1933.

Camus. *Contribution à la connaissance de la flore du Maroc: Actes du 1er congrès international de botanique tenu à Paris, à l'occasion de l'exposition universelle de 1900.* Paris: Lons le Saunier, 1900.

Cassar, A. *Influence de l'arsénotherapie sur la fréquence de la paralysie générale progressive et du tabès chez le Musulman tunisien.* Congrès de la fédération des sociétés des sciences médicales de l'Afrique du Nord, March 21–24. Tunis: Finzi, 1934.

Castries, Henri de. *Les Sources inédites de l'histoire du Maroc de 1530 à 1845. Dynastie Saadienne.* Paris: E. Leroux, 1906–1923.

Catrice, P., and G. Buchet. "Les musulmans en France: Enquête à Gennevilliers." *En Terre d'Islam*, December 1929: 336–348.

Cauvin, François. "La protection de la femme enceinte au Maroc." *Maroc médical*, no. 330, November 1952: 997–998.

Célérier, Jean. "Les mouvements migratoires des indigènes au Maroc." *Bulletin économique du Maroc* 1, no. 4 (1934): 232–238.

Champagne, Pierre. "Le Mythe de l'enfant qui dort chez la femme marocaine." Thèse de Doctorat d'État en Médecine, Bourdeaux, 1955.

Chaperon, G. "Ostéopathies à tendance ostéomalacique en milieu marocain." *Maroc médical* (March 1954): 193–226.

Charbonneau, Pierre. "L'assistance et la prévoyance sociale au Maroc." *Maroc médical* no. 350 (1954): 731–752.

Charmes, Gabriel. *Une Ambassade au Maroc.* Paris: Levy, 1887.

Charnot, A. *La Toxicologie au Maroc: Mémoires de la société des sciences naturelles du Maroc.* Rabat: Institut Scientifique Chérifien, 1945.

Chastand, Paul. *Le Protectorat français au Maroc.* Paris: Jouve, 1913.

Chatinières, Paul. *Dans le Haut Atlas marocain—Extraits du carnet de route d'un médecin d'assistance médicale indigène, 1912–1916.* Paris: Plon-Nourrit, 1919.

Chaumont, H. "L'oeuvre de Madame la Maréchale Lyautey au Maroc." *La Tribune des vieux marocains*, February 1948, 2.

Chenebault, J. "Contribution à l'étude de la tuberculose pulmonaire de l'enfant marocaine en milieu citadin." *Maroc médical*, 1948: 70–75.

Chénébeaux. "Le Bureau Marocain de Travail." CHEAM mémoire no. 861.

Chevalier, Louis. *Le Problème démographique nord-africain.* Paris: PUF, 1947.

Chevrillon, André. *Visions du Maroc*. Marseille: Detaille, 1933.

Cismigiu, F. "Facteurs de mortinatalité et dystocie en milieu marocain." *Maroc médical* no. 330 (November 1952): 971–977.

Coliac. "Intervention des sociétés indigènes de prévoyance dans la lutte contre la formation d'un proletariat indigène." *Bulletin économique du Maroc* 3, no. 13 (July 1936): 249–252.

Colin, Gabriel. *Abderrezzâq El-Jezâiri. Un Médecin arabe du XIIe siècle de l'hégire*. Montpellier: Delord-Boehen et Martial, 1905.

———. "La noria marocaine et les machines hydrauliques dans le monde arabe." *Hésperis* 14 (1921): 22–60.

———. *La Tedkira d'Abu 'l-'Alâ—Publié et traduite pour la première fois par Gabriel Colin*. Paris: Leroux, 1911.

Colombani, Jules. "À propos de l'état sanitaire du Maroc et de son prétendu caractère infecteur." *Revue générale de médecine et de chirurgie de l'Afrique du Nord et des colonies françaises* 185 (July 10, 1932): 1340–1346.

———. *L'Effort prophylactique au Maroc*. Rabat: Bonnin and Gonzalvez, 1924.

———. "Une grande figure de la croix rouge française, La Maréchale Lyautey." *Le Courrier du Maroc*, Feb. 10 (1953): 1, 3.

———. "La pénétration pacifique au Maroc: Lyautey et le médecin (1912–1925)." *Vert et Rouge: Revue de la Légion Étrangère*, no. special, "Lyautey et la Légion" (1937): 40–47.

Comité d'Action Marocaine. *Plan de réformes marocaines*. Paris: Labor, 1934.

Comte, Auguste. *The Catechism of Positivism, or Summary Exposition of the Universal Religion*. London: Kegan, 1891.

———. *Discours sur l'esprit positif*. Paris: Union Générale d'Éditions, 1963.

Couillieux. *Le Programme de la France au Maroc: L'Organisation du protectorat, les affaires au Maroc*. Paris: Larose, 1912.

Counillon, G. "Les écoles franco-musulmans de fillettes au Maroc." *Bulletin économique et social du Maroc* 8, no. 29 (April 1946): 320–327.

Cruchet, René. *La Conquête pacifique du Maroc et du Tafilalet*. Paris: Berger-Levrault, 1930.

Décor, A. "Vingt années d'activité d'une maternité en milieu marocain urbain." *Bulletin de l'Institut d'Hygiène du Maroc* 6 (1946): 15–39.

Decrop, G. "Où en est la syphilis marocaine?" *Maroc médical* (January 1950): 132–137.

Decrop, G., and Salle. *Album de documents photographiques syphiligraphie et de dermatologie marocaines*. 1921.

Dekester. *Utilisation du marocain comme infirmier indigène, par M. Dekester, médecin de l'Assistance publique, médicin adjoint á l'Hôpital Cocard, à Fez*. Marseille: Baulatier, 1923.

Delanoë, Eugénie Roubinstein. "Considerations générales sur le fonctionnement du service des femmes et enfants à l'hôpital regional de Mazagan pendant l'année 1925." *Marseille médical* 15 (May 1926).

———. "Les croyances indigènes sur la grossesse." *Paris-Maroc*, 1915.

———. "L'huile de chaulmoogra dans le traitement du trachôme." *La Clinique*, July (1928).

———. "Note sur le traitement de la syphilis chez les femmes enceintes." *Maroc médical* 3 (15 janvier 1922).

————. "La prophylaxie antitrachomateuse exercée dans le milieu indigène marocain d'une façon suivie et énergique depuis 10 ans fait baisser de moitié le nombre des trachomateux, elle diminue aussi et surtout la gravité des cas." *Revue du trachome*, July 1936.

————. "À propos de l'allaitement artificiel des nourrissons." *Presse marocaine*, April (1925).

————. "Protection de la femme et de l'enfant indigènes: Quelques questions de médecine sociale indigène à l'occasion du Ve congrès de la mutualité coloniale et des pays de protectorat." *Maroc médical* 63 (March 15, 1927): 70–73.

————. *Trente années d'activité médicale et sociale au Maroc*. Paris: Maloine, 1949.

De Lens, Aline Reveillaud. *Pratiques des harems marocains: Sorcellerie, médecine, beauté*. Paris: Geuthner, 1925.

Delon, J. " À propos du Kwashiorkor." *Presse médicale*, November 4, 1950.

Delorme. "Une inspection générale médicale au Maroc en 1908." *Archives de Médecine et de Pharmacie militaires* 60, no. 8 (August–September 1908): 97–222.

Delphin, Gaëtan. *L'Astronomie au Maroc*. Paris: Imprimerie Nationale, 1891.

————. *Fas, son université et l'enseignement supérieur musulman*. Paris: Leroux, 1889.

Denat, C. "Coutumes berbères Ichkern: Dissolution du mariage." *La Revue marocaine de droit* 5 (May 1, 1951): 202–210.

————. "Droit coutumier berbère Ichkern: Coutume de l'enfant endormi." *La Revue marocaine de droit*, April 1, 1951, 157–161.

Depont, Octave, and Xavier Coppolani. *Les Confréries religieuses musulmanes*. Algiers: Jourdan, 1897.

Dermenghem, Emile. *Le Culte des saints dans l'Islam maghrébin*. Paris: Gallimard, 1954.

Deschamps, Hubert. *Souvenirs des premiers temps du Maroc français*. Paris: Charles-Lavauzelle, 1935.

Devillars, Pierre. "L'immigration marocaine en France." *Bulletin économique et social du Maroc* 13, no. 46 (1950): 7–14.

Djaznâi, Abou-l-Hasan 'Ali al-. *Zahrat El-As (La Fleur du myrte), Traitant de la fondation de la ville de Fès; Texte arabe et traduction par Alfred Bel*. Algiers: Carbonel, 1923.

Doutté, Edmond. *Les Aissaoua à Tlemcen*. Châlons-sur-Marne: Martin Frères, 1900.

————. *En Tribu—Missions au Maroc*. Paris: Geuthner, 1914.

————. *L'Islam algérien en l'an 1900*. Algiers: Giralt, 1900.

————. *Magie et religion dans l'Afrique du Nord*. Algiers: Jourdan, 1908.

————. *Merrâkech*. Paris: Comité du Maroc, 1905.

————. *Notes sur l'Islam maghribin: Les marabouts*. Paris: Leroux, 1900.

————. "Notes sur l'Islam maghribin: Les marabouts." Pts. 1 and 2. *Revue de l'histoire des religions* 40 (1899): 343–369; 41 (1899): 289–366.

————. Préface to A. Gabriel-Rousseau, *La Mausolée des Princes Sa'adiens à Marrakech*. Paris: Geuthner, 1925.

————. *Les Tas de pierres sacrés et quelques pratiques connexes dans le Sud du Maroc*. Algiers: Imprimerie Administrative Victor Heintz, 1903.

Douzans. "Mémoire sur la nosologie marocaine avant le protectorat, 1906–08." *L'Avenir médical, Lyon* (1913–1914): 23, 26–29, 55–58, 72–3, 90–95.

Dumas, Pierre. *Le Maroc*. Grenoble: Arthaud, 1928.

Du Mazel, Dr. "Visite au maristan de Sidi Fredj à Fès." Paper presented at the exposition coloniale de Marseille. Marseille, 1922.

Durkheim, Émile. "Préface." *Année sociologique* 1 (1897–1898).

———. "La Sociologie en France." *Revue bleue*, 1900: 609–613, 647–652.

L'Echo d'Oran. "Un témoignage de la grande oeuvre française au Maroc: L'éducation de la femme marocaine, plus importante que l'action médicale pour les assistantes sociales." Vols. 11–12 (February 1951): 6.

L'Echo du Maroc. "Mort de la maréchale Lyautey—Elle sera inhumée jeudi à Rabat dans la mausolée où repose le Maréchal—La vie et l'oeuvre d'une grande française." February 10, 1953, 1, 4.

Ecochard, M. "Problèmes d'urbanisme au Maroc." *Bulletin économique et social du Maroc* 15 no. 52 (1951): 28–35.

Emily, Shareefa of Wazan [Emily Keene]. *My Life Story*. London: Arnold, 1912.

Erckmann, Jules. *Le Maroc moderne*. Paris: Challamel, 1885.

Faraj, Abdalmalik. *Relations médicales hispano-maghrébines au XIIe siècle*. Paris: Éditions Vega, 1935.

Fasi, 'Ali ibn 'Abd Allah Ibn Abi Zar al-. *Roudh el-Kartas: Histoire des souverains du Maghreb (Espagne et Maroc) et annales de la ville de Fès*. Translated by Auguste Beaumier. Paris: Imprimerie Impériale, 1860.

Fasi, 'Allal al-. *The Independence Movements in North Africa, Al-Harakat al-Istiqlaliyya*. 1947. Reprint, New York: Octagon, 1970.

Fasi, Muhammad al-. *Contes fasis*. Paris: Éditions d'Aujourd'hui, 1976, 1926.

Ferry, Edmond. *La Réorganisation marocaine (Rapport au Comité du Maroc)*. Paris: Comité du Maroc, 1905.

Fischbacher, A. "Aspects de la médecine au Maroc: Certificats." *Maroc médical* (August 1954): 808–809.

Flaubert, Gustave. *Flaubert in Egypt: A Sensibility on Tour*. Translated by Francis Steegmuller. New York: Penguin, 1996.

Foucauld, Charles de. *Reconnaissance au Maroc: Journal de route*. Paris: Société d'éditions géographiques, maritimes et coloniales, 1939.

Fourment, Pierre, and Henri Roques. "Contribution à l'étude des drogues indigènes nord-africaines—Le 'souak' ou 'Djouz' (juglans regia L.)." *Bulletin de la Société d'Histoire Naturelle de l'Afrique du Nord* (June–July 1935): 171–176.

France Outremer. "En terre qu'ils ont tant aimée (décès de madame la maréchale Lyautey)." March 1953, 2.

Garcin and Sacquépée. "La peste des Ouled Fredj (Maroc), La peste des animaux domestiques: Remarques sur la contagion de la peste et sur sa prophylaxie." *Archives de médecine et de pharmacie militaires* 62 (1913): 561–579.

Gaud, J. "Développement de l'enfant indigène au Maroc." *Bulletin économique du Maroc* 3, no. 13 (July 1936): 245–247.

Gaud, J., and E. Mage-Humbert. "La tuberculose pulmonaire au Maroc en milieu musulman." *Bulletin de l'Institut d'Hygiène du Maroc* 7 (1947): 83–99.

———. "La fête des mères." *Jeunesse* 22 (May 31, 1942).

Gaud, J., G. Houel, and G. Fayveley. "Indices tuberculiniques au Maroc." *Bulletin de l'Institut d'Hygiène du Maroc* 11, no. 2 (1951): 5–52.

Gaud, Maurice. "La mortalité infantile à Meknes." *Maroc médical* 32 (August 15, 1924): 239–241.

Gaudry, Mathea. *La Femme chaouia de l'Aurès: Étude de sociologie berbère.* Paris: Geuthner, 1929.

Gentil, Louis. *Dans le bled es siba, Explorations au Maroc, Mission de Segonzac.* Paris: Masson, 1906.

———. *Voyages d'exploration dans l'atlas marocain.* Paris: Comité de l'Afrique française, 1924.

Gentil, Louis, and Émile Perrot. *Sur les productions végétales du Maroc—Notice 10 de l'Office national des matières premières végétales—Contient en outre: (Maire, Dr. R.) Coup d'oeil sur la végétation du Maroc; (Gattefossé, J.) Les Plantes dans la thérapeutique indigène au Maroc; (Dufougeré Mme.), Sur les matières colorantes végétales employées au Maroc.* Paris: Larose, 1921.

Godard, Léon. *Description et histoire du Maroc: Comprenant la géographie et la statistique de ce pays, depuis le temps les plus anciens jusqu'à la paix de Tétouan en 1860.* Paris: Tanera, 1860.

Godebargh, M. "Deux corporations berbères à Fès: Les 'izerzain et les igerraben.'" CHEAM mémoire no. 1020.

Goichon, Amélie Marie. *La Femme de la moyenne bourgeoisie fassiya.* Paris: Librarie Orientaliste Paul Geuthner, 1929.

Gorrée, Georges. *Les Amitiés sahariennes du Père de Foucauld.* Grenoble: Arthaud, 1946.

Goyau, Georges. *Une Fondatrice d'institut missionaire. Mère Marie de la Passion et les franciscaines missionaires de Marie.* Paris: Ramlot, 1935.

Guillemin, Henri. *Biographie du Docteur Émile Mauchamp.* Chalon-sur-Saône: Imprimerie Bertrand, 1910.

Hamida, Okbani Hadj. "Les modes de preuve dans la coutume de la tribu des Aid Izdeq." *Revue marocaine de législation, doctrine et jurisprudence* 3 (1935–1936): 52–56.

Hardy, Georges, and Louis Brunot. *L'Enfant marocain: Essai d'ethnographie scolaire . . . Avec la collaboration de Mlle Burtey, Mme. Driss-Amor, Mme. De Pressigny.* Paris: Larose, 1925.

Harris, Lawrence. *With Mulai Hafid at Fez: Behind the Scenes in Morocco.* Boston: Gorham, 1910.

Herber, J. "La mortalité estivale infantile de 0 à 1 an, à Rabat." *Maroc médical* 29 (May 15, 1924): 149–150.

———. "Origine et signification des tatouages marocains." *L'Anthropologie* 37 (1927): 517–525.

———. "Tatouage et religion." *Revue de l'histoire des religions,* 1921.

———. "Tatouages curatifs au Maroc." *Revue d'ethnographie et des traditions populaires* 34–36 (1928): 179–87.

———. "Les Tatouages du pied au Maroc." *L'Anthropologie* 33: 87–102.

Houel, Guy. "La campagne de vaccination antituberculeuse." *Bulletin économique et social du Maroc* 13, no. 47 (1950): 295–296.

Huguet. "La goutte de lait de Rabat." *France-Maroc* (July 15, 1917): 22–25.

Ibn 'Arabi, Muhya ad-Din. *At-Tadbirat al-ilahiyyah fi islah al-mamalakat al-insaniyya.* Translated by Shaykh Tosun Bayrak al-Jerrahi al-Halveti. Louisville, Ky.: Fons Vitae, 1997.

Ibn Ishaq, Khalil. *Abrégé de la loi musulmane selon le rite de l'imam Malek, tra-*

duction nouvelle par G.H. Bousquet. Algiers: Editions Algériennes En-Nahda, 1956.

Ifrani, Muhammad as-Saghir ibn al-Haj Muhammad ibn 'Abdallah al-. *Nuzhat al-hadi bi akhbar muluk al-qarn al-hadi*. Edited by O. Houdas. Paris: Leroux, 1888.

Imbert, J. "La tuberculose pulmonaire de primo infection chez l'enfant." *Maroc médical* (February 1948): 64–69.

Jahandiez, Emile, and René Maire. *Catalogue des plantes du Maroc*. Algiers: Imprimerie Minerva, 1931.

Jahier, Henri, and G.-H. Bousquet. "L'enfant endormi: Notes juridiques, ethnographiques et obstétricales." *Cahiers médicaux de l'union française* 1 (1946): 9–27.

Jahier, Henri, and A. Noureddine. "De l'obstétrique et de la pédiatrie en Espagne musulmane aux Xème siècle." *Histoire de la Médecine* 5 (1952): 21–35.

Jeanselme, Edouard. *Histoire de la syphilis, son origine, son expansion: Progrès realisés dans l'étude de cette maladie depuis la fin du Xve siècle jusqu'a l'époque contemporaine*. Paris: Doin, 1931.

J. G. "Edmond Doutté 1867–1926." *Académie des sciences coloniales: Comtes-rendues des séances; Communications* 8 (1926–1927): 531–535.

Jilani, Abd al-Qadir al-. *The Book of the Secret of Secrets and the Manifestation of Lights [Kitab Sirr al-Asrar wa Mazahar al-Anwar]*. Translated by Muhtar Holland. Fort Lauderdale, Fla.: Al-Baz, 2000.

Jourdan. "Le rôle du médecin dans la société marocaine." *Presse médicale* 92 (November 12, 1913): 1293–1299.

Journal de février. "La maréchale n'est plus." February 11, 1953, 3.

Juin, Alphonse. Introduction to *Lyautey et le médecin*. Casablanca: Maroc Médical, 1954.

Kahhak, Abdelkader. "Un diplôme de médecin marocain à Fès en 1832." *Extrait de Revue de l'occident musulman et de la Méditerranée* 7 (1970): 195–210.

Kattani, Ja'far ibn Idris al-. *Al-ta'lif al-mubarak fi hukm sabun al-sharq wa sham al-buji wa sunduq an-nar al-majlub tilka min bilad al-kuffar la'anahum Allah wa hukm khiyata ahl al-dhimma qabbahahum Allah*. Fez lithograph (date unknown).

Kattani, Muhammad ibn Ja'far al-. *Kitab salwat al-anfas wa muhadathat al-akyas bi man uqbira min al-'ulama' wa al-sulaha' bi Fas*. 3 vols. Fez lithograph, 1898.

Lacapère, Georges. "La lutte contre la syphilis au Maroc." *France-Maroc* 2, no. 15 (February 1918): 54–57.

———. "La mortalité infantile au Maroc et ses rapports avec la syphilis." *Presse médicale*, January 7, 1918.

———. *La Syphilis arabe: Maroc, Algérie, Tunisie*. Paris: Doin, 1923.

Lacapère, Georges, and Charles Laurent. *Le Traitement de la syphilis par les composés arsenicaux*. Paris: Masson, 1918.

Lacascade, Renée. *Puériculture et colonisation: Étude sur la puériculture au Maroc (Aperçu du role colonisateur que peut jouer la femme médecin dans les pays d'occupation)*. Paris: Vigot Frères, 1922.

Lacour, Raymond, Jacques Varanguien de Villepin, and André Rebreyend. "La rénovation de l'Institution des Habous." In *Livre d'Or du Centenaire de la Naissance du Maréchal Lyautey*, edited by A. Brochier, 734–755. Casablanca: Imprimerie du Maghreb, 1934.

Laffont, A. "Problèmes obstétricaux et gynécologiques en Afrique du Nord." *Maroc médical*, no. 330 (November 1952): 993–996.

La Martinière, H. M. P. de. *Morocco: Journeys in the Kingdom of Fez and to the Court of Mulai Hassan, with Itineraries Constructed by the Author and a Bibliography of Morocco from 1844 and 1887*. London: Whittaker, 1889.

Laoust, Emile. *Mots et choses berbères*. Paris: Challamel, 1920.

Lapin, Pierre. "La lutte contre la tuberculose." *Maroc médical* (April 15, 1924): 112–117.

Leared, Arthur. *Morocco and the Moors: Being an Account of Travels, With a General Description of the Country and Its People*. 2nd ed. London: Sampson Low, Marston, Searle, and Rivington, 1891.

Le Chatelier, Alfred. *Les Confréries musulmanes du Hedjaz*. Paris: Leroux, 1887.

———. *L'Islam au XIXe siècle*. Paris: Leroux, 1888.

———. *Lettre à un Algérien sur la politique saharienne*. Versailles: Société anonyme des imprimeries Gérardin, 1900.

———. *Notes sur les villes et tribus du Maroc en 1890*. Angers: Imprimerie Orientale A. Burdin, 1902.

———. *Politique musulmane, I: Lettre au "Standard" par A. le Chatelier*. Tours: Arrault, 1907.

———. *Questions d'économie coloniale: Lettres à M. Eugène Étienne, Vice-President de la Chambre des Députés*. Paris: Challamel, 1902.

———. *Sud-Oranais et Maroc*. Paris, 1903.

Leclerc, Lucien. *Histoire de la médecine arabe*. 2 vols. Paris: Leroux, 1876.

———. *Kachef Er-Roumoûz (Révélation des Énigmes) d'Abd Er-Rezzaq Ed-Djezaîry ou Traité de matière arabe d'Abd Er-Rezzaq l'algérien traduit et annoté par . . .* Paris: Ballière, Leroux, 1874.

Le Coeur, Charles. "Les rites de passage d'Azemmour." *Hespéris* (1933). Volume 17, fasc. 2, 129–148.

———. *Textes sur la sociologie et l'école au Maroc*. Paris: Alcan, 1939.

Lefrançois, C. "Les travailleurs marocains en France pendant la guerre." *France-Maroc* 3 (March 15, 1917): 14–17.

Legey, Françoise. "Un centre de puériculture à Marrakech." *Archives de médecine des enfants* 10 (1924), 583–586.

———. "De l'utilisation des femmes indigènes dans les formations sanitaires." Paper presented at the Congrès de la santé publique. Marseille, 1922.

———. *Essai de folklore marocain: Lettre-Préface du Maréchal Lyautey*. Paris: Geuthner, 1926.

Legey, Françoise, and A. Décor. "L'assistance aux femmes en couches à la maternité indigène de Marrakech." *Bulletin de l'Institut d'Hygiène du Maroc*, April–June 1932, 48–61.

Lempriere, William. *Tour from Gibraltar to Tangier, Sallee, Mogodore, Santa Cruz . . . Including a Particular Account of the Royal Harem*. London, 1834.

Lepinay, Émile. "La lutte contre les maladies vénériennes au Maroc." *Maroc médical* (January 1950): 124–131.

Le Play, Frédéric. *La Réforme sociale en France déduite de l'observation comparée des peuples européens*. Paris: Plon, 1864.

———. *L'Organisation de la famille selon le vrai modèle signalé par l'histoire de toutes les races et de tous les temps.* Tours: A. Mame et fils, 1845.

Leredde, Laurent Victor. *Instructions complémentaires relatives au diagnostic et au traitement de la syphilis.* Rabat: Imprimerie du Bulletin Officiel du Gouvernement du Protectorate, 1917–1918.

Letellier, Roger. "La famille indigène devant les problèmes sociaux modernes." In *Journées sociales nord-africaines, avril 1941, Alger,* 37–56. Algiers: Imprimerie Polyglotte Africaine, Maison-Carrée, 1941.

Le Tourneau, Roger. *Fès avant le protectorat: Étude économique et sociale d'une ville de l'occident musulman.* Rabat: Editions La Porte, 1949, 1987.

———. *La Vie quotidienne à Fès en 1900.* Paris: Hachette, 1965.

Lévi-Provençal, Évariste. *Les Historiens des Chorfa: Essai sur la littérature historique et biographique au Maroc du XVIe au XXe siècle.* Paris: Larose, 1922.

Linarès, F. "Voyage au Tafilalet avec S.M. le Sultan Moulay Hassan en 1893." *Bulletin de l'Institut d'Hygiène du Maroc* 3 (1932): 91–116, and 4 (1932): 95–136.

Lyautey, Louis-Hubert-Gonzalve. *Choix de lettres.* Paris: Colin, 1947.

———. "Du rôle colonial de l'armée." *Revue des deux mondes,* vol. 157 (January 15, 1900): 308–322.

———. "Du rôle social de l'officier dans le service militaire universel." *Revue des deux mondes,* March 15, 1891: 443–459.

———. "Le rôle des services de santé et d'hygiène dans les colonies." *La Marche de France,* August 1929: 473–477.

Lyautey, Mme. *Au Maroc: Pour protéger la mère et l'enfant.* Bruxelles: Office de publicité, 1921.

———. "Les oeuvres de l'enfance au Maroc." *France-Maroc* 59 (October 1921): 177–185.

———. *Les Oeuvres de l'enfance au Maroc. Rapport présenté par Mme La Maréchale Lyautey au congrès international des oeuvres de l'enfance (Bruxelles, 22–26 Juillet 1921).* Paris: Comité de l'Afrique française, 1921.

Lyautey, Mme., and F. Huguet. "La goutte de lait de Rabat." *France-Maroc* (July 15, 1917): 22–25.

Lyautey et le médecin. Casablanca: Maroc Médical, 1954.

Mage-Humbert, E. "Aspects de la tuberculose pulmonaire chez l'enfant marocaine." *Bulletin de l'Institut d'Hygiène du Maroc* 11, nos. 1–2 (1951): 53–68.

Maneville, Roger. "De l'évolution sociale et politique des marocains en France." CHEAM mémoire, 1946.

Marmey, Charles, and Jean Marmey. "Contribution à l'étude de l'obstétrique au Maroc: Travail de la Maternité 'Maréchale Lyautey' à Rabat." *Bulletin de l'Institut d'Hygiène du Maroc* 3 (July–September 1933): 5–41.

Marmey, Jean. "Avenir obstétrical des femmes symphyséotomisées (suivant la technique de Zarate)." *Presse médicale* 62, no. 45: 956.

———. "Du choix de l'incision utérine au cours des césariennes abdominales, d'après 263 interventions pratiquées à la maternité de Rabat." *Maroc médical,* November 1952: 987–990.

Marmey J., and A. Lacroix. "Indications de la symphyséotomie de Zarate dans la pratique obstétricale marocaine d'après 56 observations." *Maroc médical,* no. 330 (November 1952): 978–986.

Maroc médical. "Les muwallidat: Leur rôle dans l'assistance obstétricale au Maroc," no. 330 (November 1952): 999–1002.

————. "Tableau des Formations d'Accouchement, de Gynécologie, de Consultations prénatales, Centres d'education sanitaire, organisés par la Direction de la Santé Publique et de la Famille au Maroc," no. 330 (November 1952): 1001.

Martin, L. "Description de la ville de Fès, Quartier de Keddan." *Revue du monde musulman* 9 (1909), 433–443, 621–642.

Massignon, Louis. "Enquête sur les corporations d'artisans et de commerçants au Maroc (1923–1924), d'après les réponses au questionnaire transmis par circulaire du 15 novembre 1923 sous le timbre de la direction des Affaires Indigènes et du Service des Renseignements." *Revue du monde musulman* 28 (1924): iii–250.

Massonnaud, A. "L'évolution des corporations depuis notre installation au Maroc: Ses repercussions économiques et politiques." *Bulletin économique du Maroc* 4, no. 15 (1937): 83–85.

Massy, René. "Contribution à l'étude des produits susceptibles d'être fournis à l'industrie et à la matière médicale par les forêts du Maroc." *C.R. des recherches effectuées en 1923, dans Bulletin de la Société des Sciences Naturelles du Maroc,* vol. 4, nos. 1 and 2: 42–45; vol. 3, nos. 1 and 2: 25–28; vol. 5: 110–113.

————. "Goudron marocain de *cedrus atlantica*: Préparation indigène; Quelques caractères physiques et chimiques." *Journal de pharmacie et de chimie* 24 (1921): 294–301.

Mathieu, Jean. "Contrôle de l'état de nutrition des indigènes musulmans d'un douar marocain suburban, 'bidonville' de Port-Lyautey." *Bulletin de l'Institut d'Hygiène du Maroc,* 4, no. 68 (1937).

————. "Notes sur les pratiques médicales indigènes à Figuig." *Maroc médical,* April 15, 1928: 125–132.

Mathieu, Jean, and Roger Maneville. *Les Accoucheuses musulmanes traditionnelles de Casablanca.* Paris: Imprimerie Administrative Centrale, 1952.

Mauchamp, Émile. "L'Allaitement artificiel des nourrissons par le lait stérilisé: Conditions—Pratique—Résultats—Indications." Doctorat en Médecine, Faculté de médecine de Paris, 1898.

————. *La Sorcellerie au Maroc, oeuvre posthume.* Paris: Dorbon-Aîné, 1911.

Mauran, Dr. "Considérations sur la médecine indigène actuelle au Maroc." *Bulletin de l'Institut des Hautes Etudes Marocains* 1 (December 1920): 83–91.

————. "L'hygiène du marocain." *Revue générale des sciences,* April 15, 1914: 306–308.

————. *Le Maroc d'aujourd'hui et de demain: Rabat; Études sociales.* Paris: Paulin, 1909.

————. *La Société marocaine: Études sociales, impressions et souvenirs, avec une lettre-préface de M. Le Générale d'Amade, et une lettre de M. Guiot.* Paris: Paulin, 1910.

Mazières, Marc de. "La situation économique du Maroc." *Bulletin de la société géographique d'Alger et de l'Afrique du Nord* 17 (1912): 161–219.

M.C. "Une visite à l'O.S.E. oeuvre de secours pour l'enfant juive." *Le Courier du Maroc,* October 23, 1954, 7.

Mercier, Ernest. *La Condition de la femme musulmane dans l'Afrique septentrionale.* Algiers: Jourdan, 1895.

Meynadier, E. "Les eaux chloro-sulfurées-sodiques de Moulay-Yacoub." *Maroc médical*, December 15, 1928: 365–368.

Michaux-Bellaire, Edouard. "Description de la ville de Fès." *Archives marocaines* 11 (1907): 252–330.

———. "La Maison d'Ouezzan." *Revue du monde musulman* (1908): 23–89.

———. *Quelques tribus de montagnes de la region du Habt.* Paris: Leroux, 1911.

———. "Les tribus arabes de la vallée du Lekkous." *Archives marocaines* 6 (1905): 233–235.

Michaux-Bellaire, Edouard, and Georges Salmon. "El-Qcar el-Kebir: Une ville de province au Maroc septentrional." *Archives marocaines* 2, no. 2 (1905): 1–228.

Millet, A. H. *Au Maroc: Ce que tout officier ou médecin doit savoir.* Paris: Imprimerie et Librairie Militaires Charles-Lauvazelle, 1921.

Millet, René. *La France au Maroc: Discours prononcé par M. René Millet, Ancien Résident Général à Tunis. Banquet du 30 novembre 1909 sous la présidence de M. Étienne, le Prince d'Arenberg (President du Comité de l'Afrique française), et Guillain, député, President du Comité du Maroc.* Paris: Comité du Maroc, 1909.

Milliot, Louis. *Démembrements du Habous: Menfa'a, Gza, Guelsa, Zina, Istighraq.* Paris: Leroux, 1918.

———. *Étude sur la condition de la femme musulmane au Maghreb (Maroc, Algérie, Tunisie).* Paris: Rousset, 1910.

Ministère des Affaires Étrangères. *Rapport général sur la situation du protectorat du Maroc au 31 juillet 1914 . . . sous la direction de M. le Résident Général Lyautey.* Rabat: Résidence Générale de la République Française au Maroc, 1914.

Montagne, Robert. *Les Berbères et le makhzen dans le sud du Maroc: Essai sur la transformation politique des berbères sédentaires.* Paris: Alcan, 1930.

———. "L'évolution moderne des pays arabes." In *Extrait des annales sociologiques*, 1–52. Paris: Alcan, 1935.

———. *Un Magasin collectif de l'Anti-Atlas: L'Agadir des Ikounka.* Paris: Larose, 1930.

———. *Naissance du prolétariat marocain, enquête collective 1948–1950.* Paris: Peyronnet, 1952.

———. "Note sur la Kasbah de Mehdiya." *Hésperis*, 1921, 93–97.

———. "Un plan d'enquêtes sociologiques—Démographie et questions sociales marocaines." *Bulletin économique du Maroc* 3 (January 1936): 75–76.

———. *Révolution au Maroc.* Paris: France Empire, 1953.

Morand, Marcel. *Études de droit musulman algérien.* Algiers: Jourdan, 1910.

———. *La Famille musulmane.* Algiers: Jourdan, 1903.

———. *Introduction à l'étude du droit musulman algérien.* Algiers: Carbonel, 1921.

Nasiri, Ahmad ibn Khalid al-. *Kitab al-Istiqsa li-Akhbar Duwwal al-Maghrib al-Aqsa.* Translated as *Kitab elistiqsa li akhbari doual elmaghrib elaqsa*, edited by Eugène Fumey. Paris: Leroux, 1906.

Nobécort, P. Preface to Charles Bouveret and Pierre Vallery-Radot, "Éléments de puériculture à l'usage des jeunes filles des écoles du Maroc." *Bulletin de l'enseignement publique du Maroc*, February 1922: 9–10.

Ockley, Simon. *An Account of South-West Barbary: Containing What Is Most Remarkable in the Territories of the King of Fez and Morocco. Written by a Person Who Had Been a Slave There a Considerable Time; and Published from His*

Authentick Manuscript. To Which Are Added Two Letters: One from the Present King of Morocco to Colonel Kirk; the Other to Sir Cloudesly Shovell: With Sir Cloudesly's Answer. London: Bowyer and Clements, 1713.

Ollive, C. "Géographie médicale: Climat de Mogador et de son influence sur la phthisie." *Bulletin de la Société de Géographie* (October 1875): 365–416.

Ouazzani, Mohamed Hassan [Muhammad Hasan al-Wazzani]. *Combats d'un nationaliste marocain.* 3 vols. Fez: Fondation Mohamed Hassan Ouazzani, 1989.

Pasquier-Bronde. "La vie économique et l'organisation du travail." In *Le Problème social nord-africaine: Compte rendu in extenso des conférences et exposés divers, Session d'Avril 1941* (Algiers), 57–74.

Péraud, Jeanne. *La Femme médecin en Afrique du Nord: Son rôle d'éducatrice.* Bordeaux: Imprimerie de l'Université, 1932.

Périer, Jean-André-Napoléon. *De l'Acclimatement en Algérie.* Paris: Baillière, 1845.

———. *De l'Hygiène en Algérie, suivi d'un mémoire sur la peste en Algérie par A. Berbrugger.* Paris: Imprimerie Royale, 1847.

———. *Le Docteur Boudin: Notice historique sur sa vie et ses travaux, lue à la Société d'Anthropologie dans la séance solonnelle du 20 juin 1867, suivie d'un index bibliographique.* Paris: Rozier, 1867.

Perrot, Emile. *Chaulmoogra et autres graines utilisables contre la lèpre.* Paris: Office national des matières premières végétales pour la droguerie, la distillerie, la pharmacie et la parfumerie, 1926.

———. *Les Matières premières usuelles d'origine végétale indigènes et exotiques.* Paris: Vigot Frères, 1906.

———. *Plantes médicinales et plantes à parfum au Maroc (Action du Comité Marocain, 1920–25).* Lons-le-Saunier: Declume, 1926.

Pesle, O. *La Femme musulmane dans le droit, la religion et les moeurs.* Rabat: Les Éditions La Porte, 1946.

Pharaon, Florian, and A. Bertherand. *Livre de la miséricorde dans l'art de guérir les maladies et de conserver la santé.* Paris: Baillière, 1856.

Pharaon, Florian, and Émile-Louis Bertherand, *Vocabulaire français-arabe à l'usage des médecins, vétérinaires, sages-femmes, pharmaciens, herboristes.* Paris: Morel, 1860.

Pierson, Antoine C. *Naissance d'une vocation: Colombani, disciple de Lyautey.* Casablanca: Presses des Imprimeries Réunies, 1956.

Pinta, R. "La lutte contre la misère au Maroc en 1945." *Bulletin économique du Maroc* 8, no. 28 (January 1946): 284–287.

Qarawani [Kayrawani], Ibn Abou Zeyd al-. *Risala ou traïté abrégé de droit malékite et morale musulmane, traduction avec commentaire et index analytique par E. Fagnan.* Paris: Geuthner, 1914.

Qurtubi, ʿArib ibn Saʿid al-Katib al-. *Le Livre de la génération du foetus et le traitement des femmes enceintes et des nouveau-nés, publié, traduit et annoté par Henri Jahier et Abdelkader Noureddine.* Algiers: Publications de la faculté mixte de médecine et de pharmacie d'Alger III, 1956.

Rapport sur l'activité des services de la direction de la santé et de l'hygiène pendant l'année 1936. Documents du Centre des Hautes Études Administratives sur l'Afrique et l'Asie Modernes [CHEAM], no. 726, 1936.

Ray, Joanny. *Les Marocains en France.* Paris: Librarie du Recueil Sirey, 1938.

———. "Quelques aspects économiques et sociaux de l'émigration nord-africaine en France." *Journées sociales nord-africaines, avril 1941* (Algiers): 89–104.

Raynaud, Lucien. *Étude sur l'hygiène et la médecine au Maroc, suivie d'une notice sur la climatologie des principales ville de l'Empire.* Paris: Baillière, 1902.

Raynaud, Lucien, Henri Soulié, and Paul Picard. *Hygiène et pathologie nord-africaines—Assistance médicale.* Paris: Masson, 1932.

Remlinger, Pierre. "Un cas de nodosités juxta-articulaires observé au Maroc chez un Européen." *Bulletin de la Société de Pathologie Exotique* 16 (1923): 346–347.

———. "Essai de nosologie marocaine." *Annales d'hygiène publique et de médecine légale*, August 1913: 129–167.

———. "La main d'oeuvre marocain en France et la propagation de la tuberculose au Maroc." *Maroc médical*, March 15, 1928.

———. "Les maladies vénériennes et la prostitution au Maroc." *Annales d'hygiène publique et de médecine légale*, February 1913: 100–106.

Remlinger, Pierre, and J. Bailly. "Cent réactions de Friedman pour le diagnostic biologique de la grossesse." *Maroc médical* 157 (1935): 261–267.

———. "Le diagnostic biologique de la grossesse en médecine indigène et devant les tribunaux musulmans." *Maroc médical*, March 15, 1934, 107–109.

Renan, Ernest. *Averroès et l'averroïsme, essai historique.* Paris: Michel Levy Frères, 1867.

———. *L'Islamisme et la science: Conférence faite à la Sorbonne le 29 mars 1883.* Paris: Calmann Levy, 1883.

———. "L'Islamisme et la science . . . L'équivoque contenu dans ces mots: Science arabe, philosophie arabe, art arabe, science musulmane, civilisation musulman. En tuant la science, l'Islam s'est tué lui-même et s'est condamné dans le monde à une complète infériorité." Conférence à la Sorbonne, Paris, March 29, 1883.

———. *Le Livre de Job, traduit de l'hébreu par Ernest Renan.* Paris: Levy, 1858.

———. "Mahomet et les origines de l'Islamisme." *Revue des deux mondes* 12 (December 15, 1851): 1063–1101.

———. "Nouvelles considérations sur le caractère général des peuples sémitiques et en particulier sur leur tendance au monothéisme." *Journal asiatique* 5, no. 13: 214–282, 417–450.

———. *Système comparé et histoire générale des langues sémitiques.* Paris: Imprimerie Impériale, 1855.

Renard, Suzanne. "L'aide aux Mères." *Jeunesse*, June 29, 1941.

Renaud, H. P. J. "La connaissance de l'heure 'En pieds d'ombre' chez les musulmans marocains." *La Nature*, August 15, 1939: 109–110.

———. "L'enseignement des sciences exactes et l'édition d'ouvrages scientifiques au Maroc avant l'occupation européenne." *Hespéris* 14 (1932): 78–89.

———. "État de nos connaissances sur la médecine ancienne au Maroc: Programme d'études et sources d'investigations." *Bulletin de l'Institut des Hautes Études Marocains* 1 (December 1920): 71–83.

———. "Médecine et médecins marocains au siècle de Moulay Ismail." In *Extrait des Annales de l'Institut d'Études Orientales, Tome III, Annee 1937*, 89–109. Paris: Librairie Larose, 1937.

———. "Un registre d'inventaire et de prêt de la bibliothèque de la mosquée 'Ali ben Youssef à Marrakech, date de 1111H./1700 J.C." *Hésperis* 31 (1994): 55–59.

Renaud, H. P. J., and G. S. Colin. *Documents marocains pour servir à l'histoire du "Mal franc," textes arabes, publiés et traduits avec une introduction.* Paris: Publications de l'Institut des Hautes Études Marocaines, 1935.

————. *Tuhfat Al-Ahbab, Glossaire de la matière médicale marocaine, Texte, traduction et notes critiques, Publication de l'Institut des Hautes Études Marocaines.* Paris: Geuthner, 1934.

La Revue marocaine de droit. "Juridictions chérifiennes, Tribunal d'Appel du Chrâa, Audience du 24 Qaada 1368, Répudiation—répudiation par le tamlik—irrévocabilité—Vocation héréditaire des ex-conjoints (non)—Dernière maladie—Maladie accidentale—affection chronique—Capacité juridique—Mention Adoulaire—Preuve du contraire—Certificat Médical—Médecin non-musulman—Témoignage ou expertise: Caractère d'information de la science—Déclarations devant l'adoul—Attestation de l'identité du malade" (17 September, 1949)." February 1, 1951, 76–91.

————. "Jurisprudence chérifienne, Tribunal d'Appel du Chrâa, Arrêté du 29 rabia I 1368 (29 janvier 1949), Désaveu de paternité—serments d'anathème (lican)—Conditions d'admission." July 1, 1949, 123–127.

————. "Jurisprudence chérifienne, Tribunal d'Appel du Chrâa (Arrêté du 8 Joumada I 1368—8 mars 1949), Filiation—Durée de la conception, Partage—Survenance d'héritier—Rescision." November 1, 1949, 168–170.

————. "Juridictions chérifiennes, Tribunal d'Appel du Chrâa, Audience du 24 Qaada 1368" [September 17, 1949]. Vol. 2 (February 1, 1951): 76–91.

————. "Jurisprudence chérifienne, Tribunaux du chrâa, Mariage (nullité)—Prohibition d'une cinquième co-épouse. Filiation—Filiation putative—conditions." October 1, 1949, 142–146.

Ricard, Robert. "Médecine et médecins à Arzila (1508–1539)." *Hésperis.* Vol. 26 (1939): 171–178.

Rinn, Louis. *Marabouts et Khouan: Étude sur l'Islam en Algérie.* Algiers: Jourdan, 1884.

Rivière, Pierre-Louis. *Traités, codes, lois et règlements du Maroc (Dahirs, arrêtés viziriels et résidentiels, ordres, ordonnances, circulaires, instructions et avis), 1912–1923.* 3 vols. Paris: Recueil Sirey, 1923.

Saint, Andrée. *Les Oeuvres de protection de l'enfance européenne et indigène au Maroc.* Rabat: Protectorat de la République Française au Maroc, 1933.

Salmon, Georges. "Le culte de Moulay Idris et la mosquée des Chorfa à Fès." *Archives marocaines* 3, no. 3 (1905): 413–429.

————. "Essai sur l'histoire politique du nord-marocain." *Archives marocaines* 2, no. 1 (1905): 1–99.

————. "Notes sur les superstitions populaires dans la region de Tanger." *Archives marocaines* 1 (1904): 262–272.

Salmon, Georges, and Edouard Michaux-Bellaire. "Les tribus arabes de la vallée du Lekkous." *Archives marocaines* 3 and 4 (1906): 219–397.

Salzes. "Quelques cas de syphilis nerveuse chez les indigènes de l'Afrique du Nord." *Journal des praticiens*, March 9, 1912.

Samné, Georges. *De l'Assistance considérée comme un moyen de colonisation: L'assistance au Maroc . . . rapport présenté au congrès coloniale française, tenu à Paris le 29 mai 1904.* Paris: Jules Rousset, Librairie médicale et scientifique, 1904.

Sanguy, C. "Remarques sur la mortalité infantile musulmane: Ses causes et ses remèdes." *Maroc médical*, no. 269 (1946): 206.

Secret, Edmond. "Rites de magie thermale: La journée d'un berbère à Moulay Yacoub." *Maroc médical*, January–February 1947: 37–43.

———. *Les Sept printemps de Fès: Des airs, des eaux, des lieux; Fès, capitale thermale*. Amiens, 1990. Self-published.

Segonzac, Edouard Marie René, marquis de. *Au Coeur de l'Atlas: Mission au Maroc, 1904–1905*. Paris: Larose, 1910.

———. *Excursion au Sous avec quelques considérations préliminaires sur la question marocaine*. Paris: Chalamel, 1901.

———. *Voyages au Maroc (1899–1901)*. Paris: Colin, 1903.

Semach, Y. D. "Le Saint d'Ouezzan, Ribbi Amran ben Divan, et les saints juifs du Maroc." *Bulletin de l'enseignement publique du Maroc*, March 1937 and June 1938.

Sfrioui, A. "Les rites de naissance à Fès." *Maroc médical*, no. 330 (November 1952): 1007–1010.

Sicault, G. "La protection médico-social de l'enfance au Maroc." *Maroc médical*, February 1948: 41–43.

"Stations climatiques et hydrothermales du Maroc." *Maroc médical*, 15 November 1929: 583–604.

Steiner, M. "Medizinisher Brief aus Marokko Tangier, August 1908." *Wiener Klinische Rundschau* 40 (October 1908): 639–640.

Surdon, Georges. *Esquisses de droit coutumier berbère marocain: Conférences données au cours préparatoire au service des affaires indigènes pendant l'année 1927–1928*. Rabat: Moncho, 1928.

———. *Institutions et coutumes des berbères du Maghreb (Maroc-Algérie-Tunisie-Sahara), Leçons de droit coutumier berbère*. Tangier and Fez: Les Éditions Internationales, 1938.

Tharaud, Jérome, and Jean Tharaud. *Fès ou les bourgeois de l'Islam*. Paris: Plon, 1951.

Thévenin, D. "Du climat de Mogador sous le rapport des affections pulmonaires." *Bulletin de la Société de Géographie* (April 1868): 335–339.

Trillat, Paul. "Évolution de l'obstétrique au XXe siècle." *Maroc médical*, no. 330 (November 1952): 859–861.

Valeton, Paul. *Le Marabout de Sidi Ben Achir (à Salé): Ses rapports avec l'assistance publique*. Marseille: Publications du Service de la Santé et de l'Hygiène publiques au Maroc, 1922.

Van Gennep, Arnold. *Les Rites de passage—Étude systématique des rites de la porte et du seuil, de l'hospitalité, de l'adoption, de la grossesse et de l'accouchement, de la naissance, de l'enfance, de la puberté, de l'initiation, de l'ordination, du couronnement, des fiançailles et du mariage, des funérailles, des saisons, etc.* Paris: Nourry, 1909.

Wazzani, Muhammad Hasan al-. "L'eau de Boufekrane et son angoissant problème," *L'Action du peuple*, June 3, 1937.

———. "Notre nationalisme." *L'Action du peuple*, no. 48, July 15, 1937.

———. "Le problème de la misère." *L'Action du peuple*, April 22, 1937.

Weisgerber, F. *Au Seuil du Maroc moderne*. Rabat: Les Éditions la Porte, 1947.

———. *Casablanca et les Chaouia en 1900*. Casablanca: Réunies, 1935.

———. "Pathologie et thérapeutique marocaines." *Revue générale des sciences*, May 30, 1903: 567–573.

Westermarck, Edward. *Marriage Ceremonies in Morocco.* London: Macmillan, 1914.

———. *Ritual and Belief in Morocco.* 2 vols. London: Macmillan, 1926.

Worms, M. G. *Exposé des conditions de l'hygiène et de traitement propres à préve-nir les maladies et à diminuer la mortalité dans l'armée en Afrique, et spécialement dans la province de Constantine, suivi d'une théorie nouvelle de l'intermittence, et de la nature ainsi que du siège des maladies des pays chauds.* Paris: Baillière, Libra-rie de l'académie royale de médecine, 1838.

Xicluna. "Le Fetoua des 'oulama de Fès." *Archives marocaines* 3 (1905): 141–143.

Zeys, Paul. "Case 7, 11 Août 1924 (10 moharrem 1343), Jugement du Tribunal cou-tumier des Aït Seghrouchen d'Immouzer prononçant le divorce par consentement mutual." *Revue marocaine de législation, doctrine, jurisprudence chérifiennes* 1 (1935): 17.

———. "Répression du vagabondage des jeunes marocains: Redressement et sauvetage de l'enfance indigène en danger moral." *Questions nord-africains: Revue des pro-blèmes sociaux de l'Algérie, de la Tunisie, et du Maroc* 4 (November 25, 1935): 60–87, 6 (July 15, 1936): 47–71.

SECONDARY PRINTED SOURCES, BOOKS, AND ARTICLES

Abi-Mershed, Osama W. *Apostles of Modernity: Saint-Simonians and the Civilizing Mission in Algeria.* Stanford, Calif.: Stanford Univ. Press, 2010.

Abu-Lughod, Janet. "The Islamic City: Historic Myth, Islamic Essence, and Con-temporary Relevance." *International Journal of Middle East Studies* 19 (1987): 155–176.

———. *Rabat: Urban Apartheid in Morocco.* Princeton, N.J.: Princeton Univ. Press, 1980.

Abun-Nasr, Jamil M. *A History of the Maghrib in the Islamic Period.* Cambridge: Cambridge Univ. Press, 1987.

Ackerknecht, Erwin. *Medicine at the Paris Hospital, 1794–1848.* Baltimore: Johns Hopkins Univ. Press, 1967.

Adas, Michael. *Machines as the Measure of Men: Science, Technology, and Ideologies of Western Dominance.* Ithaca, N.Y.: Cornell Univ. Press, 1989.

Akhmisse, Mustapha. *Histoire de la médecine au Maroc: Des origines au protectorat.* Casablanca: Imprimerie Eddar El Beida, n.d.

———. *Rites et secrets des marabouts à Casablanca.* Casablanca: SEDIM, 1984.

———. *Les Septs dormants de Marrakech.* Casablanca: Dar Kortoba, 1994.

Allouche, I. S. "Lettres chérifiennes inédites relatives à l'assassinat du Dr. Mauchamp et à l'occupation d'Oujda en 1907." In *Actes du XXIe congrès international des orientalistes,* 302–304. Paris: Imprimerie Nationale, 1948.

———. "Un plan des canalisations de Fès au temps de Mawlay Isma'il d'après un texte inédit, avec une étude succincte sur la corporation des Kwadisiyya." *Hespéris* 18, no. 1 (1934): 49–63.

Amster, Ellen. "Abd al-Salam." In *Encyclopedia of Islam* 3, Vol. 1, edited by Kate Fleet, Gudrun Krämer, Denis Matringe, John Nawas, and Everett Rowson, 16–17. London: Brill, 2011.

———. "'The Harem Revealed' and the Islamic-French Family: Aline de Lens and a French Woman's Orient in Lyautey's Morocco." *French Historical Studies* 32, no. 2 (Spring 2009): 279–312.

Arabi, Oussama. "Orienting the Gaze: Marcel Morand and the Codification of Le Droit Musulman Algérien." *Journal of Islamic Studies* 11, no. 1(2000): 43–72.

Arnold, David. *Colonizing the Body: State Medicine and Epidemic Disease in Nineteenth-Century India.* Berkeley and Los Angeles: Univ. of California Press, 1993.

———. Introduction to *Warm Climates and Western Medicine: The Emergence of Tropical Medicine, 1500–1900.* Amsterdam and Atlanta: Rodopi, 1996.

Asad, Talal. *Formations of the Secular: Christianity, Islam, Modernity.* Palo Alto, Calif.: Stanford Univ. Press, 2003.

Ayache, Albert. *Le Mouvement syndical au Maroc,* Vol. 1, 1919–1942. Paris: L'Harmattan, 1982.

Baker, Alison. *Voices of Resistance: Oral Histories of Moroccan Women.* Albany: SUNY Press, 1998.

Bakker, Jogien. *The Lasting Virtue of Traditional Healing: An Ethnography of Healing and Prestige in the Middle Atlas of Morocco.* Amsterdam: Vrije Universiteit Univ. Press, 1993.

Bamford, Paul. *Fighting Ships and Prisons: The Mediterranean Galleys of France in the Age of Louis XIV.* Minneapolis: Univ. of Minnesota Press, 1973.

Bargach, Jamila. *Orphans of Islam: Family, Abandonment, and Secret Adoption in Morocco.* Oxford: Rowman and Littlefield, 2002.

Barnes, David. *The Making of a Social Disease: Tuberculosis in Nineteenth-Century France.* Berkeley and Los Angeles: Univ. of California Press, 1995.

Bazin, Hervé. *The Eradication of Smallpox: Edward Jenner and the First and Only Eradication of a Human Infectious Disease.* London and San Diego: Academic Press, 2000.

Bazzaz, Sahar. *Forgotten Saints: History, Power, and Politics in the Making of Modern Morocco.* Cambridge, Mass.: Center for Middle East Studies, Harvard University, 2010.

———. "Reading Reform beyond the State: Salwat al-Anfas, Islamic Revival, and Moroccan National History." *Journal of North African Studies* 13, no. 1 (March 2008): 1–13.

Beck, Herman. "Sultan Isma'il and the Veneration of Idris I at Mawlay Idris in the Djabal Zarhun." In *The Sacred Centre as the Focus of Political Interest,* edited by Hans Bakker, 53–65. Groningen, Netherlands: Egbert Forsten, 1992.

Bellakhdar, Jamal. *La Pharmacopée marocaine traditionnelle: Médecine arabe ancienne et savoirs populaires.* Paris: Ibis, 1997.

Ben-Ami, Issachar. *Haaretset Haqedoshim beqereb Yehudei Maroqo.* Jerusalem: Magnes, 1984.

Bennison, Amira. *Jihad and Its Interpretations in Pre-Colonial Morocco: State-Society Relations during the French Conquest of Algeria.* London: Routledge, 2002.

Ben Talha, Abdelouahed. *Moulay-Idriss du Zerhoun: Quelques aspects de la vie sociale et familiale.* Rabat: Éditions Techniques Nord-Africaines, 1965.

Benton, Lauren. *Law and Colonial Cultures: Legal Regimes in World History, 1400–1900.* Cambridge: Cambridge Univ. Press, 2002.

Berkey, Jonathan P. "Circumcision Circumscribed: Female Excision and Cultural Accommodation in the Medieval Near East." *International Journal of Middle East Studies* 28 (1996): 19–38.

Berque, Jacques. *Al-Yousi: Problèmes de la culture marocaine au XVIIeme siècle.* Paris: Mouton, 1958.

El Bezzaz, Mohammed Amine. "La chronique scandaleuse du pèlerinage marocain à la Mecque au XIXème siècle." *Hespéris-Tamuda*, 20–21 (1982–1983): 319–331.

Bhabha, Homi K. *The Location of Culture.* London: Routledge, 1994.

Bidwell, Robin. *Morocco under Colonial Rule: French Administration of Tribal Areas, 1912–1956.* London: Cass, 1973.

Boddy, Janice. *Wombs and Alien Spirits: Women, Men, and the Zar Cult in Northern Sudan.* Madison: Univ. of Wisconsin Press, 1989.

———. *Civilizing Women: British Crusades in Colonial Sudan.* Princeton, N.J.: Princeton Univ. Press, 2007.

Bonnemain, Bruno. "Le professeur Émile Perrot: Sept ans de collaboration avec la Quinzaine coloniale (1907–1914)." *Revue d'histoire de la pharmacie* 56, no. 360 (2009): 457–468.

Bookin-Weiner, Jerome. "Corsairing in the Economy and Politics of North Africa." In *North Africa: Nation, State and Region*, edited by G. Joffé, 3–33. London: Routledge, 1993.

Boubrik, Rahal. *Saints et société en Islam: La confrérie ouest-saharienne Fâdiliyya.* Paris: CNRS, 1999.

Bourdieu, Pierre. *Outline of a Theory of Practice.* Cambridge: Cambridge Univ. Press, 1977.

Bourqia, Rahma. "Don et théâtralité: Réflexion sur le rituel du don (hadiyya) offert au Sultan au XIXe siècle." *Hespéris-Tamuda* 31 (1993): 61–75.

Bourqia, Rahma, and Susan Miller. *In the Shadow of the Sultan: Culture, Power, and Politics in Morocco.* Cambridge, Mass.: Harvard Univ. Press, 1999.

Brandt, Allen. *No Magic Bullet: A Social History of Venereal Disease in the United States since 1880.* New York: Oxford Univ. Press, 1987.

Brett, Michael."Legislating for Inequality in Algeria: The Sénatus-Consulte of 14 July 1865." *Bulletin of the School of Oriental and African Studies* 15, no. 3 (1988): 440–461.

Britel, Farid, and Jacques Rigaud. *Le Mécénat au Maroc.* Casablanca: Sochepress, 2001.

Brown, Kenneth. *People of Salé: Tradition and Change in a Moroccan City, 1830–1930.* Cambridge, Mass.: Harvard Univ. Press, 1976.

Brown, Peter. *The Cult of the Saints: Its Rise and Function in Latin Christianity.* Chicago: Univ. of Chicago Press, 1981.

Burckhardt, Titus. *Fez: City of Islam.* Translated by William Stoddart. Cambridge: Islamic Texts Society, 1992.

———. *An Introduction to Sufism.* New York: Thorsons, 1997.

Bürgel, Christoph. "Secular and Religious Features of Medieval Arabic Medicine." In *Asian Medical Systems: A Comparative Study*, edited by C. Leslie, 44–62. Berkeley and Los Angeles: Univ. of California Press, 1976.

Burke, Edmund, III. "The Image of the Moroccan State in French Ethnographic Literature: A New Look at the Origin of Lyautey's Berber Policy." In *Arabs and Berbers*, edited by Ernest Gellner and Charles Micaud, 175–200. London: Duckworth, 1973.

———. "La mission scientifique au Maroc: Science sociale et politique dans l'âge d'impérialisme." *Bulletin économique et social du Maroc* (1971): 37–56.

———. "The Political Role of the Moroccan Ulema, 1860–1912." In *Scholars, Saints, and Sufis: Muslim Religious Institutions since 1500*, edited by N. Keddie, 91–125. Berkeley and Los Angeles: Univ. of California Press, 1972.

———. *Prelude to Protectorate in Morocco: Precolonial Protest and Resistance.* Chicago: Univ. of Chicago Press, 1976.

———. "The Sociology of Islam: The French Tradition." In *Islamic Studies: A Tradition and Its Problems*, edited by Malcolm H. Kerr, 73–88. Malibu: Undena, 1980.

Burton, Antoinette. "The White Woman's Burden: British Feminists and 'The Indian Woman,' 1865–1915." In *Western Women and Imperialism: Complicity and Resistance*, edited by Nupur Chaudhuri and Margaret Strobel, 137–157. Bloomington: Indiana Univ. Press, 1992.

Bu Rugbah, Sa'id. *Dawr al-waqf al-hayah al-thaqafiyah bi al-Maghrib fi 'ahd al-dawla al-'Alawiya.* Rabat: Al-Mamlakah al-Maghribiyah, Wizarat al-Awqaf wa al-Shu'un al-Islamiya, 1996.

Caille, J. *La Mission du Capitaine Burel au Maroc en 1808.* Paris: Arts et Métiers Graphiques, 1953.

Callahan, Bryan Thomas. "Syphilis and Civilization: A Social and Cultural History of Sexually-Transmitted Disease in Colonial Zambia and Zimbabwe, 1890–1960." PhD diss., Johns Hopkins University, 2002.

Campbell, Donald. *Arabian Medicine and Its Influence on the Middle Ages*, 2 volumes. London: Kegan Paul, Trench, Trubner, 1926.

Capelli, Irene. "Risk and Safety in Context: Medical Pluralism and Agency in Childbirth in an Eastern Moroccan Oasis." *Midwifery* 27, no. 6 (December 2011): 781–785.

Chakrabarty, Dipesh. *Provincializing Europe: Postcolonial Thought and Historical Difference.* Princeton, N.J.: Princeton Univ. Press, 2000.

Chittick, William. *Faith and Practice of Islam: Three Thirteenth-Century Sufi Texts.* Albany: SUNY Press, 1992.

———. *Science of the Cosmos, Science of the Soul: The Pertinence of Islamic Cosmology to the Modern World.* Oxford: Oneworld, 2007.

Chodkiewicz, Michel. *Seal of the Saints: Prophethood and Sainthood in the Doctrine of Ibn 'Arabi.* Cambridge: Islamic Texts Society, 1993.

Chrifi-Alaoui, El-Hassane. "Typologie du récit légendaire du saint judéo-musulman au Maroc." In *From Iberia to Diaspora: Studies in Sephardic History and Culture*, edited by Yedida Kalfon Stillman and Norman A. Stillman, 393–396. Leiden: Brill, 1998.

Christelow, Allen. *Muslim Law Courts and the French Colonial State in Algeria.* Princeton, N.J.: Princeton Univ. Press, 1985.

Clancy-Smith, Julia. "Islam, Gender, and Identities in the Making of French Algeria, 1830–1962." In Clancy-Smith and Gouda, *Domesticating the Empire*, 154–174.

———. *Rebel and Saint: Muslim Notables, Populist Protest, Colonial Encounters (Algeria and Tunisia), 1800–1904.* Berkeley and Los Angeles: Univ. of California Press, 1994.

Clancy-Smith, Julia, and Frances Gouda, eds. *Domesticating the Empire: Race, Gender, and Family Life in French and Dutch Colonialism.* Charlottesville: Univ. Press of Virginia, 1998.

Clapier-Valadon, Simone. *Les Médecins français d'outre-mer.* Paris: Anthropos, 1982.

Coleman, William. *Death Is a Social Disease: Public Health and Political Economy in Early Industrial France*. Madison: Univ. of Wisconsin Press, 1982.

Comaroff, Jean. *Body of Power, Spirit of Resistance: The Culture and History of a South African People*. Chicago: Univ. of Chicago Press, 1985.

———. "Medicine: Symbol and Ideology." In *The Problem of Medical Knowledge: Examining the Social Construction of Medicine*, edited by Peter Wright and Andrew Treacher, 49–68. Edinburgh: Edinburgh Univ. Press, 1982.

Comaroff, Jean, and John Comaroff. "The Madman and the Migrant: Work and Labor in the Historical Consciousness of a South African People." *American Ethnologist* 14, no. 2: 191–209.

Combs-Schilling, Elaine. *Sacred Performances: Islam, Sexuality, and Sacrifice*. New York: Columbia Univ. Press, 1989.

Conklin, Alice. *A Mission to Civilize: The Republican Idea of Empire in France and West Africa, 1895–1930*. Stanford, Calif.: Stanford Univ. Press, 1997.

Conrad, Lawrence. "Arab-Islamic Medicine." In *Companion Encyclopedia to the History of Medicine*, edited by W. F. Bynum and Roy Porter, 676–727. London: Routledge, 1995.

———. "Epidemic Disease in Formal and Popular Thought in Early Islamic Society." In *Epidemics and Ideas: Essays on the Historical Perception of Pestilence*, edited by Terence Ranger and Paul Slack, 77–100. Cambridge: Cambridge Univ. Press, 1992.

Corbin, Alain. *Women for Hire: Prostitution and Sexuality in France after 1850*. Cambridge, Mass.: Harvard Univ. Press, 1990.

Cornell, Vincent. "The Logic of Analogy and the Role of the Sufi Shaykh in Post-Marinid Morocco." *International Journal of Middle East Studies* 15 (1983): 67–83.

———. *Realm of the Saint: Power and Authority in Moroccan Sufism*. Austin: Univ. of Texas Press, 1998.

Crapanzano, Vincent. *The Hamadsha: A Study in Moroccan Ethnopsychiatry*. Berkeley and Los Angeles: Univ. of California Press, 1973.

Crinson, Mark. *Modern Architecture and the End of Empire*. Aldershot, UK: Ashgate, 2003.

Crissey, John Thorne, and Lawrence Charles Parish. *The Dermatology and Syphilology of the Nineteenth Century*. New York: Praeger, 1981.

Crone, Patricia. *God's Rule: Government and Islam*. New York: Columbia Univ. Press, 2004.

Curtin, Philip. *Death by Migration: Europe's Encounter with the Tropical World in the Nineteenth Century*. Cambridge: Cambridge Univ. Press, 1989.

Dahane, Mohamed. "Itinéraire ethnographique de Montagne dans les années vingt." In *La Sociologie musulmane de Robert Montagne*, edited by François Pouillon and Daniel Rivet, 55–67. Paris: Maisonneuve et Larose, 2000.

Delaney, Carol. *The Seed and the Soil: Gender and Cosmology in Turkish Village Society*. Berkeley and Los Angeles: Univ. of California Press, 1991.

Delanoë, Nelcya. *La Femme de Mazagan*. Paris: Seghers, 1989.

Deshen, Shlomo. "Urban Jews in Sherifian Morocco." *Middle East Studies* 20 (1984): 212–223.

Dols, Michael W. *Majnun: The Madman in Medieval Society*. Oxford: Clarendon Press, 1992.

Donzelot, Jacques. *The Policing of Families*. New York: Pantheon, 1979.

Doumato, Eleanor Abdella. *Women, Islam, and Healing in Saudi Arabia and the Gulf.* New York: Columbia Univ. Press, 2000.

Dumont, M. "The Long and Difficult Birth of Symphyseotomy from Séverin Pineau to Jean-René Sigault." *Journal de gynécologie, obstétrique et biologie de la reproduction* 18, no. 1 (1989): 11–21.

Dunn, Ross. "Bu Himara's European Connexion: The Commercial Relations of a Moroccan Warlord." *Journal of African History* 21, no. 2 (1980): 235–253.

———. *Resistance in the Desert: Moroccan Responses to French Imperialism, 1881–1912*. Madison: Univ. of Wisconsin Press, 1977.

Ech-Channa, Aicha. *Miseria: Témoignages*. 5th ed. Casablanca: Le Fennec, 2010.

Eickelman, Dale. *Moroccan Islam: Tradition and Society in a Pilgrimage Center*. Austin: Univ. of Texas Press, 1976.

Elgood, Cyril. "Tibb-Ul-Nabbi or Medicine of the Prophet: Being a Translation of Two Works of the Same Name." *Osiris* 13 (1962): 33–192.

Eliade, Mircea. *The Sacred and the Profane: The Nature of Religion*. New York: Harcourt, 1959.

Ellis, Jack. *The Physician-Legislators of France: Medicine and Politics in the Early Third Republic, 1870–1914*. Cambridge: Cambridge Univ. Press, 1990.

El Shakry, Omnia. *The Great Social Laboratory: Subjects of Knowledge in Colonial and Postcolonial Egypt*. Stanford, Calif.: Stanford Univ. Press, 2007.

Elwitt, Sanford. *The Third Republic Defended: Bourgeois Reform in France, 1880–1914*. Baton Rouge: Louisiana State Univ. Press, 1986.

Ensel, Remco. *Saints and Servants in Southern Morocco*. Leiden: Brill, 1999.

Evans, Richard. *Death in Hamburg: Society and Politics in the Cholera Years, 1830–1910*. New York: Oxford Univ. Press, 1987.

Evans-Pritchard, E. *The Sociology of Comte: An Appreciation*. Manchester: Manchester Univ. Press, 1970.

Fabian, Johannes. *Remembering the Present: Painting and Popular History in Zaire*. Berkeley and Los Angeles: Univ. of California Press, 1996.

Fahmy, Khaled. *All the Pasha's Men: Mehmed Ali, His Army, and the Making of Modern Egypt*. Cambridge: Cambridge Univ. Press, 1997.

Farmer, Paul. *Pathologies of Power: Health, Human Rights, and the New War on the Poor*. Berkeley and Los Angeles: Univ. of California Press, 2003.

Fawzi, Abdulrazak. *Fihris majmu'at al-kutub wa-al-dawriyat al-'arabiyah fi Jami'at Harvard*. Boston: Hall, 1983.

———. *The Kingdom of the Book: The History of Printing as an Agency of Change in Morocco between 1865 and 1912*. London: Mansell, 1979.

Feierman, Steven. "Colonizers, Scholars, and the Creation of Invisible Histories." In *Beyond the Cultural Turn: New Directions in the Study of Society and Culture*, edited by Victoria Bonnell and Lynn Hunt, 200–209. Berkeley and Los Angeles: Univ. of California Press, 1999.

———. "Concepts of Sovereignty among the Shambaa." PhD diss., Northwestern University, 1972.

———. "Healing as Social Criticism in the Time of Colonial Conquest." *African Studies* 54, no. 1 (1995): 73–88.

Feierman, Steven, and John Janzen, eds. *The Social Basis of Health and Healing in Africa.* Berkeley and Los Angeles: Univ. of California Press, 1992.

Fleck, Ludwig. *The Genesis and Development of a Scientific Fact.* Chicago: Univ. of Chicago, 1979.

Foucault, Michel. *The Birth of Biopolitics: Lectures at the Collège de France, 1978–1979.* Edited by Michel Senellart. Translated by Graham Burchell. New York: Picador, 2008.

———. *The Birth of the Clinic: An Archaeology of Medical Perception.* New York: Vintage, 1994.

———. *The History of Sexuality: An Introduction.* Translated by Robert Hurley. New York: Vintage, 1990.

Franke, Peter. "Khidr in Istanbul: Observations on the Symbolic Construction of Sacred Spaces in Traditional Islam." In *On Archaeology of Sainthood and Local Spirituality in Islam: Past and Present Crossroads of Events and Ideas; Yearbook of the Sociology of Islam 5,* edited by Georg Stauth, 36–56. Piscataway, N.J.: Transaction Publishers / Rutgers Univ. Press, 2004.

Friedman, Ellen. *Spanish Captives in North Africa in the Early Modern Age.* Madison: Univ. of Wisconsin Press, 1983.

Fuchs, Rachel. *Poor and Pregnant in Paris: Strategies for Survival in the Nineteenth Century.* New Brunswick, N.J.: Rutgers Univ. Press, 1992.

Gallagher, Nancy. *Medicine and Power in Tunisia, 1780–1900.* Cambridge: Cambridge Univ. Press, 1983.

———. *Egypt's Other Wars: Epidemics and the Politics of Public Health.* Syracuse, N.Y.: Syracuse Univ. Press, 1990.

Geertz, Clifford. *Islam Observed: Religious Development in Morocco and Indonesia.* Chicago: Univ. of Chicago Press, 1968.

Gellner, Ernest. *Saints of the Atlas.* London: Weidenfeld and Nicholson, 1969.

Gershovich, Moshe. *French Military Rule in Morocco: Colonialism and Its Consequences.* London: Cass, 2000.

Ghoti, Mohamed. *Histoire de la médecine au Maroc: Le XXe siècle.* Casablanca: Imprimerie Idéale, 1995.

Giblin, James. "Trypanosomiasis Control in African History: An Evaded Issue." *Journal of African History* 31 (1990): 59–80.

Giladi, Avner. *Infants, Parents, and Wet Nurses: Medieval Islamic Views on Breastfeeding and Their Social Implications.* Leiden: Brill, 1999.

Good, Byron. "The Heart of What's the Matter: The Structure of Medical Discourse in a Provincial Iranian Town." PhD diss., University of Chicago, 1977.

Good, Byron, and Mary-Jo DelVecchio Good. "The Comparative Study of Greco-Islamic Medicine: The Integration of Medical Knowledge into Local Symbolic Contexts." In *Paths to Asian Medical Knowledge,* edited by Charles Leslie and Allan Young, 257–271. Berkeley and Los Angeles: Univ. of California Press, 1992.

Good, Mary-Jo DelVecchio. "Of Blood and Babies: The Relationship of Popular Islamic Physiology to Fertility." *Social Science and Medicine* 14B (1980): 147–156.

Goodman, Lenn Evan. *Ibn Tufayl's Hayy ibn Yaqzan.* Los Angeles: GeeTeeBee, 1991.

Goubert, Jean-Pierre. *The Conquest of Water: The Advent of Health in the Industrial Age.* Translated by Andrew Wilson. Princeton, N.J.: Princeton Univ. Press, 1989.

Gran, Peter. "Medical Pluralism in Arab and Egyptian History: An Overview of Class Structures and Philosophies of the Main Phases." *Social Science and Medicine* 13B (1979): 339–348.

Green, Monica. *Making Women's Medicine Masculine: The Rise of Male Authority in Pre-Modern Gynaecology.* Oxford: Oxford Univ. Press, 2008.

Greenwood, Bernard, "Cold or Spirits? Ambiguity and Syncretism in Moroccan Therapeutics." In *The Social Basis of Health and Healing in Africa*, edited by Steven Feierman and John Janzen, 285–314. Berkeley and Los Angeles: Univ. of California Press, 1992.

Gruner, Roger. *Du Maroc traditionnel au Maroc moderne, 1912–1956: Histoire Du Protectorat.* Paris: Nouvelles éditions latines, 1984.

Guerin, Adam. "Racial Myth, Colonial Reform, and the Invention of Customary Law in Colonial Morocco." *Journal of North African Studies* 16, no. 3 (September 2011): 361–380.

Gutas, Dmitri. *Greek Thought, Arabic Culture: The Graeco-Arabic Translation Movement in Baghdad and Early 'Abbasid Society (2nd–4th/8th–10th Centuries).* London: Routledge, 1998.

Halevi, Leor. *Muhammad's Grave: Death Rites and the Making of Islamic Society.* New York: Columbia Univ. Press, 2007.

Halstead, John. *Rebirth of a Nation: The Origins and Rise of Moroccan Nationalism, 1912–1944.* Cambridge, Mass.: Center for Middle Eastern Studies, Harvard University, 1969.

Hamarneh, Sami. "The First Known Independent Treatise on Cosmetology in Spain." *Bulletin of the History of Medicine* 39 (1965): 309–25.

Hammoudi, Abdellah. "Construction de l'ordre et usage de la science coloniale: Robert Montagne, penseur de la tribu et de la civilisation." In Rivet and Pouillon, *La Sociologie musulmane de Robert Montagne*, 265–288.

———. *Master and Disciple: The Cultural Foundations of Moroccan Authoritarianism.* Chicago: Univ. of Chicago Press, 1997.

Hart, David. "An Awkward Chronology and a Questionable Genealogy: History and Legend in a Saintly Lineage in the Moroccan Central Atlas, 1397–1702." *Journal of North African Studies* 6, no. 2 (Summer 2001): 95–116.

———. "Making Sense of Moroccan Tribal Sociology and History." *Journal of North African Studies* 6, no. 2 (Summer 2001): 11–28.

———. "Moroccan Dynastic *Shurfa'*-hood in Two Historical Contexts: Idrisid Cult and 'Alawid Power." *Journal of North African Studies* 6, no. 2 (Summer 2001): 81–94.

Hayden, Deborah. *Pox: Genius, Madness, and the Mysteries of Syphilis.* New York: Basic Books, 2003.

Headrick, Daniel. *The Tentacles of Progress: Technology Transfer in the Age of Imperialism.* New York: Oxford Univ. Press, 1988.

Heck, Paul L. *Sufism and Politics.* Princeton, N.J.: Markus Wiener, 2007.

Hoisington, William A., Jr. *The Casablanca Connection: French Colonial Policy, 1936–1943.* Chapel Hill: Univ. of North Carolina Press, 1984.

———. *Lyautey and the French Conquest of Morocco.* New York: St. Martin's, 1995.

Holden, Stacey E. *The Politics of Food in Modern Morocco.* Gainesville: Univ. of Flordia Press, 2009.

Homerin, T. "Ibn Taimiya's *Al-Sufiya wa-al-Fuqara*." *Arabica* 32 (1985): 219–244.

Hourani, Albert. *Arabic Thought in the Liberal Age, 1798–1939*. Cambridge: Cambridge Univ. Press, 1983.

Houroro, Faouzi M. *Sociologie politique coloniale au Maroc: Cas de Michaux-Bellaire*. Casablanca: Afrique Orient, 1988.

Hunt, Lynn. *The Family Romance of the French Revolution*. Berkeley and Los Angeles: Univ. of California Press, 1992.

Hunt, Nancy Rose. *A Colonial Lexicon of Birth Ritual, Medicalization, and Mobility in the Congo*. Durham, N.C.: Duke Univ. Press, 1999.

Inhorn, Marcia. *Quest for Conception: Gender, Infertility, and Egyptian Medical Traditions*. Philadelphia: Univ. of Pennsylvania Press, 1994.

Janzen, John. *The Quest for Therapy in Lower Zaire*. Berkeley and Los Angeles: Univ. of California Press, 1978.

Kantorowicz, Ernst. *The King's Two Bodies: A Study in Mediaeval Political Theology*. Princeton, N.J.: Princeton Univ. Press, 1957.

Karamustafa, Ahmet. *God's Unruly Friends: Dervish Groups in the Islamic Middle Period, 1200–1550*. Oxford: Oneworld, 2006.

Katz, Jonathan. *Murder in Marrakesh: Émile Mauchamp and the French Colonial Adventure*. Bloomington: Indiana Univ. Press, 2006.

———. "The 1907 Mauchamp Affair and the French Civilising Mission in Morocco." *Journal of North African Studies* 6, no. 1 (Spring 2001): 143–166.

Keddie, Nikki R. *An Islamic Response to Imperialism: Political and Religious Writings of Sayyid Jamal al-Din al-Afghani*. Berkeley and Los Angeles: Univ. of California Press, 1968.

———. *Sayyid Jamal ad-Din "Al-Afghani": A Political Biography*. Berkeley and Los Angeles: Univ. of California Press, 1972.

Keller, Richard. *Colonial Madness: Psychiatry in French North Africa*. Chicago: Univ. of Chicago Press, 2007.

Kenbib, Muhammad. "Les années de guerre de Robert Montagne (1939–1944)." In Rivet and Pouillon, *La Sociologie musulmane de Robert Montagne*, 185–209.

———. "Structures traditionnelles et protections étrangères au Maroc au XIXe siècle." *Hespéris* 22 (1984): 79–101.

Khalloufi, Mohammad Essaghir al-. *Bouhmara du jihad à la compromission: Le Maroc oriental et le Rif de 1900 à 1909*. Rabat: Imprimerie El Maarif Al Jadida, n.d.

Knut, Vikor. *Sufi and Scholar on the Desert Edge: Muhammad b. 'Ali al-Sanusi and His Brotherhood*. Evanston, Ill.: Northwestern Univ. Press, 1995.

Kodesh, Neil. *Beyond the Royal Gaze: Clanship and Public Healing in Buganda*. Charlottesville: Univ. of Virginia Press, 2010.

Kraemer, Joel L. "Maimonides and the Spanish Aristotelian School." In *Christians, Muslims, and Jews in Medieval and Early Modern Spain*, edited by Mark D. Meyerson and Edward D. English, 40–68. Notre Dame, Ind.: Univ. of Notre Dame Press, 1999.

Kugle, Scott. *Rebel between Spirit and Law: Ahmad Zarruq, Sainthood, and Authority in Islam*. Bloomington: Indiana Univ. Press, 2006.

———. *Sufis and Saints' Bodies: Mysticism, Corporeality, and Sacred Power in Islam*. Chapel Hill: Univ. of North Carolina Press, 2007.

Kuhn, Thomas. *The Structure of Scientific Revolutions.* Chicago: Univ. of Chicago, 1970.

Kurzman, Charles, ed. *Modernist Islam, 1840–1940: A Sourcebook.* Oxford: Oxford Univ. Press, 2002.

Lal, Maneesha. "The Politics of Gender and Medicine in Colonial India: The Countess of Dufferin's Fund, 1885–1888." In *Bulletin of the History of Medicine* 68 (1994): 29–66.

Landau-Tasseron, Ella. "The 'Cyclical Reform': A Study of the *Mujaddid* Tradition." *Studia Islamica* 70 (1989): 79–117.

Laroui, Abdallah. *L'Histoire du Maghreb: Un essai de synthèse.* Casablanca: Centre Culturel Arabe, 1995.

———. *Les Origines sociales et culturelles du nationalisme marocain, 1830–1912.* Casablanca: Centre Culturel Arabe, 1993.

Laskier, Michael. *The Alliance Israelite Universelle and the Jewish Communities of Morocco, 1862–1962.* Albany: SUNY Press, 1983.

Latour, Bruno. *We Have Never Been Modern.* Cambridge, Mass.: Harvard Univ. Press, 1991.

Léonard, Jacques. "Women, Religion, and Medicine." In *Medicine and Society in France: Selections from the "Annales: Economies, Sociétés, Civilizations,"* edited by Robert Forster and Orest Ranum, translated by Elborg Forster and Patricia M. Ranum, 24–47. Vol. 6. Baltimore: Johns Hopkins Univ. Press, 1989.

Lévi-Strauss, Claude. *The Savage Mind.* Chicago: Univ. of Chicago Press, 1966.

Lewis, I. M., Ahmed al-Safi, and Sayyid Hurreiz, eds. *Women's Medicine: The Zar-Bori Cult in Africa and Beyond.* Edinburgh: Edinburgh Univ. Press for the International African Institute, 1991.

Lings, Martin. *Muhammad: His Life Based on the Earliest Sources.* Rochester, Vt.: Inner Traditions, 1983.

———. *A Sufi Saint of the Twentieth Century: Shaikh Ahmad al-'Alawi; His Spiritual Heritage and Legacy.* Cambridge: Islamic Texts Society, 1993.

Lorcin, Patricia M. E. *Imperial Identities: Stereotyping, Prejudice, and Race in Colonial Algeria.* London: Tauris, 1995.

———. "Imperialism, Colonial Identity, and Race in Algeria, 1830–1870: The Role of the French Medical Corps." *Isis* 90 (1999): 653–679.

Luccioni, Joseph. "L'élaboration du dahir berbère du 16 mai 1930." *Revue de l'occident musulman et de la Méditerranée* 38 (1984): 75–81.

Lukes, Steven. *Emile Durkheim: His Life and Works; A Historical and Critical Study.* Stanford, Calif.: Stanford Univ. Press, 1985.

Lyons, Maryinez. *The Colonial Disease: A Social History of Sleeping Sickness in Northern Zaire, 1900–1940.* Cambridge: Cambridge Univ. Press, 1992.

Makdisi, George. *The Rise of Colleges: Institutions of Learning in Islam and the West.* Edinburgh: Edinburgh Univ. Press, 1981.

Manuni, Muhammad al-. *Madhahir yaqdha al-maghrib al-hadith.* 2 vols. Casablanca: Sharika an-nashr wa al-tawzia' al-mudarris, 1985.

Marçais, Georges, *Manuel d'art musulman: L'architecture Tunisie, Algérie, Maroc, Espagne, Sicile.* Paris: Picard, 1926–1927.

———. *Tunis et Kairouan.* Paris: Librairie Renouard, 1937.

Marcovich, Anne. "French Colonial Medicine and Colonial Rule: Algeria and Indochina." In Roy Macleod and Milton Lewis, *Disease, Medicine, and Empire: Perspectives on Western Medicine and the Experience of European Expansion*, 103–117. London: Routledge, 1988.

Maxwell, Anne. *Colonial Photography and Exhibitions: Representatives of the "Native" and the Making of European Identities*. London: Leicester Univ. Press, 1999.

McClellan, James E., III, and François Regourd. "The Colonial Machine: French Science and Colonization in the Ancien Regime." *Osiris* (15) 2000: 31–50.

Merleau-Ponty, Maurice. *The Phenomenology of Perception*. 1962. Excerpted in *Beyond the Body Proper: Reading the Anthropology of Material Life*, edited by Margaret Lock and Judith Farquahar, 133–149. Durham, N.C.: Duke Univ. Press, 2007.

Mernissi, Fatima. "Women, Saints, and Sanctuaries in Morocco." In *Unspoken Worlds: Women's Religious Lives*, 112–121. Belmont, Calif.: Wadsworth, 1989.

Messick, Brinkley. *The Calligraphic State: Textual Domination and History in a Muslim Society*. Berkeley and Los Angeles: Univ. of California Press, 1993.

Meyerhof, Max. "Esquisse d'histoire de la pharmacologie et botanique chez les musulmans d'Espagne." *Al Andalus* 3 (1935): 1–41.

Meyerhof, Max, and D. Joannides. *La Gynécologie et l'obstétrique chez Avicenne (Ibn Sina) et leur rapports avec celles des Grecs*. Cairo: Schindler, 1940.

Micouleau-Sicault, Marie-Claire. *Les Médecins français au Maroc: Combats en urgence (1912–1956)*. Paris: L'Harmattan, 2000.

Miège, Jean-Louis. *Le Maroc et l'Europe, 1830–1894*. 4 vols. Paris: PUF, 1963.

———. *Lyautey: Paroles d'action*. Rabat: Editions la Porte, 1995.

Miller, Susan Gilson. *Disorienting Encounters: Travels of a Moroccan Scholar in France in 1845–1846; The Voyage of Muhammad As-Saffar*. Berkeley and Los Angeles: Univ. of California Press, 1992.

———. "Sleeping Fetus." In *Encyclopedia of Women in Islamic Cultures*, vol. 5, edited by Suad Joseph, 421–424. Leiden: Brill, 2003–2007.

Mitchell, Timothy. *Colonising Egypt*. Cambridge: Cambridge University Press, 1988.

———. *Questions of Modernity*. Minneapolis: Univ. of Minnesota Press, 2000.

Morsy, Soheir. *Gender, Sickness, and Healing in Rural Egypt: Ethnography in Historical Context*. Boulder, Colo.: Westview, 1993.

Moulin, Anne Marie. "Les Instituts Pasteur de la Méditerranée arabe: Une religion scientifique en pays d'Islam." In *Santé, médecine et société dans le monde arabe*, edited by Elisabeth Longuenesse, 129–164. Paris: L'Harmattan, 1995.

———. "Tropical without the Tropics: The Turning-Point of Pastorian Medicine in North Africa." In *Warm Climates and Western Medicine: The Emergence of Tropical Medicine, 1500–1900*, edited by David Arnold, 160–180. Amsterdam and Atlanta: Rodopi, 1996.

Moussaoui, Driss, and Michel Roux Dessarps. *Histoire de la médecine au Maroc et dans les pays arabes et musulmans*. Casablanca: Imprimerie Najah El Jadida, 1995.

Murata, Sachiko. *The Tao of Islam: A Sourcebook on Gender Relationships in Islamic Thought*. Albany: SUNY Press, 1992.

Musallam, Basim. *Sex and Society in Islam*. Cambridge: Cambridge Univ. Press, 1983.

Nasr, Seyyed Hossein. *An Introduction to Islamic Cosmological Doctrines*. Albany: SUNY Press, 1993.

———. *Islamic Art and Spirituality*. Lahore: Suhail Academy, 1997.

———. *Science and Civilization in Islam*. Cambridge: Harvard University Press / Islamic Texts Society, 1987.

Nékrouf, Younès. *Une Amitié orageuse: Moulay Ismaïl et Louis XIV*. Paris: Albin Michel, 1987.

Nicolet, Claude. "Jules Ferry et la tradition positiviste." In *Jules Ferry: Fondateur de la République*, edited by François Furet, 23–47. Paris: EHESS, 1985.

Noiriel, Gérard. *État, nation et immigration: Vers une histoire du pouvoir*. Paris: Belin, 2001.

———. "République et exclusion en France à la fin du XIXe siècle." In *Les Exclus en Europe*, edited by A. Gueslin and D. Kalifa, 267–273. Paris: Éditions de l'Atelier, 1998.

Nora, Pierre. "Between Memory and History: *Les Lieux de mémoire*." *Representations* 26 (Spring 1989): 7–24.

Nordman, Daniel. "Les expéditions de Moulay Hassan: Essai statistique." *Hespéris-Tamuda* 19 (1980–1981): 123–152.

Obermeyer, Carla Makhlouf. "Pluralism and Pragmatism: Knowledge and Practice of Birth in Morocco." *Medical Anthropology Quarterly* 14, no. 2: 180–201.

Osborne, Michael. *Nature, the Exotic, and the Science of French Colonialism*. Bloomington: Univ. of Indiana Press, 1994.

———. "Resurrecting Hippocrates: Hygienic Sciences and the French Scientific Expeditions to Egypt, Morea, and Algeria." In *Warm Climates and Western Medicine: The Emergence of Tropical Medicine, 1500–1900*, edited by David Arnold, 80–98. Amsterdam and Atlanta: Rodopi, 1996.

Owusu-Ansah, David. "Prayer, Amulets, and Healing." In *The History of Islam in Africa*, edited by Nehemia Levtzion and Randall L. Pouwels, 477–488. Athens: Ohio Univ. Press, 2000.

Packard, Randall. *White Plague, Black Labor: Tuberculosis and the Political Economy of Health and Disease in South Africa*. Berkeley and Los Angeles: Univ. of California Press, 1989.

Pandolfo, Stefania. "Detours of Life: Space and Bodies in a Moroccan Village." *American Ethnologist* 16, no. 1: 3–23.

———. "The Thin Line of Modernity: Some Moroccan Debates on Subjectivity." In *Questions of Modernity*, edited by Timothy Mitchell, 115–147. Minneapolis: Univ. of Minnesota Press, 2000.

Pascon, Paul, "Le rapport 'secret' d'Edmond Doutté: Situation politique du Houz, 1er janvier 1907." *Hérodote* 1978:132–159.

Pedersen, Susan. *Family, Dependence, and the Origins of the Welfare State: Britain and France, 1914–1945*. Cambridge: Cambridge Univ. Press, 1993.

Pelis, Kim. *Charles Nicolle: Pasteur's Imperial Missionary; Typhus and Tunisia*. Rochester, N.Y.: Univ. of Rochester Press, 2006.

Pennell, C. R. "Lineage, Genealogy and Practical Politics: Thoughts on David Hart's Last Work." *Journal of North African Studies* 6, no. 2 (Summer 2001): 2–10.

———. *Morocco since 1830: A History*. New York: New York Univ. Press, 2000.

Penz, Charles. *Les Captifs français du Maroc au XVIIe siècle (1577–1699)*. Rabat: Institut des Hautes Études Marocaines, 1944.

Perho, Irmeli. *The Prophet's Medicine: A Creation of the Muslim Traditionalist Scholars*. Helsinki: Finnish Oriental Society, 1995.

Philips, Abu Ameenah Bilal. *Ibn Taymeeyah's Essay on the Jinn (Demons)*. Riyadh: Tawheed, 1989.

Pickering, Andrew. *The Mangle of Practice: Time, Agency, and Science*. Chicago: Univ. of Chicago Press, 1995.

Pickering, Mary. *Auguste Comte: An Intellectual Biography*. Vol 2. Cambridge: Cambridge Univ. Press, 2009.

———. "Auguste Comte." In *The Wiley-Blackwell Companion to Major Social Theorists*, edited by George Ritzer and Jeffrey Stepnisky, 30–60. Malden, Mass.: Wiley-Blackwell, 2011.

Pitt, Alan. "The Cultural Impact of Science in France: Ernest Renan and the *Vie de Jésus*." *Historical Journal* 43, no. 1 (2000): 79–101.

Porch, Douglas. *The Conquest of Morocco*. New York: Knopf, 1983.

Powers, David. *Law, Society, and Culture in the Maghrib, 1300–1500*. Cambridge: Cambridge Univ. Press, 2002.

———. "Orientalism, Colonialism, and Legal History: The Attack on the Muslim Family Endowments in Algeria and India." *Comparative Studies in Society and History* 31, no. 3 (1989): 539–543.

Prakash, Gyan. "Body Politic in Colonial India." In *Questions of Modernity*, edited by Timothy Mitchell, 189–222. Minneapolis: Univ. of Minnesota Press, 2000.

Proschan, Frank. "Syphilis, Opiomania, and Pederasty: Colonial Constructions of Vietnamese (and French) Social Diseases." *Journal of the History of Sexuality* 11, no. 4 (2002): 610–636.

Pyenson, Lewis. "Pure Learning and Political Economy: Science and European Imperialism in the Age of Imperialism." In *New Trends in the History of Science: Proceedings of a Conference Held at the University of Utrecht*, edited by R. P. W. Visser, H. J. M. Bos, L. C. Palm, and H. A. M. Snelders, 209–78. Amsterdam: Rodopi, 1989.

Rabinow, Paul. *French Modern: Norms and Forms of the Social Environment*. Chicago: Univ. of Chicago Press, 1989.

Radtke, Bernd, John O'Kane, Knut S. Vikor, and R. S. O'Fahey. *The Exoteric Ahmad ibn Idris: A Sufi's Critique of the Madhahib and the Wahhabis*. Leiden: Brill, 2000.

Ramsey, Matthew. *Professional and Popular Medicine in France, 1770–1830: The Social World of Medical Practice*. Cambridge: Cambridge Univ. Press, 1988.

Ranger, Terence. "Godly Medicine: The Ambiguities of Medical Mission in Southeast Tanzania." *Social Science and Medicine* 15, no. 3 (1981): 261–277.

Rivet, Daniel. *Lyautey et l'institution du protectorat français au Maroc, 1912–1925*. 3 vols. Paris: L'Harmattan, 1996.

Rivet, Daniel, and François Pouillon, eds. *La Sociologie musulmane de Robert Montagne*. Paris: Maisonneuve and Larose, 2000.

Rosenberg, Charles E. *The Cholera Years: The United States in 1832, 1849, and 1866*. 1962. Reprint, Chicago: Univ. of Chicago Press, 1987.

Rosenthal, E. I. J. *Political Thought in Medieval Islam: An Introductory Outline*. Cambridge: Cambridge Univ. Press, 1968.

Ross, Eric. *Sufi City: Urban Design and Archetypes in Tuba*. Rochester, N.Y.: Univ. of Rochester Press, 2006.

Rousselle, Maxime. *Médecins, chirurgiens et apothicaires français au Maroc (1577–1907)*. 1996. Self-published.

Ruedy, John. *Modern Algeria: The Origins and Development of a Nation*. Bloomington: Indiana Univ. Press, 1992.

Russell, Alexander David, and Abdullah al-Mamun Suhrawardy. *A Manual of the Law of Marriage from the Mukhtasar of Sidi Khalil*. Lahore: Law Pub. Co., 1979.

Said, Edward. *Orientalism*. New York: Vintage, 1979.

Savage-Smith, Emilie, and Peter Pormann. *Medieval Islamic Medicine*. Edinburgh: Edinburgh Univ. Press, 2007.

Schahien, Abdul Salam. "Die Geburtshilflich-gynäkologischen Kapitel aus der Chirurgie des Abulkasim, ins Deutsche übersetzt und kommentiert." PhD thesis, Friedrich-Wilhelms-Universität zu Berlin, 1937.

Scham, Alan. *Lyautey in Morocco: Protectorate Administration, 1912–1925*. Berkeley and Los Angeles: Univ. of California Press, 1970.

Schayegh, Cyrus. *Who Is Knowledgeable Is Strong: Science, Class, and the Formation of Modern Iranian Society, 1900–1950*. Berkeley and Los Angeles: Univ. of California Press, 2009.

Scheper-Hughes, Nancy, and Margaret Lock. "The Mindful Body: A Prolegomenon to Future Work in Medical Anthropology." *Medical Anthropology Quarterly* 1, no. 1 (1987): 6–41.

Schiebinger, Londa. *Plants and Empire: Colonial Bioprospecting in the Atlantic World*. Cambridge, Mass.: Harvard Univ. Press, 2004.

Schimmel, Annemarie. *And Muhammed Is His Messenger: The Veneration of the Prophet in Islamic Piety*. Chapel Hill: Univ. of North Carolina Press, 1985.

———. "Aspects of Mystical Thought in Islam." In *The Islamic Impact*, edited by B. Haines, Y. Haddad, and E. Findly, 113–136. Syracuse, N.Y.: Syracuse Univ. Press, 1984.

Schneider, William. *Quality and Quantity: The Quest for Biological Regeneration in Twentieth-Century France*. Cambridge: Cambridge Univ. Press, 1990.

Schroeter, Daniel. *Merchants of Essaouira: Urban Society and Imperialism in Southwestern Morocco, 1844–1886*. Cambridge: Cambridge Univ. Press, 1988.

Sebti, Abdelahad. "Chroniques de la contestation citadine: Fès et la révolte des tanneurs (1873–1874)." *Hespéris-Tamuda* 29 (1992): 283–312.

Segalla, Spencer D. *The Moroccan Soul: French Education, Colonial Ethnology, and Muslim Resistance, 1912–1956*. Lincoln: Univ. of Nebraska Press, 2009.

Serels, M. Mitchell. "Aspects of the Effects of Jewish Philanthropic Societies in Morocco." In *From Iberia to Diaspora: Studies in Sephardic History and Culture*, edited by Yedida Kalfon Stillman and Norman A. Stillman, 102–112. Leiden: Brill, 1999.

Shapiro, Louise. *Housing the Poor of Paris, 1850–1902*. Madison: Univ. of Wisconsin Press, 1985.

Shatzmiller, Maya. *The Berbers and the Islamic State: The Marinid Experience in Pre-Protectorate Morocco*. Princeton, N.J.: Wiener, 2000.

Sijelmassi, Abdelhai. *Les Plantes médicinales du Maroc*. Casablanca: Éditions le Fennec, 1993.

Simou, Bahija. *Les Réformes militaires au Maroc de 1844 à 1912*. Rabat: Université Mohammed V, Publications de la faculté des lettres et des sciences humaines, 1995.

Siraisi, Nancy. *Avicenna in Renaissance Italy: The Canon and Medical Teaching in Universities after 1500*. Princeton, N.J.: Princeton Univ. Press, 1987.

———. *Medieval and Early Renaissance Medicine: An Introduction to Knowledge and Practice*. Chicago: Univ. of Chicago Press, 1990.

Sirriyeh, Elizabeth. *Sufis and Anti-Sufis: The Defence, Rethinking, and Rejection of Sufism in the Modern World*. London: Curzon, 1999.

Slomka, Jacquelyn. "Medicine and Reproduction in Urban Morocco." PhD diss., University of Michigan, 1986.

Sonbol, Amira El Azhary. *The Creation of a Medical Profession in Egypt, 1800–1922*. Syracuse, N.Y.: Syracuse Univ. Press, 1991.

Sournia, Jean-Charles. "L'intervention chirurgicale et l'obstétrique." In *À l'ombre d'Avicenne: La médecine au temps des califes: Exposition présentée du 18 novembre 1996 au 2 mars 1997*, edited by Éric Delpont, 109–113. Ghent: Snoeck-Ducaju and Zoon, 1996.

Spadola, Emilio. "The Scandal of Ecstasy: Communication, Sufi Rites, and Social Reform in 1930s Morocco." *Contemporary Islam* (2008): 119–138.

Spink, M. S. "Arabian Gynaecological, Obstetrical, and Genito-Urinary Practice, Illustrated from Abulcasis." *Proceedings of the Royal Society of Medicine* 30 (1937): 653–670.

Stearns, Justin K. *Infectious Ideas: Contagion in Premodern Islamic and Christian Thought in the Western Mediterranean*. Baltimore: Johns Hopkins Univ. Press, 2011.

Stillman, Yedida Kalfon, and Norman A. Stillman. *From Iberia to Diaspora: Studies in Sephardic History and Culture*. Leiden: Brill, 1999.

Stöber, Georg. *"Habous Public" in Marokko: Zur wirtschaftlichen Bedeutung religiöser Stiftungen im 20. Jahrhundert*. Marburg: Im Selbstverlag der Marburger Geographischen Gesellschaft, 1986.

Stoler, Ann Laura. "Carnal Knowledge and Imperial Power: Gender, Race, and Morality in Colonial Asia." In *Gender at the Crossroads of Knowledge: Feminist Anthropology in the Postmodern Era*, edited by Micaela di Leonardo, 51–202. Berkeley and Los Angeles: Univ. of California Press, 1991.

———. *Race and the Education of Desire: Foucault's History of Sexuality and the Colonial Order of Things*. Durham, N.C.: Duke Univ. Press, 1995.

———. "Rethinking Colonial Categories: European Communities and the Boundaries of Rule." *Comparative Studies in Society and History* 31, no. 1 (1989): 134–161.

Swearingen, William. *Moroccan Mirages: Agrarian Dreams and Deceptions, 1912–1986*. London: Tauris, 1998.

Taussig, Michael. *Colonialism, Shamanism, and the Wild Man: A Study in Terror and Healing*. Chicago: Univ. of Chicago Press, 1987.

Tazi, Loubna, Jamila El Baghdadi, Sarah Lesjean, Camille Locht, Philip Supply, Michel Tibayrenc, and Anne-Laure Bañuls. "Genetic Diversity and Population Structure of *Mycobacterium tuberculosis* in Casablanca, a Moroccan City with High Incidence of Tuberculosis." *Journal of Clinical Microbiology* 42, no. 1: 461–466. January 2004.

Thompson, Elizabeth. *Colonial Citizens: Republican Rights, Paternal Privilege, and Gender in French Syria and Lebanon.* New York: Columbia Univ. Press, 2000.

Trumbull, George R. *An Empire of Facts: Colonial Power, Cultural Knowledge, and Islam in Algeria, 1870–1914.* Cambridge: Cambridge Univ. Press, 2009.

Turner, Victor. *Revelation and Divination in Ndembu Ritual.* Ithaca, N.Y.: Cornell Univ. Press, 1975.

Ullmann, Manfred. *Islamic Medicine.* Edinburgh: Edinburgh University Press, 1997.

———. *Die Medizin im Islam.* Leiden: Brill, 1970.

van den Belt, Henk. "Spirochaetes, Serology and Salvarsan: Ludwik Fleck and the Construction of Medical Knowledge about Syphilis." PhD thesis, Landbouwuniversiteit Wageningen, 1998.

Van Hollen, Cecilia. *Birth on the Threshold: Childbirth and Modernity in South India.* Berkeley and Los Angeles: Univ. of California Press, 2003.

Vaughan, Meghan. *Curing Their Ills: Colonial Power and African Illness.* Stanford, Calif.: Stanford University Press, 1991.

———. "Syphilis in Colonial East and Central Africa: The Social Construction of an Epidemic." In *Epidemics and Ideas: Essays on the Historical Perception of Pestilence*, edited by Terence Ranger and Paul Slack, 269–302. Cambridge: Cambridge Univ. Press, 1992.

von Osten, Marian. "Architecture without Architects: An Anarchist Approach." *e-flux* 5, no. 6 (2009).

Watenpaugh, Keith David. *Being Modern in the Middle East: Revolution, Nationalism, Colonialism, and the Arab Middle Class.* Princeton, N.J.: Princeton Univ. Press, 2006.

Waterbury, John. *North for the Trade: The Life and Times of a Berber Merchant.* Berkeley and Los Angeles: Univ. of California Press, 1972.

Wegener, Frederick. "Edith Wharton on French Colonial Charities for Women: An Unknown Travel Essay." *Tulsa Studies in Women's Literature* 17, no. 1 (Spring 1998): 11–36.

Weiner, Dora. *The Citizen Patient in Revolutionary and Imperial Paris.* Baltimore: Johns Hopkins Univ. Press, 1993.

Weisser, Urusla. *Zeugung, Vererbung und Pränatale Entwicklung in Der Medizin Des Arabisch-Islamischen Mittelalters.* Erlangen: Verlagsbuchhandlung Hannelore Lüling, 1983.

White, Luise. *Speaking with Vampires: Rumor and History in Colonial Africa.* Berkeley and Los Angeles: Univ. of California Press, 2000.

———. "'They Could Make Their Victims Dull': Gender and Genres, Fantasies and Cures in Colonial Southern Uganda." *American Historical Review* 100 (December 1995): 1379–1402.

Wilder, Gary. *The French Imperial Nation-State: Negritude and Colonial Humanism Between the Two World Wars.* Chicago: Univ. of Chicago Press, 2005.

Williams, Roger. *The Horror of Life.* Chicago: Univ. of Chicago Press, 1980.

Wilson, Lindsay. *Women and Medicine in the French Enlightenment: The Debate over "Maladies des Femmes."* Baltimore: Johns Hopkins Univ. Press, 1993.

Winichakul, Thongchai. *Siam Mapped: A History of the Geo-Body of the Nation.* Honolulu: Univ. of Hawaii Press, 1994.

Wolper, Ethel. *Cities and Saints: Sufism and the Transformation of Urban Space in Medieval Anatolia.* University Park: Pennsylvania State Univ. Press, 2003.

World Health Organization. *New Trends and Approaches in the Delivery of Maternal and Child Care in Health Services.* WHO Technical Report series. Geneva: WHO, 1976.

Wright, Gwendolyn. *The Politics of Design in French Colonial Urbanism.* Chicago: Univ. of Chicago Press, 1991.

Yakhlef, Mohamed. "La Municipalité de Fès à l'époque du Protectorat, 1912–1956." Doctorat d'État, Université Libre de Bruxelles, 1990. (3 vols.)

Yegenoglu, Meyda. *Colonial Fantasies: Towards a Feminist Reading of Orientalism.* Cambridge: Cambridge Univ. Press, 1998.

Zouanat, Zakia. *Ibn Mashish: Maître d'al-Shadhili.* Casablanca: Imprimerie Najah El Jadida, 1998.

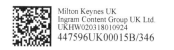

Milton Keynes UK
Ingram Content Group UK Ltd.
UKHW020318010924
447596UK00015B/346